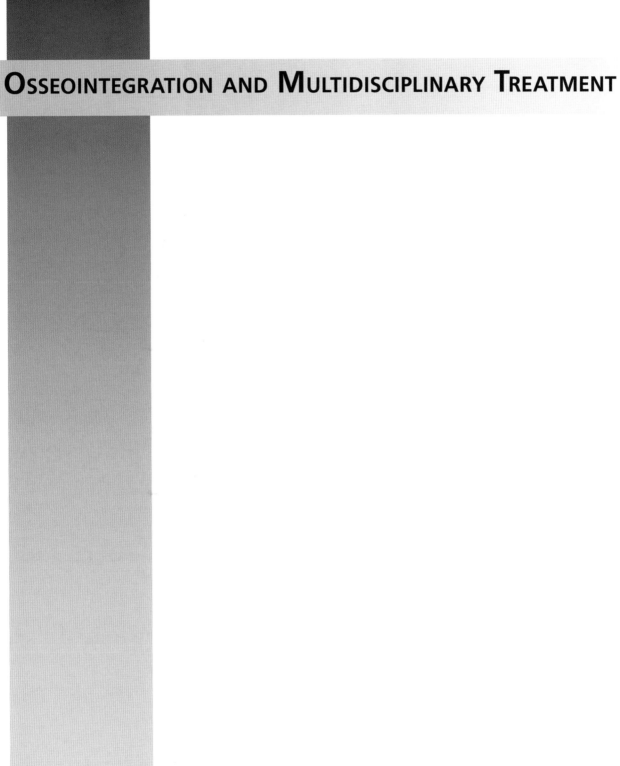

OSSEOINTEGRATION AND MULTIDISCIPLINARY TREATMENT

OSSEOINTEGRATION AND MULTIDISCIPLINARY TREATMENT

Coordinator: Carlos Eduardo Francischone

Carlos Eduardo Francischone
Daniella A. D. Matos
Helcio Ganda Lira
José Bernardes das Neves
Luis G. Peredo-Paz
Luis Rogério Duarte
Reinaldo R. P. Janson

Hugo Nary Filho
Glécio V. Campos
Reginaldo M. Migliorança
Renato Savi de Carvalho
Carlos E. Francischone Junior

Paulo Malo
Maria B. Papageorge
Robert J. Chapman
Ziad Jaboult

Chicago, Barcelona, Beijing, Berlin, Bukarest, Istanbul,
London, Milan, Moscow, New Delhi, Paris, Prague,
São Paulo, Tokyo, Warsaw

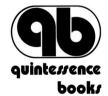

quintessence
books

Title in Portuguese:	Osseointegração e o Tratamento Multidisciplinar
Title in English:	Osseointegration and Multidisciplinary Treatment
Author:	Carlos Eduardo Francischone *et al.* drfrancischone@yahoo.com.br
Translation:	Paulo H. O. Rossetti
Revision:	Paulo H. O. Rossetti Carlos Eduardo Francischone
Eletronic Editorialization:	Adriano V. Zago
Cover:	Gilberto R. Salomão

© 2008 Quintessence Editora Ltda.

ISBN: 978-85-87425-76-8

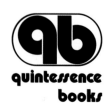
quintessence
books

Rua Machado de Assis, 142 – Vila Mariana
04106-000 – São Paulo – SP
Tel.: (11) 5539-3183
E-mail: quintedit@terra.com.br

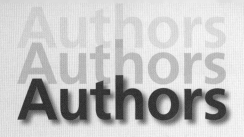
Authors

Carlos Eduardo Francischone,
DDS, MSc, PhD
- Titular Professor
  Department of Restorative
  Dentistry, Endodontics and
  Dental Materials
  Bauru School of Dentistry
  Sao Paulo University
  Bauru, Brazil
- Titular Professor
  Department of Oral Implan-
    tology
  Sagrado Coração University
  – Bauru, Brazil

Daniella Andaluza Dias Matos,
DDS, MSc
- Clinical Professor
  Undergraduate Course in
  Dentistry and Specialization
  Course on Prosthodontics
  Para University Center
  Para, Brazil
- Master of Science in Implan-
  tology, USC, Brazil

Helcio Ganda Lira, DDS, MSc
- Chairman, Oral Implantology
  Discipline
  Naval Central Clinics,
  Rio de Janeiro, Brazil

José Bernardes das Neves, DDS,
MSc, PhD
- Member of the American
  Academy of Osseointegration
- Master of Science in Implan-
  tology, USC, Brazil

Luis Guillermo Peredo-Paz,
DDS, MSc
- Clinical Professor, Oral Im-
  plantology and Periodontics
  Course – Santa Cruz Dentis-
  try College, Bolivia
  Santa Cruz de La Sierra, Boli-
  via
- Master of Science in Implan-
  tology, USC, Brazil

Luis Rogério Duarte, DDS, MSc,
PhD
- Clinical Professor, Specializa-
  tion Course on Oral Implan-
  tology – School of Dentistry
  Bahia Federal University
  Bahia, Brazil
- Master of Science on Implan-
  tology, USC, Brazil

Reinaldo R. P. Janson, DDS, MSc
- Private Practice
  Bauru, Sao Paulo, Brazil
- Master of Science on Implan-
  tology, USC, Brazil

Maria B. Papageorge, DMD, MS
- Professor and Chairman
- Director of Advanced Education in Oral and Maxillofacial Surgery
  Tufts University School of Dental Medicine
  Boston, Massachusetts

Robert J. Chapman, DMD
- Professor and Chair
  Departments of Prosthodontics and Operative Dentistry
  Tufts University School of Dental Medicine
  Boston, Massachusetts

Ziad Jaboult, DDS, MSc, PhD
- Professor
  Department of Implantology
  New York University
  New York, USA

Paulo Malo, DDS
- President – Malo Clinics International – Lisbon, Portugal

Isabel Lopes, DDS
- Member of Malo Clinics International – Lisbon, Portugal

Raul Costa, DDS
- Member of Malo Clinics International – Lisbon, Portugal

Hugo Nary Filho, DDS, MSc, PhD
- Titular Professor
  Department of Oral and Maxillofacial Surgery
  Sagrado Coração University
  Bauru, Brazil

Renato Savi de Carvalho, DDS, MSc
- Professor – Department of Oral Implantology
  Sagrado Coração University
  Bauru – São Paulo – Brazil

- Master of Science on Implantology, USC – Brazil

Reginaldo M. Migliorança, DDS, MSc
- Clinical Professor, Specialization Course on Oral Implantology
- Director, Malo Clinics, Campinas, Sao Paulo, Brazil

Marcos R. P. Janson, DDS, MSc
- Private Practice
  Bauru, Sao Paulo, Brazil

Carlos Eduardo Francischone Jr., DDS, MSc
- Professor – Department of Oral Implantology
  Sagrado Coração University,
  Bauru, Sao Paulo, Brazil
- Master of Science on Implantology, USC, Brazil

Glécio Vaz de Campos, DDS
- Specialist in Periodontics and Dental Prosthetics
- Lecturer, Plastic Periodontal Microsurgery Course, Coordinator Associação Paulista dos Cirurgiões Dentistas (APCD) Sao Paulo, Brazil
- Introducer, Plastic Periodontal Microsurgery Technique in Brazil

Laércio W. Vasconcelos, DDS, PhD
- Director, Brånemark Osseointegration Center
  Sao Paulo, Brazil

Paulo Henrique Orlato Rossetti, DDS, MSc, PhD
- Master of Science and Doctorade Courses,
  Oral Rehabilitation Program
  Bauru School of Dentistry
  Sao Paulo University,
  Bauru, Sao Paulo, Brazil

Contributors

Contributors
Contributors

Ana Paula Rabello de Macedo Costa, DDS
- Professor
  Discipline of Orthodontics
  Brazilian Dental Association
  Bauru, Brazil

Ana Carolina Francischone, DDS, MSc
- Master of Science on Restorative Dentistry.
  Bauru School of Dentistry, Sao Paulo University, Brazil
- Private Practice
  Bauru, Sao Paulo, Brazil

Marcelo de Sá Zamperlini, DDS, MSc
- Master of Science on Implantology, Sao Leopoldo Mandic University, Brazil
- Professor, Specialization Course on Implantology, ABO, Campinas, Brazil

Gisseli Bertozzi Ávila, DDS, MSC
- Specialist on Implantology
- Master of Science on Implantology, Sao Leopoldo Mandic University

Euloir Passanezzi, DDS, MSc, PhD
- Titular Professor
  Department of Periodontics
  Bauru School of Dentistry
  Sao Paulo University
  Bauru, Brazil

Adriana Campos Passanezzi Sant'Ana, DDS, MSc, PhD
- Professor
  Department of Periodontics
  Bauru School of Dentistry
  Sao Paulo University
  Bauru, Brazil
- Professor – Specialization Course in Periodontics
  Bauru School of Dentistry
  Sao Paulo University
  Bauru, Brazil

José Antonio de Siqueira Laurenti, DDS
- Private Practice, Bauru, Sao Paulo, Brazil

Thiago Martins de Mayo, DDS
- Master of Science in Implantodontics
  Sao Leopoldo Mandic University, Brazil

- Specialist on Implantology
  HRAC-USP, Bauru, São Paulo,
  Brazil

Mariza Akemi Matsumoto,
DDS, MSc, PhD
- Professor
  Department of Oral and
  Maxillofacial Surgery
  Disciplines of Histology and
  Pathology
  Sagrado Coração University
  Bauru, Sao Paulo, Brazil

Ivete de Mathias Sartori, DDS, PhD
- Private practice, Bauru,
  Sao Paulo, Brazil

Ricardo Falcão Tuler, DDS, MSc
- Professor – Department of Oral
  and Maxillofacial Surgery
  Sagrado Coração University,
  Bauru, Sao Paulo, Brazil

Fabrício Francischone, MD
- Ribeirão Preto School of
  Medicine
  Ribeirão Preto University
  Ribeirão Preto, Sao Paulo, Bra-
  zil

José Gilmar Batista, DDS, PhD
- Private practice, Bauru,
  Sao Paulo, Brazil

Laura P. G. Paleckis, DDS, PhD
- Private Practice
  Araçatuba, Sao Paulo, Brazil

Gustavo Petrilli, DDS
- Associated Member of
  Brånemark   Osseointegration
  Center, Sao Paulo, Brazil

Luciano Dumalak Saters, CDT,
DDS
- Oral Art Dental Laboratory
  Bauru, Sao Paulo, Brazil

This book is dedicated to my father Sebastião (*in memorian*) and my mother Milthes, to my wife Ana Luiza, and to my children Carlos Eduardo, Ana Carolina and Fabrício, who allowed me to sacrifice much of our family activities and devote myself to Dentistry and patients.

To Professor Per-Ingvar Brånemark, for his constant lessons in life and profession.

To the Sao Paulo and Sagrado Coração Universities, where I could develop my scientific and instructive activities on Restorative Dentistry and Oral Implantology, respectively.

To Sagrado Coração University at Bauru by the opportunity of making the Oral Implantology course a reality. This course provided their postgraduate students with the opportunity to prepare part of the material of this book.

Thank you

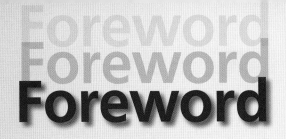

Introduction to Osseointegrated Oral Rehabilitation

The edentulous patient is an oral invalid, a condition similar to the defect situation after amputation of any other part of the body.

Accordingly, it is imperative to respect the functional consequences of loss of teeth and provide not only anatomical substitutes, but also respect the necessity of restoring incorporation of the prosthetic replacement within the physical and psychological function of the patient. Thus, whereas the articulator could be an important tool for somatic restoration of a third dentition it is equally decisive to provide cognitive perception so that the neuromuscular harmony of maxillo-facial function is provided.

This is where Osseointegration can make an important contribution to the final result of rehabilitation.

A carefully planned and multidisciplinary based therapeutic protocol, interacting with the patients expectations and realities, is strongly motivated. The provision of a third dentition is expected to last a lifetime. Unprejudiced consultation between clinical disciplines, – all the time with the patient's comments and consent – is a prerequisite for a predictable prognosis whatever methods are finally chosen.

It is imperative, that the clinical procedures are provided by clinicians with adequate experience, not only of routine techniques, but particularly with knowledge of alternative solutions, if the preoperative planning can not be realized in some decisive aspects when the actual anatomy is exposed.

It is equally crucial to be able to discuss selection of interactive alternatives between surgery and prosthetics before a final decision is made – remembering that it could have a decisive influence on the quality of life for the patient.

Another aspect is the ambition of using procedures which expose the patient to minimal surgery as well as individualized harmonious occlusion, carefully and successively adjusted over time, as the directly bone anchored teeth are being recognized by the multicapabel brain via osseoperception.

The neurophysiological function of how dynamic load is transferred from a rigid metallic body – a fixture – to a much less rigid bone tissue, remodelled to the specific situation, is still incompletely understood.

However, parallel studies on amputated limbs with Osseointegrated prostheses, provide important additional information on how to adjust anchorage and prosthetics to optimize function.

In the future, advanced neuro physiological analytical methods will be available to understand how to secure undisturbed function in a situation, that was not genetically intended.

Even now, decisive factors can be identified by listening to the patient and talking to experienced colleagues.

Parafunctional situations require individual analysis – including psychological considerations – of how to adjust the anatomy of the third dentition with respect to transfer of load across the interface between maxilla and mandible, but also between fixture and bone at different levels of dimension.

Prestige and prejudice are certainly counterproductive, particularly since we are still in a very early phase of identifying choice of safe and optimal surgical methods for the individual patient and reliable,

affordable prosthetic devices, with the option of future adaptation to possible changes in maxillofacial topography and function.

In close cooperation between basic and clinical disciplines there is a strong indication and motivation – also related to cost of treatment – to simplify procedures within obvious respect for the safetly of the patient.

Consequences – good or bad – of minor or major alternations – in hardware or software in clinical systems should be openly documented and reported after adequate time of relevant observation in consecutive series of patients.

The final advice to the patient should be based on respect for the basic philosophy in health care, that less is more and that re-establishing quality of life for the edentulous patient is not necessarily requiring the most sophisticated scientific clinical procedures but instead giving priority to what is safe, simple and predictable. Long term documented clinical function without negative effects should be the decisive intention for selection of the restorative procedure.

In many cases careful exploration of the anatomy of available local bone for anchorage of the necessary dimensions and adequate numbers of fixtures will reveal opportunities for anchorage without resorting to grafting of bone tissue or other major surgical procedures.

Careful detailed radiographic diagnosis of the 3-dimensionally defect jaw bone topography is always required, and collaboration with diagnostic radiology is a prerequisite for unprejudiced selection of minimalistic surgical procedures and precision, harmonious prosthetics for the benefit of the patient.

P-I Brånemark

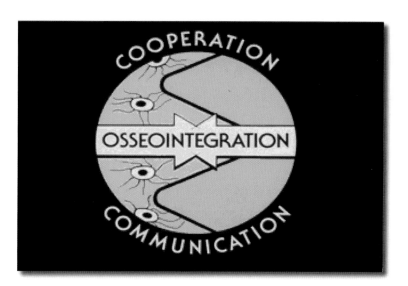

Contents

1

INTRODUCTION

Carlos Eduardo Francischone

The biological phenomenon of osseointegration was discovered by Per-Ingvar Brånemark in 1965, being widely applied in different areas of Dentistry and Medicine. Based on the rationale of anchorage or prosthesis retention form, it has provided new alternatives and provoked radical changes in treatment planning and prosthetic resolutions for single, partial and total edentulism cases, establishing rigorous and well-defined surgical and prosthetic protocols. The Osseointegration is one of the most significant advances occurred in the first half of the past century. It has generated high success rates that praise its use.

From the very beginning and clinical application, osseointe-gration was seen as an anchorage tool for fixed or removable prostheses. Thus, implants were installed in jaws to create retention and function, underestimating esthetics. Over the years, a more in depth understanding of, and the technological development related to components and devices used for implant prostheses, fulfilled this aspect with satisfactory results.

The fundamentals of implants were introduced in the United States by 1982 and came to Brazil in 1987, resuming itself to installation and prosthesis confection. Due to its widespread use sustained on solid concepts, as well as its importance to osseointegration in dentistry, other specialties rather than Implantology could benefit from it. Professionals from areas such as Oral and Maxillofacial Surgery, Orthodontics, and Periodontics were the first to join Implantology, followed by Operative Dentistry, Gerodontology and Advanced Diagnostic Methods, Esthetics and more recently, Audiology, Nutrition and Physiology.

At this time, as a clinical and research professor during 34 years, I could not forget to give my testimonial on it. In the year of 1972, I was incorporated to the teaching staff of Bauru School of Dentistry, Sao Paulo University-Brazil at the Department of Operative Dentistry, headed by Professor Dr. Jose Mondelli. Concomitant to my academic activities, I began my professional activities in a private practice. Later, in 1973, it came about the opportunity to attend a graduate course (Master of Science degree). Professor Mondelli suggested that I should attend to the Program of Oral Rehabilitation, starting cooperation between Operative Dentistry, Periodontics and Prosthodontic areas. Since then, he has highlightened the importance of a muldisciplinary knowledge for the undergraduate student. His philosophy stated that dental students should learn to diagnose, plan and provide a functional restorative and esthetic treatment according to its appropriate sequence, timing, and involvement. In 1984, a book entitled *"Dentistica Restau-*

radora – tratamentos clinicos integrados" was launched reflecting the philosophical principles of this Department. In the words of Professor Mondelli : " Theory and technique must be learnt, acquired, developed, and improved all together. It is virtually impossible to demonstrate or prove something that you cannot recognize theoretically or conceive by yourself. The real professor is recognized for his didactic planning and knowledge. He shows his qualifications during patient treatment, examining, planning, and conversations with students, involving them into the decision making process, at the same time that acquires clinical experience."

My professional career was developed bearing this philosophy in mind. When I realized, implantology suddenly became part of my dental practice. This was also suggested by Prof. Mondelli in 1990. So soon I understood that Implantology could not be separated from basic disciplines. At this time, I was introduced to Prof. Per-Ingvar Brånemark by Dr. Laércio W. Vasconcelos. Imagining all possibilities, Brånemark sent us to the cities of Spokane and Washington, in the USA, to begin our training on advanced surgeries for oromaxilofacial reconstruction with Prof. Phillip Worthington, as well as in orthodontics associated to implantology, with Prof. Kenji Higuchi. Also, we still had contact with maxillofacial prosthesis, under the guidance of Prof. Jeffrey Rubstein.

Modern dentistry was evolving into an interdisciplinary practice, and implantology became part of this change. A global vision in the treatment planning is of utmost importance, because a satisfactory esthetic and functional result can only be achieved through involvement of different clinical specialties, as well as patient comprehension and collaboration. The development of integrated procedures is related to a treatment planning based on a correct diagnosis and therapeutic sequence, eliminating all existing etiological factors, restoring form and function, resulting in the homeostasis of the stomatognathic system.

As a clinical professor, I saw a demand for an implantology discipline on the dentistry graduate course of Sagrado Coração University in 1996. The purpose of it was to provide knowledge of osseointegration to dental students, enabling them to plan their treatments with one more option: the anchorage for implant prosthesis. This was the first Brazilian University to adopt it on dental course. Today, I am very proud of that because many universities have understood its clinical impact and incorporated implantology on their dental practice.

The same was verified in the postgraduate scenario, being necessary to initiate a Master Degree Course in Oral Implantology. We started the first course in 1998. In addition to osseointegration, we decided to emphasize the multidisciplinary treatment planning, closely supervised by Prof. Brånemark, through his lectures and demonstrations of intra and extra-oral techniques for osseointegration. Since its installation at the Sagrado Coração University, the Associated Brånemark Osseointegration Center has sharing experiences with foreign universities, rehabilitating patients through modern technologies. At this Center, we are inspired by the philosophy of Prof. Brånemark: "The success and development of osseointegration largely depends on collaboration, cooperation and communication among people in the healthcare area".

The incorporation of Prof. Brånemark to our clinical team, the chance to rehabilitate several handicapped patients and the necessity of doing more for the benefit of them motivated him to settle the P-I Brånemark Institute in Bauru. Certainly, this fact will turn Bauru into an international reference center on osseointegration.

On February 2007, the Sagrado Coração University began to offer its PhD program with a 3-year duration for Brazilian and foreign students.

The year of 2005 will be unforgettable for all health professionals involved with osseointegration: forty-years ago, Brånemark installed the first fixtures on his patients. With our mentor, Brazil is proud of held the Congress World Celebration- 40 Years of Osseointegration, at the city of Sao Paulo. This is the appropriate moment to launch *Osseointegration and Multidisciplinary Treatment*. The book expresses a rehabilitation philosophy toward osseointegration, strongly reflected by research, practice, and team concepts, aiming to regain patient self-esteem through osseointegrated implants.

To conceive this book, we invited Brazilian and foreign professionals engaged on this philosophy, along with postgraduate students of the Master Degree Course in Oral Implantology at the Sagrado Coração University. They represented the core of this book, providing the real sense of Implantology and Trans and Multidisciplinary Treatment.

During its fiftheenth chapters, we attempted to demonstrate several rehabilitation possibilities, ranging from the simplest to more complex alternatives, as well as the interactive role of implantology with the other disciplines. Its purpose was to optimize functional, esthetic and psychological results.

Technical, surgical, and prosthetic strategies from different disciplines are presented here with their basic concepts applied to osseointegration.

The chapter on provisional or transitional restorations has shown its importance on implantology, not only to facilitate treatment, but also to evaluate its course and predict the final results. This becomes paramount when treating patients with high esthetic demands.

The chapters that illustrate esthetic rehabilitations show the great challenge and importance of these to dental professionals. In this regard, it is necessary to consider the *white esthetics*, related to dental crowns, and the *red esthetics*, related to gingival tissue. If one can conclude that esthetics represents the overall balance, both must be in harmony with facial appearance and to each other.

The two chapters on soft tissue management related to smile esthetics, show the importance of evaluating periodontal phenotype, and how it can contributes to more positive and safe surgical procedures. The classical techniques on periodontal surgery have shown highly satisfactory results to obtain an harmonious gingival architecture. Periodontal microsurgery, first developed to obtain wound healing by primary intention through minimally invasive procedures, has broadened new parameters to optimize results on red esthetics and its transition to white esthetics.

Also, there are two interrelated chapters to periodontal

surgery; the first assesses tooth substitution for implant. The second verifies the role of different implant systems on periimplant microflora. New insights on complex questions such as the periodontium, periimplantitis and dental plaque are highlightened.

Reflections on immediate implant function after removal of teeth associated or not with periodontal infections must be done by clinical professionals. The judicious analysis of bone quantity and quality, initial stability, implant design and patient demand and expectations can elicit its use. Esthetics is another aspect to be pointed out, because any deviation or complication from the original planning can cause irreversible damage to patients.

Three well illustrated chapters address two different possibilities for rehabilitation of the atrophic maxilla: reconstructions techniques using autogenous grafts, with intra and extra-oral donor sites, and anchorage techniques by means of zygomatic fixtures.

After, the chapter on procedures and planning of implant positioning toward esthetics and function shows the importance of three-dimensional implant installation. Orthodontics techniques not only made possible but also facilitated the ideal implant placement, improving prognosis and final esthetic and functional treatment results.

The chapter on craniofacial reconstruction for mandibular defects shows the necessity to integrate medical and dental specialties to satisfactory rehabilitate handicapped patients. These patients may present with anatomic defects due to surgical resection of benign or malign neoplasms, or damage caused by jaws disease. When possible, the final objective of reconstructing dentition must be considered according to the surgical planning related to form restoration. Once an anatomic configuration has been established, implant installation provides a solid foundation for dental reconstruction and esthetics. Only through an interdisciplinary treatment can well-successfully results be obtained on craniofacial reconstructions, regaining patient self-esteem and quality of life.

Two additional chapters on the treatment of atrophied maxillary arches were introduced in this book, bringing more significant treatment alternatives. The All-on-4 concepts are clearly defined regarding the type of maxillary atrophy. Thus, the All-on-4 Standard, All-on-4 Zygoma, as well as the All-on-Hybrid can be used to their plenitudes. The surgical procedures are dramatically simplified in the All-on-4 Standard modality, increasing the number of treated patients and reducing the use of more advanced techniques, such as bone grafts and zygomatic implants. Also, flapless surgical procedures for implant placement are exposed, aided by the virtual computerized 3-D navigation, known as the Nobel-Guide. This technology allows implant placement and prosthesis delivery in the same session within one hour.

The last chapter presents a classification created by the author on different types of implant prostheses, with the aim to facilitate communication understanding, and intereaction between surgeons, dental technicians, prosthodontists, and patients as well.

Professor José Alberto de Souza Freitas, Chairman of the Hospital for Rehabilitation of Craniofacial Anomalies (USP – Bauru) immortalized his thoughts when said: "It is a privilege to live together with a patient...because we learn a message of faith, life and optimism... Reconstruct a smile is equivalent to psychologically interact with all family members. Thus, the professional with the mission of building smiles is the same that moulds behaviors. It is the same that builds the dreams. To rehabilitate a smile is much more than a job. Is to love and dedicate all existence to the well-being of someone, to the happiness of the individual. Finally, is to be an everyday smile builder".

Technology has changed the world drastically; it is impressive how we can communicate across the oceans in less than seconds, but is still interesting to observe that a pleasant smile may take too much time to be developed.

A thorough comprehension of osseointegration and the multidisciplinary treatment possibilities, along with the development of new systems and devices, will permit functional and esthetic rehabilitations with better and faster results in the Oral Implantology. Personally, I would resume all the stated above in one simple but essential paragraph: **"The smile is the supreme expression of felicity!".**

Carlos Eduardo Francischone
drfrancischone@yahoo.com.br

2

PROVISIONAL/TRANSITIONAL RESTORATIONS IN OSSEOINTEGRATION

Carlos Eduardo Francischone
Renato Savi de Carvalho

Introduction

The concept of provisional/transitional (personal communication by Dr. Renato de Andrade) restorations in dentistry has been modified over the years. Initially, the idea was to provide relative comfort while waiting for the definitive treatment. This condition sometimes overlooked important characteristics necessary to the success of provisional restorations. Recently, new and important aspects were attributed to this type of reconstruction, being debated trough the profession, to optimize the rehabilitation treatment. The provisional/transitional restorations are a prerequisite for success. Thus, all the time spent on the basic tenets of provisional/transitional restorations is invaluable, since it directly influences the excellence of definitive prosthetic reconstruction.[20,35,25,26]

The overall planning and some drawbacks during treatment can delay the placement of definitive restorations. This will lead to long-term use of provisionals. Even thus, they should not be fabricated for short-term usage, because it is important to maintain the patient health for longer periods of time.

Conventional Prostheses

Several factors need to be respected to satisfy prosthodontic and patient demands:

Biological Factors

Pulp protection – the provisional restoration must seal and protect the pulp organ from external injuries, as well as providing healing capacity soon after tooth preparation.[18,28]

Periodontal health – the maintenance of periodontal health depends on the correct contour, finishing, superficial texture and fit of restorations. These characteristics will influence impression making and prosthesis cementation.[17,22]

Tooth positioning stability and occlusal relationships – tooth preparation leads to structural changes, resulting in loss of occlusal or adjacent tooth contacts. The provisional restoration must reestablish them to stabilize dynamic forces during tooth contact.

Mechanical Factors

Function – it must serve as the definitive restoration, enabling the patient to perform mastication and all necessary excursive mandibular movements that require occlusal contacts.

Resistance to removal and bulk strength – when removed should not be damaged because it must return to the oral cavity.[16,27]

Esthetic Factors

Provisional restorations must be similar to natural teeth in terms of shade, mold, contour and superficial texture. This will provides a satisfactory esthetic appearance until the definitive treatment be completed.

Implant-supported Prostheses

In addition to the all stated above, provisional implant restorations play a key role in determining another aspects:

Previous preparation

The adequacy of oral cavity before implant placement is paramount to a good treatment prognosis. Several dental specialties must interact in this phase, providing appropriate sites for implant installation. The suppression of infectious diseases, orthodontic movements, dental restorations, surgeries, and elimination of periodontal pockets previous to provisional restorations will provide surgeons with ideal treatment conditions.

Predictability and fingerprint of the definitive restoration

An well-executed provisional restoration serves as a surgical template for implant placement, being the clinician able to establish the number and the three-dimensional positioning of fixtures. Furthermore, during the osseointegration period, it must provides important aspects for the definitive treatment, such as: and idea of tooth size and positioning, muscular support, horizontal and vertical dental relationships, occlusal vertical dimension, and the high lip line. In case of existing prostheses serving as surgical guides, they should be duplicated and previous disinfected until the procedure (Fig. 2-1). Once considered satisfactory, the provisional restoration is an important diagnostic tool that provides valuable information on the definitive treatment for clinicians and patients.

Fig. 2-1. Predictability, surgical guide and the prototype of the definitive restoration.

2-1A. Acrylic resin provisional prosthesis to substitute tooth 21 presenting satisfactory configuration.

2-1B. Duplicated prosthesis in white acrylic resin adapted to the stone model.

2-1C. Surgical guide finished with occlusal extensions and the removal of palatine portion at implant site.

2-1D. Implant placement surgery. A 2mm twist drill prepares the hole according to the surgical guide.

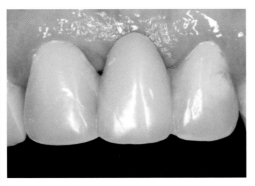

2-1A

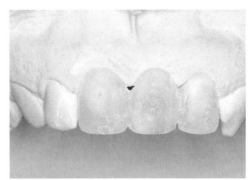

2-1B

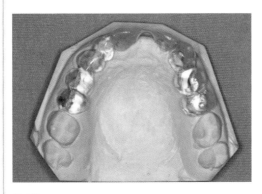

2-1C

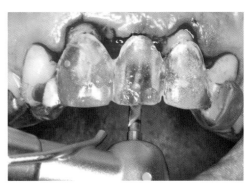

2-1D

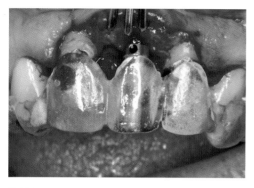

2-1E

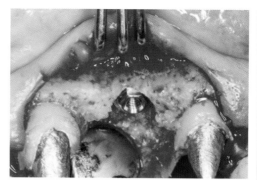

2-1F

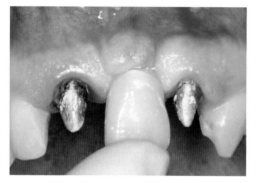

2-1G

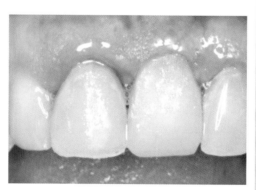

2-1H

2-1E. Guide pin inserted into the hole. Visualization facilitated by the surgical guide.

2-1F. Implant inserted according to the three-dimensional positioning of the surgical guide.

2-1G. Provisional restoration generating pressure around soft tissue for gingival conditioning.

2-1H. Gingival architecture configuration 7 days after gingival conditioning.

Maintaining or reestablishing occlusal vertical dimension

During the fabrication of definitive prostheses, implant provisional restorations can contribute to maintain vertical dimension, connected or not with dental elements. In larger restorations comprising both arches with loss of vertical dimension or occlusal breakdown due to inadequate complete dentures, implant-supported provisional prostheses can reestablish vertical dimension. Also, they will serve to evaluate whether this new jaw relationship is adequate, being further modified if necessary, due to the reversibility of these prostheses (Fig. 2-2).

2

Fig. 2-2. Reestablishment of occlusal vertical dimension, transferred to a semi-adjustable articulator.

2-2A to C. Maxillary implants, occlusal view (A), with provisional fixed prosthesis screwed onto abutments (B) after occlusal, esthetic and phonetic adjustments. Observe the relationship between fixed prosthesis, facial muscles and lip support (C).

2-2D and E. The provisional prosthesis can be used to register the occlusal relationships and relate the master casts in a semi-adjustable articulator. The definitive rehabilitation must be very similar to the provisional restoration. Centric relation position is registered with fast-set silicone impression material.

2-2F to H. Sequential steps in definitive prosthesis fabrication: metallic infra-structure (F), and metalloceramic fixed prosthesis (G).

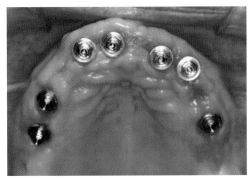
2-2A

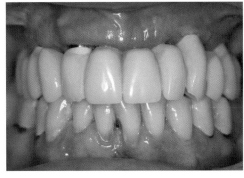
2-2B

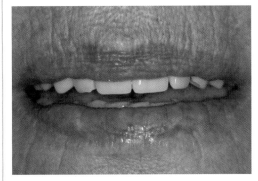
2-2C

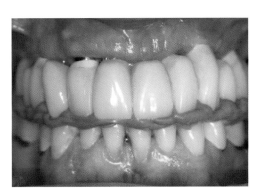
2-2D

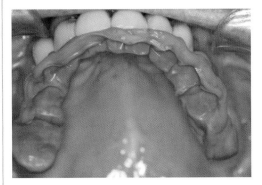
2-2E

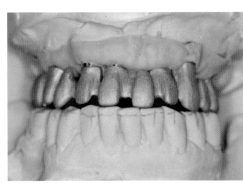
2-2F

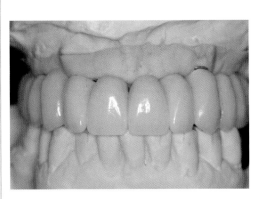
2-2G

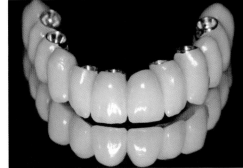
2-2H

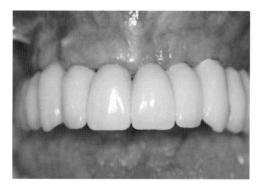

2-2I

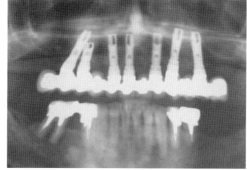

2-2J

2-2I and J. Clinical and radiographic view of definitive fixed prosthesis screwed onto the implants.

2-2K and L. The final restoration provided good muscular and lip support, similar to that obtained with the provisional crowns (Fig. 2-2C). Also, the patient smile line is equilibrated with the final prosthesis.

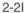

2-2K

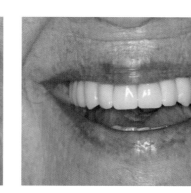

2-2L

Convenience Form

It is defined as the group of procedures that facilitates the performance of surgery, provides patient comfort and optimizes final results.

TOOTH, TUBERTOSITY-SUPPORTED PROVISIONAL FIXED PROSTHESIS

During the osseointegration treatment, provisional restorations have an strategic importance for certain patients; for example, when there remains some tooth to be extracted, and the patient will have a complete removable denture for a period, this can alter self-esteem and generate behavioral changes in some persons. As a treatment strategy, the clinician can maintain one or two teeth in position as long as they do not interfere with important implant positioning. Using these teeth or one tooth and the tuberosity, it is possible to construct a total fixed prosthesis. This will provide comfort, easy handling, more patient collaboration, and even implant and soft tissue protection when remaining roots are buried. In this case, patients do not have to wear a complete denture, avoiding the necessity of periodical relining with soft materials. Our clinical experience has shown surprising results on the use of provisional fixed prosthesis constructed over one or two teeth and supported by the tuberosity (Figs. 2-2 and 2-3). After implant uncovering and abutment installation, another provisional fixed prosthesis is fabricated onto the implants or the definitive prosthesis is made. At this stage, the remaining teeth must be extracted.

Basically, there are three techniques involving remaining tooth or root as abutments:

❑ *As terminal abutments for provisional crowns cemented with temporary materials:* the major drawback in this technique is the lack of retention due to cement nature, causing discomfort and anxiety to the patient (Fig. 2-3).

Fig. 2-3. Fixed prosthesis cemented onto teeth and tuberosity-supported.

2-3A. Initial view. Maxillary arch with two remaining teeth (21 and 27).

2-3B. Tooth 21 was extracted. Tooth 27 received a full coverage preparation and telescopic cast crown.

2-3C. Try-in of cast metal infra-structure in the mouth. The bar rests on the prepared teeth and the tuberosity on the opposite side.

2-3D. After veneering the prosthesis with termopolymerized acrylic resin, the telescopic unit is cemented on tooth 27. It will remain undisturbed during the healing period of osseointegration to protect the implants, providing esthetics and function. Depending on the treatment stage, periodical relinings and alveolar ridge remodeling are possible.

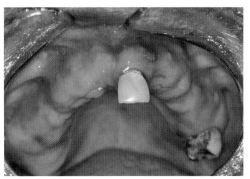

2-3A

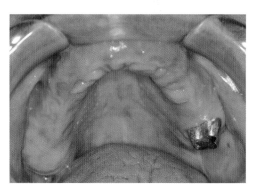

2-3B

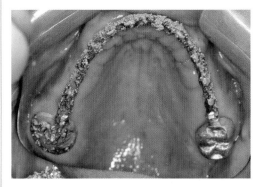

2-3C

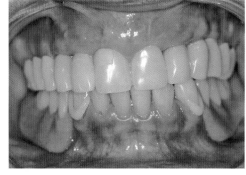

2-3D

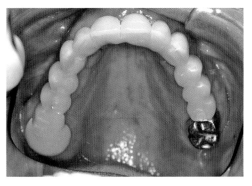

2-3E

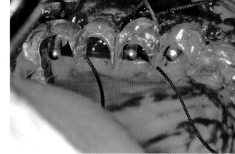

2-3F

2.3E. Occlusal view of provisional prosthesis after cementation.

2.3F and G. First-stage surgery for implant placement (F), and implant uncovering (G) after osseointegration period.

2.3H. Definitive fixed prosthesis screwed onto implants.

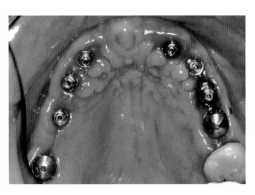

2-3G

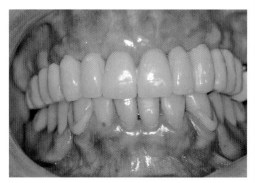

2-3H

❏ *Transforming root abutments into implant abutments:* this is done by means of a cast dowel incorporating an implant abutment that can be cemented with zinc phosphate, glass ionomer or resin luting agents. The fixed prosthesis receives a provisional or definitive prosthetic cylinder screwed into de root (Fig. 2-4). Initially, this approach was performed with custom made components. Today, replicas are made of stainless steel being machined and adapted to the dowel pattern.

❏ *Transforming root into implant abutments (simplified technique):* an implant abutment is directly cemented into the pulp chamber of the compromised tooth. First, the pulp chamber is enlarged; additional retention is created on the chamber walls with a round or inverted cone bur. Next, an abutment replica is reduced to the desired height. Care is taken to

Fig. 2-4. Provisional fixed prosthesis screwed onto remaining root.

2-4A. Residual molar root prepared to receive a dowel.

2-4B and C. Cast dowel incorporating an abutment replica.

2-4D. Surgery for removal of remaining teeth. Strategic implants were exposed, as well as the cast cemented on the molar residual root. They will serve as abutments for the provisional fixed prosthesis.

2-4E and F. Direct prosthesis relining with autopolymerized acrylic resin to capture the prosthetic cylinder. This provisional crown is finished and polished using conventional techniques.

2-4G. Finished and polished prosthesis after incorporating prosthetic cylinders.

2-4H. Provisional prosthesis in position. It can be modified anytime during treatment.

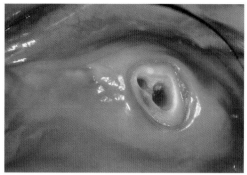

2-4A

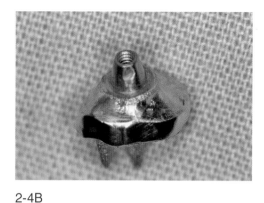

2-4B

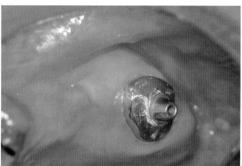

2-4C

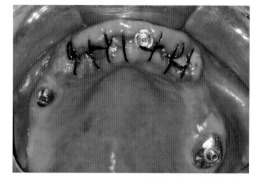

2-4D

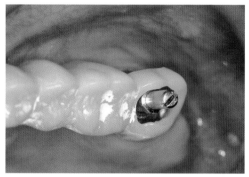

2-4E

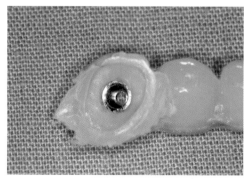

2-4F

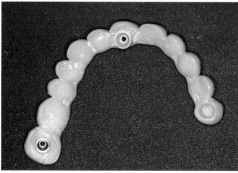

2-4G

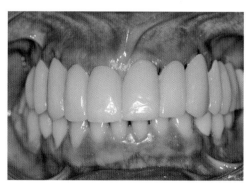

2-4H

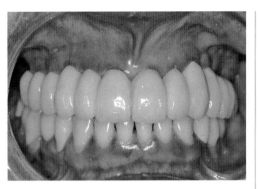

2-4I

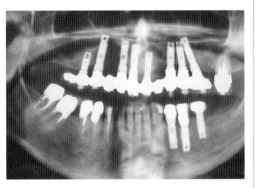

2-4J

2-4I. Definitive prosthesis installed after implant osseointegration.

2.4J. Panoramic view. Note the situation of tooth 27 after installing the definitive fixed prosthesis..

not interfere with the occlusal plane of the definitive prosthesis. After, retentive grooves are made on the abutment replica. Abutments are cemented with a composite resin or resin cement. The prosthetic cylinder is mounted on the abutment and incorporated to the fixed prosthesis with acrylic resin (Fig. 2-5). Occlusal adjustments are performed and the provisional is screwed to the root-modified implant abutment. Bracing and support can be achieved around the maxillary tuberosity on the opposite side of this prosthesis abutment.

This technique has several advantages:

❏ Reduced costs;

❏ Easy of fabrication;

❏ A screw-retention mechanism;

❏ Easy handling by the clinician and the dental technician;

❏ Patient safety; tooth does not "drop off" from mouth.

Fig. 2-5. Provisional fixed prosthesis screwed onto remaining root containing an abutment replica.

2-5A. Pulp chamber of tooth 17 prepared to receive an abutment replica.

2-5B. Retentive grooves are prepared on the abutment walls before cementation.

2-5C. Abutment replica cemented with resin luting agent.

2-5D. Abutment adapted and screwed to implant analogue.

2-5E. It is necessary to reline the prosthesis with acrylic resin to capture the prosthetic cylinder.

2-5F. Final aspect of provisional prosthesis.

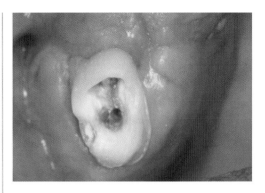

2-5A

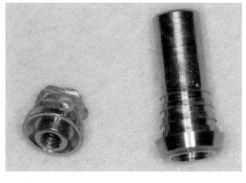

2-5B

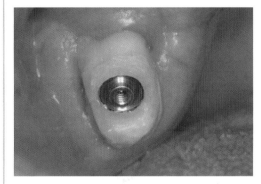

2-5C

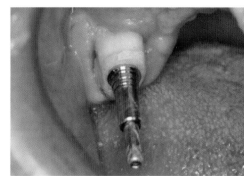

2-5D

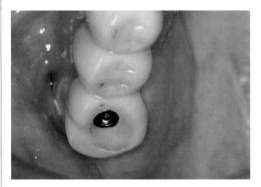

2-5E

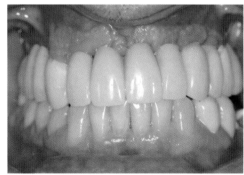

2-5F

Gingival conditioning and contouring

Provisional restorations have a fundamental role in areas with esthetic demands.[8,15,21,29] After tooth removal, gingival scalloped architecture is substituted for a flat tissue configuration due to the loss of interdental papilla (Fig. 2-6A). Implant placement and osseointegration cannot by themselves restore the integrity of gingival contours (Fig. 2-6B). For this, it is necessary to redirect periimplant gingival margins, developing its primary appearance.[11] This can be achieved through successive tissue compression and relining provided by provisional restorations, at weekly time intervals, until obtaining a concave regular arch form similar to the original shape (Figs. 2-6C to H). Provision- al restorations are the architects of gingival shape and contour[18] determining excellence in esthetics, providing an harmonious transition from white to red esthetics.

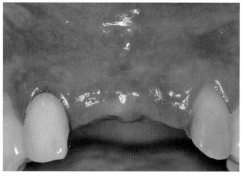

2-6A

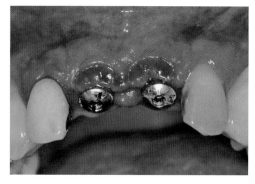

2-6B

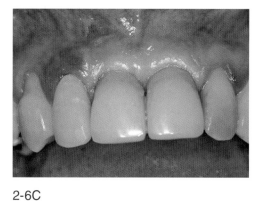

2-6C

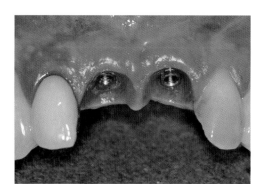

2-6D

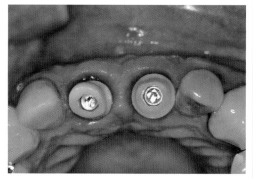

2-6E

2-6F

Fig. 2-6. Gingival contouring with provisional restorations

2-6A. Labial aspect after loss of maxillary central incisors. There is no dental papilla and the gingival tissue has a flat configuration.

2-6B. Gingival tissue after cicatrization. Note deficient esthetics after healing abutment connection.

2-6C. Initial gingival contouring. Tissue compression with provisional restorations shows ischemic areas.

2-6D. Final aspect after 4 weeks.

2-6E. Note the formation of gingival scalloping and dental papillae after crown removal.

2-6F. Custom made alumina abutments screwed to implants. Observe gingival papilla and the space between abutment and free gingival margin (periimplant sulcus), leading to an adequate emergency profile to the final prosthetic crowns.

2-6G and H. Porcelain crowns adapted to the master cast and cemented onto alumina abutments. Observe the presence of gingival contour and dental papilla.

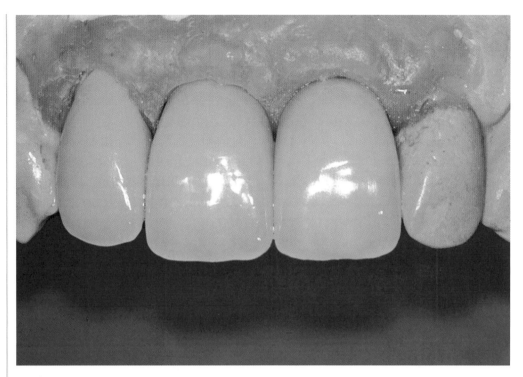

2-6G

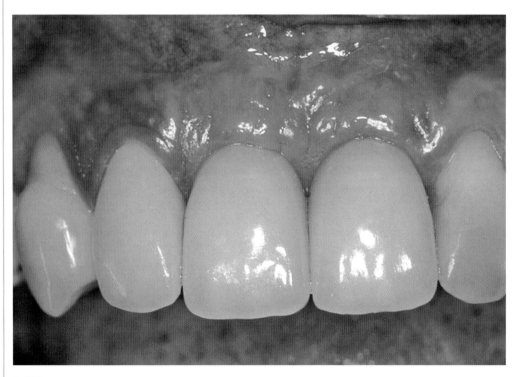

2-6H

Precise transference of gingival emergency profile to the master cast

To assure high quality dental restorations, it is necessary to capture not only implant or abutment position, but also surrounding gingival tissue. If the dental technician can not transfer this configuration to the master cast, all time and effort spent on it will be worthless. Similar to the gingival conditioning, provisional restorations do exert a fundamental role in this transference. After achieving an adequate gingival architecture, they would be used to customize impression pre-fabricated copings, since they can not capture detailed gingival information. When periimplant healing is completed, the gingival tissue has a poor configuration (Fig. 2-7A). As already described, it will be modified by pressure with the provisional restoration (Fig. 2-7C). After complete conditioning (Fig. 2-7D), impressions can be taken.

The provisional restoration is removed from the oral cavity and connected to an abutment replica. Next, crown and replica are immersed in heavy-body silicone material (Figs. 2-7 E and F). After silicone polymerization, the provisional crown is removed (Fig. 2-7G), an impression coping is connected and the empty spaces (corresponding to the gingival tissue architecture) are filled with autopolymerized acrylic resin (Fig. 2-7H). Thus, a high fidelity custom-made impression coping is obtained, because now it represents the same gingival conditioning obtained with the provisional restoration in the mouth.[11] Resin excess are removed and the coping is connected to the implant abutment for impression making (Figs. 2-7I and J). After pouring the impression in high quality dental stone, the technician will have a precise master cast for porcelain application, which reflects perfect interaction between implant and periimplant gingival tissue (Figs. 2-7K and L).

Fig. 2-7. Precise transference of gingival emergency profile.

2-7A. Gingival tissue ready to be manipulated after second stage surgery.

2-7B. Periapical radiograph showing osseointegration.

2-7C. Gingival conditioning with provisional restoration

2-7D. Adequate manipulation of gingival tissue after conditioning. Note periimplant papilla and scalloped configuration.

2-7E and F. Provisional crown adapted to the Ceraone implant analog (E), immersed in heavy-body silicone impression material (F).

2.7G and H. After crown removal, a space is formed into the silicone mold (G). An impression coping is connected to the implant analog, and the space is filled with autopolymerized acrylic resin (H).

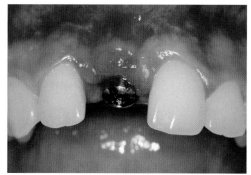
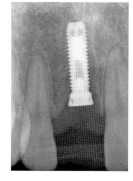

2-7A

2-7B

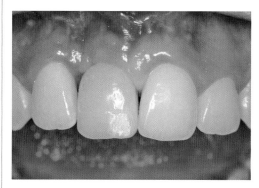
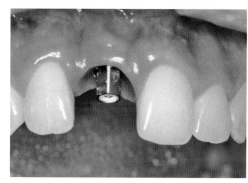

2-7C

2-7D

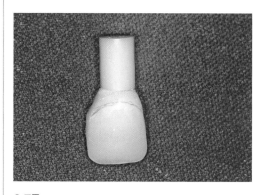
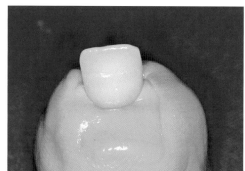

2-7E

2-7F

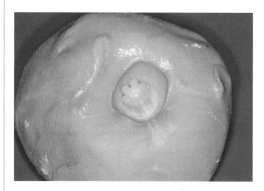
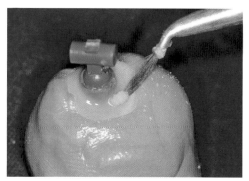

2-7G

2-7H

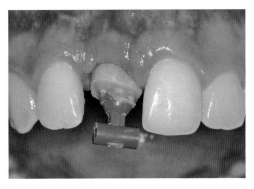

2-7I

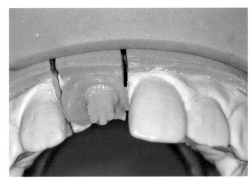

2-7J

2-7I. Custom made impression coping adapted to the implant abutment, ready for transference.

2-7J. Master cast showing adequate transference of gingival emergency profile.

2-7K and L. Porcelain crown onto the master cast (K); and in the mouth (L). Note the correct relationship of restoration and gingival tissues.

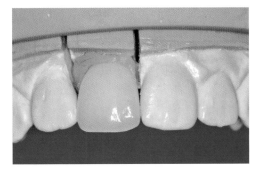

2-7K

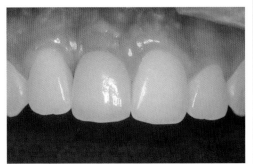

2-7L

Protection during osseointegration

In the two-stage surgical technique, undisturbed implant healing is paramount to achieve osseointegration. Tooth and tuberosity-supported provisional restorations represent mechanical barriers to possible damage in these sites, assuring better implant prognosis, as already described (Figs. 2-3 to 2-5).

Serving as a guide to repositioning implants through segmentation techniques

The correct three-dimensional positioning of osseointegrated implants (bucco-lingual, mesio-distal and apico-coronal) is of utmost importance to obtain adequate prosthetic resolutions. Sometimes, mal-positioned implants difficult or prevent prosthesis fabrication.

The dental technician has to decide whether to remove them or not during laboratory work. In some instances, segmentation techniques (osseous block osteotomies with implant repositioning) can be used to ameliorate this problem. Many implants scheduled for removal could serve as abutments (Fig. 2-8).

Fig. 2-8. Implant repositioning after segmented osteotomies in accordance with provisional crowns

2-8A. Frontal view. Note the more coronal implant position on the right side creating an esthetic compromise.

2-8B. Frontal view of provisional prosthesis. Note the unbalance between the right lateral and central incisive gingival margins.

2-8C. Segmented surgery on the master cast. The right maxillary segment is more apically repositioned to compensate for marginal discrepancies.

2-8D. Lateral view of segmented surgery. A resin verification jig (Duralay) was fabricated to guide correct implant positioning.

2-8E. Provisional prosthesis relined in the mouth. Observe the dramatic change on the final aspect.

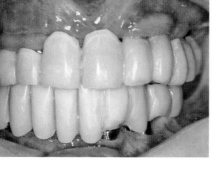

2-8A

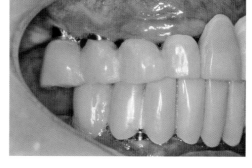

2-8B

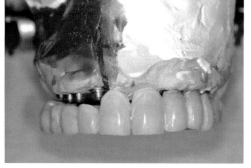

2-8C

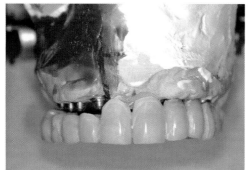

2-8D

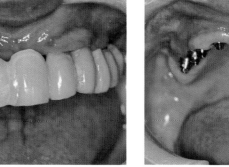

2-8E

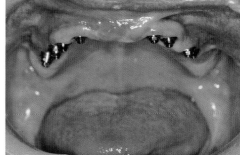

2-8F

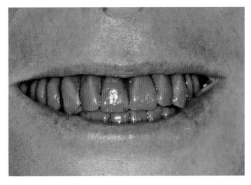

2-8G

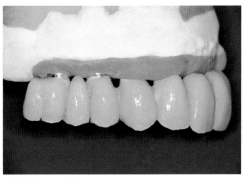

2-8H

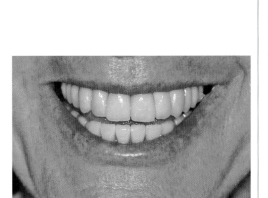

2-8I

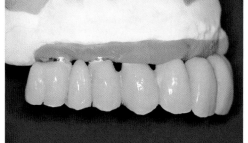

2-8J

2-8G. Wax-up try-in; it represents the prototype of final restoration. Observe the leveling of cervical line from right to left margins.

2.8H. Definitive restoration screwed on the master cast

2-8I and J. Final prosthesis delivered. Observe harmonious interaction between high lip line, patient smile line and cervical crown positioning.

Provisional restorations on immediate function

The increased success of immediate or functional implant loading have encouraged clinicians and researchers to broad its initial applications from complete dentures[13] to partial and single-tooth implant restorations.[1,3,5,12,19] Thus, unitary provisional restorations have been extremely necessary in areas of high esthetic demands. In addition to provide time needed for osseointegration, they develop the gingival tissue contour during this period. This approach represents less chairside time in the final prosthetic phase, avoiding gingival conditioning and contouring. The procedures for immediate loading and provisional restorations can be performed in healed extraction sockets (Fig. 2-10) or soon after tooth extraction[24] (Fig. 2-9).

Fig. 2-9. Provisional restoration for immediate function

2-9A and B. Periapical radiograph (A) and labial view of longitudinal fractured tooth 22. Note the absence of fistule.

2-9C. Exposed root showing the longitudinal fracture.

2-9D. After extraction, the socket was cleaned and inflamed tissue properly removed. Labial plate is intact. This detail is important for implant placement.

2-9E. Alveolar socket instrumentation before implant placement.

2-9F. Bone chips harvested from buccal area.

2-9G. The harvested bone collected.

2-9H. Harvested bone filling the space between implant and alveolar socket.

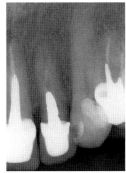
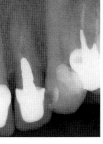
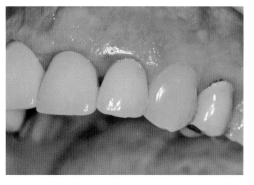

2-9A

2-9B

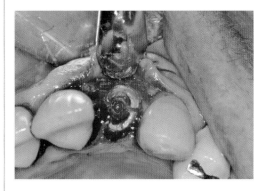
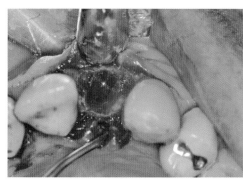

2-9C

2-9D

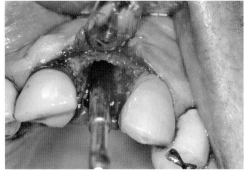
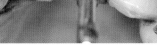
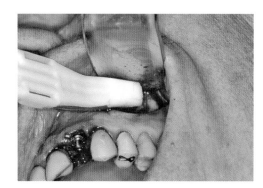

2-9E

2-9F

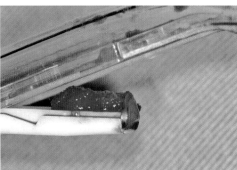
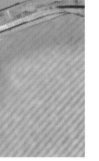
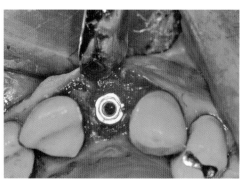

2-9G

2-9H

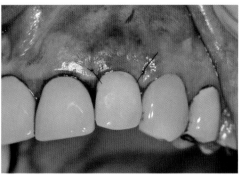

2-9I

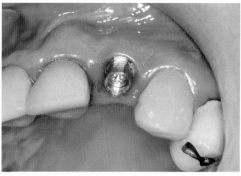

2-9J

2-9I. Provisional restoration in position soon after implant placement and suture.

2-9J and K. After 6 months, the abutment is installed (J). the abutment-implant junction (J) is verified with a periapical radiograph (K). observe good marginal quality.

2-9L. Frontal view of definitive restoration.

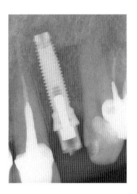

2-9K

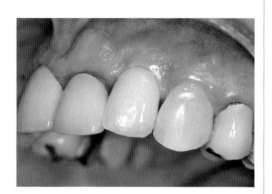

2-9L

Previous sculpture of gingival architecture

Provisional restorations have exerted a decisive role on esthetics not only in the prosthetic phase after surgery, but also in the early stages of implant treatment.[2,14] They can be regarded as important tools to predict what could be achieved until final prosthesis insertion. Edentulous alveolar ridges exhibit loss of gingival scalloping. Even after receiving implants, this tissue needs to be esthetically managed to assure excellent final results.[6] Such treatment could be done on pre and post-immediate surgical phases, reducing time to obtain favorable esthetics (Fig. 2-10). Technological innovations have changed routine surgical and prosthetic protocols to optimize treatment with dental implants. The time interval from pre-implant surgery, its insertion and prosthesis installation, along with the biological and esthetic improvements has been considerably reduced. The concept of one-stage implant systems summarizes it. Due to the lack of an implant-abutment junction, less inflammation will occur around periimplant tissue and bone levels can be successfully maintained. More conservative surgical approaches with less soft tissue manipulation enhance esthetical results. The exposed transmucosal portion provides retention and support for the provisional restorations, as well as the creation of gingival contours, assuring an easier and faster installation of definitive prosthesis. In this way, gingival conditioning may be unnecessary (Fig. 2-10). For these situations, provisional restorations can be fabricated from duplicated diagnostic wax-up or through prefabricated crown forms (Fig. 2-10N).

Fig. 2-10. Gingival sculpture.

2-10A. Initial view showing loss of central incisors and gingival architecture.

2-10B. Occlusal view showing good bone thickness.

2-10C and D. Round diamond bur used to create an scalloped gingival tissue.

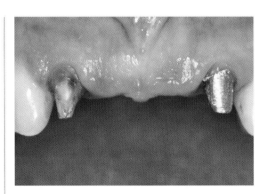

2-10A

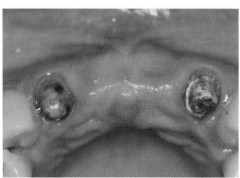

2-10B

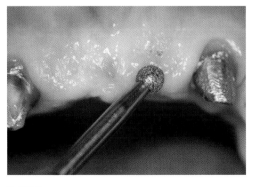

2-10C

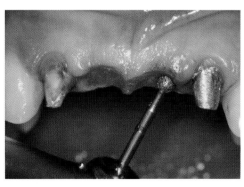

2-10D

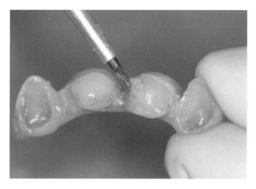

2-10E

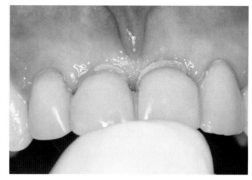

2-10F

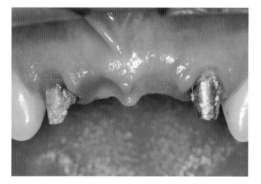

2-10G

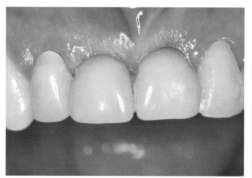

2-10H

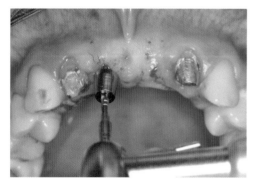

2-10I

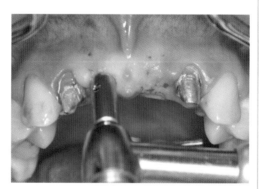

2-10J

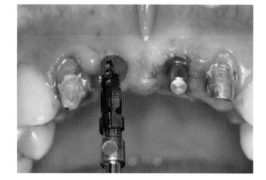

2-10K

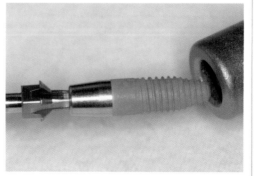

2-10L

2-10E. Acrylic resin added to the pontic intaglio surface. This will favor tissue reepithelization.

2-10F. Provisional prosthesis showing mild tissue compression.

2-10G and H. Clinical aspect 30 days after gingival sculpting.

2-10I. Implant surgery without flap reflection. Observe bur guide during perforation.

2-10J. Gingival punch removing local tissue with osseous exposition.

2-10K. A 3.75mm-conical bur for alveolus preparation (left). Guide pin positioned on perforation (right).

2-10L. Non-submerged one-stage implant with 4.3mm-diameter and 13mm-length.

2-10M. Implants inserted on their respective alveolar sockets.

2-10N. Try-in of prefabricated crown forms.

2-10O. Crowns are cemented after implant installation, maintaining proper contour, shape and gingival esthetics during osseointegration period.

2-10P. Postoperative view 60 days after surgery. Note the adequacy of gingival contour.

2-10Q and R. The definitive restoration is finished (Q). Try-in of porcelain crowns in the mouth.

2-10S and T. Detailed view showing health and good contour of gingival papilla.

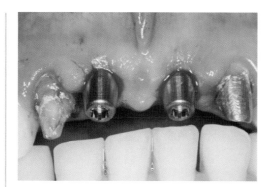

2-10M

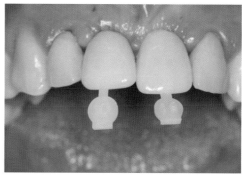

2-10N

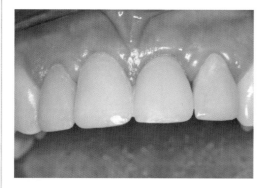

2-10O

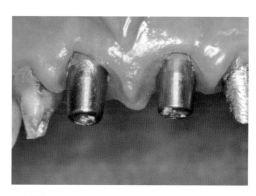

2-10P

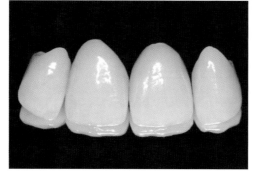

2-10Q

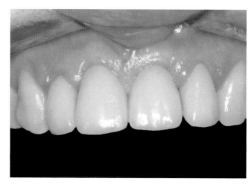

2-10R

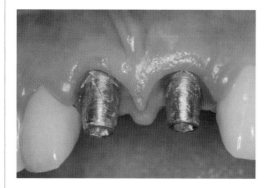

2-10S

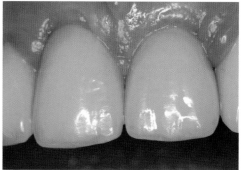

2-10T

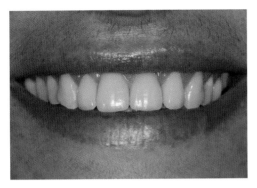

2-10U

2-10V

2-10U. The patient's smile shows good transition from red to white esthetics. This was only achieved by adequate contour, shape and emergence profile, as well as the same height between implant and adjacent tooth.

2-10V. Periapical radiograph showing adequate bone level. It provides satisfactory esthetic results for dental papilla.

2-10X. Grid according to Levin, showing anterior teeth in golden proportion, intercanine distance, smile width and buccal corridor.[10] The ideal width of the upper central incisor is found with the following equation:

$$CW = K \times SW$$

where:
CW = width of the central incisor,
K = 0.155,
SW = smile width.[10,18]

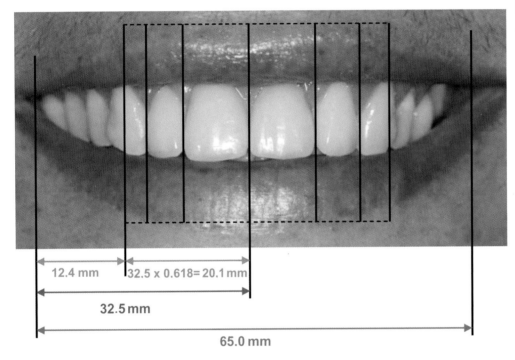

12.4 mm   32.5 x 0.618= 20.1 mm

32.5 mm

65.0 mm

2-10X

ADO´s factors

HOW TO IMPROVE LONG-TERM SUCCESS OF OSSEOINTEGRATED PROSTHETIC REHABILITATIONS

According to Dr. P-I Brånemark, harmonious occlusion is the key for long-term success of osseointegrated oral rehabilitation. It stands for:

Adjusting of
Dimension and distribution of
Occlusal
Stress and strain

We can call it **third stability of the implant**.

It is also known that primary and secondary implant stability are fundamental to achievement of osseointegration. Now, we introduce the term **Tertiary Stability** to define other factors responsible for long-term osseointegration. The tertiary stability is related to the **Ado´s Factor**.

The following events must be considered when ADO's factors are applied:

- ❑ well-fitted and contoured provisional restorations;
- ❑ shallow cusps (≤ 15 degrees);
- ❑ mutually protected occlusion;
- ❑ bucco-lingual reduction in occlusal table;
- ❑ lingualized occlusion;
- ❑ anterior guidance with minimal posterior disocclusion;
- ❑ canine disocclusion, increasing palatal concavity as necessary;
- ❑ maximum number of centric contacts on each tooth;
- ❑ avoidance of sophisticated devices;
- ❑ successive and selective occlusal adjustment of crown surfaces as soon as implants are recognized by brain (osseoperception).

Maintenance of periimplant gingival tissue health

Regardless of esthetic compromise, provisional restorations have a great influence on the periimplant tissue health. Similar to conventional prosthesis, they maintain form and positioning of free gingival margins. This further facilitates impression transfer and prosthesis installation.[4,9] However, adequate contour, superficial texture, and good marginal fit are mandatory. Usually, they can be found in all treatment modalities. When used to modify or maintain gingival appearance, Mondelli[18] considers them as "the architects" of form and contour (Fig. 2-11).

Fig. 2-11. Maintenance of periimplant gingival health.

2-11A. Gingival scalloped aspect maintained by provisional restorations.

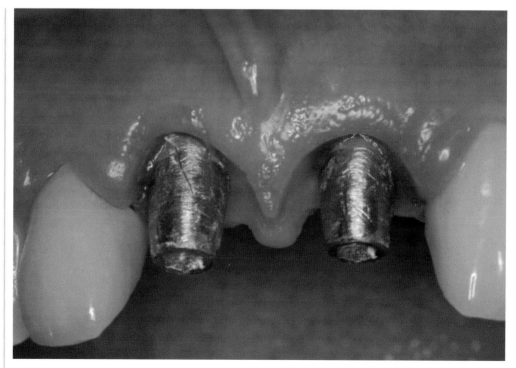

2-11A

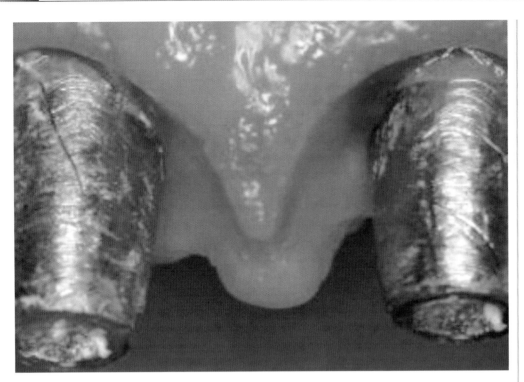

2-11B

2-11B. Larger view showing adequate periimplant gingival health and architecture. This establishes harmonious transition with the definitive crowns.

References

1. ABBOUD, M.; KOECK, B.; STARK, H.; WAHL, G.; PAILLON, R. Immediate loading of single-tooth implants in the posterior region. *Int J Oral Maxillofac Implants.* 2005 Jan-Feb; 20(1):61-8.

2. BIGGS, W.F.; LITVAK JR., A.L. Immediate provisional restorations to aid in gingival healing and optimal contours for implant patients. *J Prosthet Dent.* 2001 Aug; 86(2):177-80.

3. BLOCK, M.; FINGER, I.; CASTELLON, P.; LIRETTLE, D. Single tooth immediate provisional restoration of dental implants: technique and early results. *J Oral Maxillofac Surg.* 2004 Sep; 62(9):1131-8.

4. BRAL, M. Periodontal considerations for provisional restorations. *Dent Clin North Am.* 1989 Jul; 33(3):457-77.

5. CALVO GUIRADO, J.L.; SAEZ YUGUERO, R.; FERRER PEREZ, V.; MORENO PELLUZ, A. Immediate anterior implant placement and early loading by provisional acrylic crowns: a prospective study after a one-year follow-up period. *J Ir Dent Assoc.* 2002; 48(2):43-9.

6. CHEE, W.W. Provisional restorations in soft tissue management around dental implants. *Periodontol 2000.* 2001; 27:139-47.

7. COELHO, A.B.; MIRANDA, J.E.S.; PEGORARO, L.F. Single-tooth implants: A procedure to make a precise, flexible gengival contour on the mastercast. *J. Prosthet Dent.* 1997, 78(1):109-110.

8. DAVARPANAH, M.; MARTINEZ, H.; CELLETTI, R.; TECUCIANU, J.F. Three-stage approach to aesthetic implant restoration: emergence profile concept. *Pract Proced Aesthet Dent.* 2001 Nov-Dec; 13(9):761-7; quiz 768, 721-2.

9. FERENCZ, J.L. Maintaining and enhancing gingival architecture in

fixed prosthodontics. *J Prosthet Dent.* 1991 May; 65(5):650-7.

10. FRANCISCHONE, A.C.; MONDELLI J. The science of beautiful smile. *Rev Estética. Dental Press Int.,* 2007; 4(2):97-106.

11. FRANCISCHONE, C.E.; VASCONCELOS, L.W.; BRÅNEMARK, P-I. *Osseointegration and esthetics in single tooth rehabilitation.* São Paulo: Quintessence, 2000.

12. GROISMAN, M.; FROSSARD, W.M.; FERREIRA, H.M.; MENEZES FILHO, L.M.; TOUATI, B. Single-tooth implants in the maxillary incisor region with immediate provisionalization: 2-year prospective study. *Pract Proced Aesthet Dent.* 2003 Mar; 15(2):115-22, 124; quiz 126.

13. JAFFIN, R.A.; KUMAR, A.; BERMAN, C.L. Immediate loading of dental implants in the completely edentulous maxilla: a clinical report. *Int J Oral Maxillofac Implants.* 2004 Sep-Oct; 19(5):721-30.

14. KINSEL, R.P.; LAMB, R.E. Development of gingival esthetics in the edentulous patient prior to dental implant placement using a flangeless removable prosthesis: a case report. *Int J Oral Maxillofac Implants.* 2002 Nov-Dec; 17(6):866-72.

15. MACINTOSH, D.C.; SUTHERLAND, M. Method for developing an optimal emergence profile using heat-polymerized provisional restorations for single-tooth implant-supported restorations. *J Prosthet Dent.* 2004 Mar; 91(3):289-92.

16. MOJON, P.; HAWBOLT, E.B.; MACENTEE, M.I. A comparison of two methods for removing zinc oxide-eugenol provisional cement. *Int J Prosthodont.* 1992; 5:78.

17. MONDAY, J.J.L.; BLAIS, D. Marginal adaptation of provisional acrylic resin crowns. *J Prosthet Dent.* 1985; 54:194.

18. MONDELLI, J. *Estética e Cosmética em Clínica Integrada Restauradora.* São Paulo: Ed. Santos, 2003.

19. MOULDING, M.B.; TEPLITSKY, P.E. Intrapulpal temperature during direct fabrication of provisional restorations. *Int J Prosthod.* 1990; 3:299.

20. NORTON, M.R. A short-term clinical evaluation of immediately restored maxillary TiOblast single-tooth implants. *Int J Oral Maxillofac Implants.* 2004 Mar-Apr; 19(2):274-81.

21. PASHLEY, E.L. et al. The sealing properties of temporary filling materials. *J Prosthet Dent.* 1988; 60:292.

22. POGGIO, C.E.; SALVATO, A. Bonded provisional restorations for esthetic soft tissue support in single-implant treatment. *J Prosthet Dent.* 2002 Jun;87(6):688-91.

23. ROBINSON,F.B.;HOVIJITRA,S.Marginal fit of direct temporary crowns. *J. Prosthet Dent.* 1982; 47:390.

24. ROSENTIEL, S.F.; LAND, M.F.; FUJIMOTO, J. *Contemporary Fixed Prosthodontics.* Mosby, 2000, Chap. 15, p.380-415.

25. SCHIROLI, G. Immediate tooth extraction, placement of a Tapered Screw-Vent implant, and provisionalization in the esthetic zone: a case report. *Implant Dent.* 2003; 12(2):123-31.

26. SCOTTI, R. et al. The *in vitro* color stability of acrylic resins for provisional restorations. *Int J Prosthod.* 1997; 10:164.

27. SELTZER, S.; BENDER, I.B. The dental pulp: biologic considerations in dental procedures. 3 ed., Philadelphia: JB Lippincott, 1984, p.191.

28. TERATA, R. et al. Characterization of enamel and dentin surfaces after removal of temporary cement-effect of temporary cement on tensile bond strength of resin luting agent. *Dent Mater J.* 1994; 13:148.

29. TJAN, A.H.L. et al; Temperature rise in the pulp chamber during fabrication of provisional crowns. *J Prosthet Dent.* 1989; 62:622.

30. VOGEL, R.C. Enhancing implant esthetics with ideal provisionalization. *J Indiana Dent Assoc.* 2002 Fall; 81(3):11-4.

3

CAN DIFFERENT IMPLANT SYSTEMS INFLUENCE THE QUALITY OF PERIIMPLANT ORAL MICROFLORA?

Daniela A. D. Matos

Although similar in appearance, periimplant and gingival tissues are not truly identical. Histological evidence shows the absence of periodontal ligament and cementum around dental implants. Also, connective tissue fibers do not run perpendicular to the implant surface. The lack of tissue insertion on dental implants facilitates bacterial plaque accumulation, influx of salivary components and higher probing depths. Thus, the periimplant sulcus is more susceptible to inflammatory disease and bleeding on probing than the dentogingival complex.

Most of partially edentulous patients with implant-supported prostheses harbor almost the same microflora existing on dentate individuals.[11] Periodontal pockets represent the habitat of microorganisms with potential to colonize the periimplant sulcus. In this regard, periodontopathic bacteria found on gingival pockets constitutes a risk factor for periimplantitis.[10,36]

The microbiological contents of periimplant and periodontal tissues have been investigated by the same research methods used in Periodontology.[13,25,41,48,49] Main focus has been to study the pathogenesis and possible treatments of periimplant infeccions.

Studies indicate that periimplant microflora has a similar content found on periodontitis: a high proportion of motile microorganisms, anaerobic gram-negative bacteria and spirochetes. Thus, some aspects need to be highlighted, such as: prevention of microorganism development, adequate control of gingival health, prevention of deep periimplant pockets and the use of implants and abutments with smooth surfaces. Periodontal risk factors like smoke and poor oral hygiene can increase the chance of periimplantitis, because periodontitis susceptibility is highly indicative of periimplantitis[51,52] which varies according to type and superficial implant characteristics.

However, the high prevalence of certain bacterial species does not indicate that they are the primary causal factor of the disease, because the establishment of an inflammatory condition with loss of tissue insertion determines an adequate habitat for other microorganisms. According to Heydenrijk et al. (2002) we still do not known the major role of specific microorganisms on the etiology of compromised implants due to infectious diseases, i.e., whether the indigenous flora causes the disease or it is generated owing to a favorable ambient.

Implants with specific characteristics may enhance osseointe-gration in poor quality bone during initial healing phase, due to an increase on its superficial area. However, the maintenance of periimplant mucosal health becomes more critical because these are very irregular implant surfaces, which facilitates plaque accumulation and further development of periimplant tissue inflammation.

Nevertheless, these different surfaces neither influence the microflora colonizing supra and subgengival plaque, maturation or the microbial succession[16,28,35,46] exerting their role on the number of bacterial cells during the initial period of plaque formation. Qualitative differences on microflora occurs due to the dental status rather than differences on superficial implant characteristics.[40,55]

The classic Brånemark recommended approach (total fixed mandibular prosthesis screwed in a two-stage implant system) becomes a treatment option with high predictability and success rates.[11,12,39] Nowadays, the great challenge is to simplify available treatment and reduce time period necessary to prosthesis installation.

The Brånemark Novum concept developed in 1980 was conceived for rehabilitation with implant and teeth on the same day. It relies on the good mechanical capacity of mandibular bone as well as the functional principles necessary to the success of osseointegration. It consists of three dental implants placed on the interforaminal region stabilized with a titanium substructure screwed to the abutments. A prefabricated metallic bar (supra-structure) with artificial teeth is seated onto the substructure. This system has provided success rates comparable to the initial two-stage approach,[8,15,39] depending on adequate patient selection and precision of surgical technique.

The use of a two-stage implant system leads to gap formation at the implant-abutment junction. These areas have a potential for microorganism accumulation.[1,24,25] On the other hand, one-stage implants do not present this problem due to the absence of such interface near to the osseous tissue.

Microbiological aspects

The remaining teeth act as bacterial reservoirs in the oral cavity for surface implant colonization;[28,34,38] in addition, there is evidence of microorganism carriage from periodontal sites to periimplant areas of partially edentulous patients.[17,49]

On the other hand, the oral microflora existing on implant surface of totally edentulous patients is very similar to that before implant placement. Thus, bacterial species that compose plaque have an important role as disease indicators and, although several types of microorganism can be found in the oral cavity, not all present pathogenic characteristics.

Actinobacillus actinomycetemcomitans, *Porphyromonas gingivalis*, and *Prevotella intermedia* are considered important microorganisms in the oral cavity, and usually are associated to pathological tissue alterations.

According to its morphological characteristics, microorganisms are gram-negative rods, anaerobic, non-motile, assacharolytic, and unsporulated (*Prevotella intermedia* can metabolize sugar). The *Actinobacillus actinomycetemcomitans ssp.* and *Porphyromonas gingivalis* show pleomorphism, i.e., the capacity to alter phenotypic expression.[47,54]

The colonies of *Actinobacillus actinomycetemcomitans* are round, shining, have a 1mm-diameter convex surface and irregular borders. Although divided in five serotypes, only a and b serotypes are more frequent in the oral cavity, being these one of the few species that can colonize oral mucosa and dental plaque. The *Porphyromonas gingivalis* species show brown to black pigmentation, being primarily found on the subgingival plaque, lateral borders of tongue, oral mucosa and tonsils. Within the associated virulence factors are the production of type I and IV collagenases, lipopolysaccharide, endotoxins and the presence of fimbriae. Porphyromonas gingivalis is rarely found on health sites, being associated with deep pockets.

Prevotella intermedia also show small and round colonies, with smooth or convex surfaces, opaque or translucent, with a brown to black pigmentation. These microorganisms are much related to sites with bleeding on probing. Some of its several virulence factors include lipopolysaccharide, acid phosphatase, alkaline phosphatase enzymes, fibroblast inhibitor factor.[47,54] The absence of *Prevotella intermedia* on completely edentulous individuals is temporary. After few years of edentulism, these microorganisms can be found on the oral mucosa after being identified in saliva.[9] On the other hand, *Actinobacillus actinomycetemcomitans* species are not found in totally edentulous patients due to a change in the oral microflora after tooth loss, being the habitat difficult to colonize.[9,29] This change can also interfere with colonization of implant surfaces on the same patients.

Many authors[1,37,48] agree that not only periimplant and gingival tissues are similar, but also natural teeth and periimplant sulcus microflora because even pathogenic microorganisms as-

sociated to periodontal disease may be localized around osseointegrated implants or contribute to treatment failure. Still, some authors[25,37,38,48] state that probing depth is the most specific clinical parameter to identify microorganisms such as *Porphyromonas gingivalis*, *Prevotella intermedia*, *Fusobacterium nucleatum* and *Actinobacillus actinomecetemcomitans*, since the presence of these species is directly related to the depth of periimplant or periodontal pocket.[45]

The pathologic alterations found in the periimplant region occur due to the breakdown between local microflora and host resistance. In this way, the previous history of periimplant or periodontal disease, host general health conditions, diabetes, smoking, genetic traits and the use of drugs are factors known to alter periimplant bacterial colonization.[3,17,22,28,31,34,42,45,49]

The importance of microbiological study techniques

The development of molecular biology techniques for identification of specific bacterial plaque colonizing microorganisms has been a fundamental role in diagnosis and treatment of pathologic soft tissue alterations, since the current methods showed some drawbacks, such as: necessity of viable microorganisms, being adequate in number for identification, lack of individual species recognition, higher costs, more knowledge, time, and experience, factors already known to compromise results obtained, making them less confidence.

Polimerase Chain Reaction Technique (PCR) has been shown an important research tool to generate faster results, been capable to identify bacteria in less than four hours, demonstrating high sensitivity and specificity as well.[2,32,44,53] This technique has been the choice to study specific microorganisms related to soft tissues due to its advantages and safe outcomes. Thus, studies on colonizing microflora in the periimplant region have been conducted with this technology associated to clinical parameters found in Periodontics. According to Lang et al. (1994) and Bapoo-Mohamed et al. (1996) it is a fair clinical procedure to indicate or follow-up periimplant tissue stability or pathological reactions.

The chance to detect potentially pathogenic microorganisms increases with higher probing depths values of periimplant sulcus. Thus, deeper sites are required for the collection of periimplant or periodontal bacterial plaque samples, due to their anaerobic and virulence potential. This can be done with sterile paper points which by capillary action absorb plaque and microorganisms of interest. According to some authors,[18] there is no significant difference regarding to sample quality for the intervals of 5 and 60 seconds, but it is not recommended to take a sample with less than 10 seconds.

Due to the imperative role of osseointegration in dentistry, an increasing interest has grown on the features and behavior of periimplant marginal mucosa, as well as for related factors such as microflora characterization in health and disease condition, although in 1984 some authors[43] had already observed that microflora related to implants is quite complex, with higher concentrations of cocci in health periimplant sulcus. However, with the increase on inflammatory state and sulcus depth, the diversity of bacterial species diminishes and a high percentage of spirochetes and motile organisms can be found.

The following steps are necessary to the PCR technique:

❑ periimplant bacterial plaque sampling must be done after removal of fixed implant-supported prosthesis;

❑ the soft tissues around implants must be isolated with gauze. Supragingival bacterial plaque or calculus is removed with sterile cotton pellets or teflon curettes. The objective is not to contaminate subgingival samples (Fig. 3-1);

❏ after, six sites are measured around dental implants (Fig. 3-2) to warrant that deeper sulci will have their content removed with an sterile paper point nº 40 introduced and maintained for 10 seconds (Fig. 3-3).

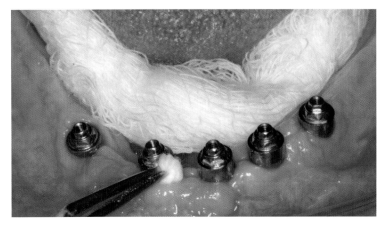

3-1

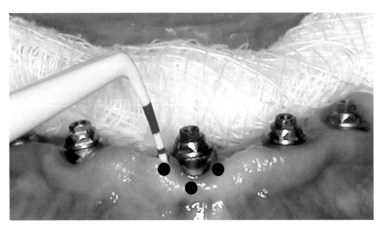

3-2

Fig. 3-1. Removal of supragingival bacterial plaque with a sterile cotton pellet.

Fig. 3-2. Periimplant probing depths been measured.

Fig. 3-3. Sampling of subgingival bacterial plaque with a sterile paper point.

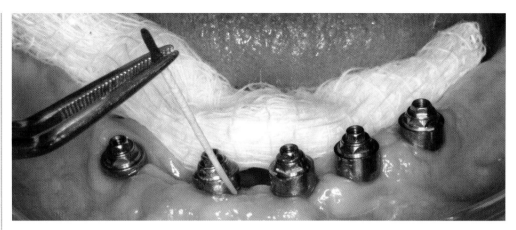

3-3

❏ Immediately after sample collection, it must be stored in plastic cryotubes at -20°C, until the start of DNA extraction.

DNA extraction

To each microtube is necessary to add 100μL of TAS (50mM tris-HCl pH 8.0; 50mM EDTA 150mM NaCl); 10μL SDS 10% (Sodium dodecyl sulfate) and 2μL of Proteinase K (20mg/mL). The tubes are left in water bath for one hour at 60°C. After, 50μL of phenol and 50μL of chlorophormium are added to each tube. Tubes are microcentrifuged for 3 minutes at 10.000rpm, removing the supernatant. To the supernatant 50μl of chlorophormium is added, centrifugating it for 3 minutes at 10.000rpm, being this process repeated twice. The final product receives 3M sodium acetate and 100% ethanol to precipitate the genomic DNA of each sample, now stored overnight at 4°C (Fig. 3-4).

After that, samples are centrifuged for 10minutes at 10.000rpm and the supernatant discarded. To the precipitate is added 50μL of 70% ethanol, centrifuged for 3 minutes at 10.000rpm, discarding supernatant. Then, samples are stored at 37°C for 5 minutes and receive 50μL T.E. (10mM tris-HCl pH 8.0; 1mM EDTA pH 8.0). Next, samples are stored in the refrigerator for further analysis through PCR technique (Fig. 3-5).

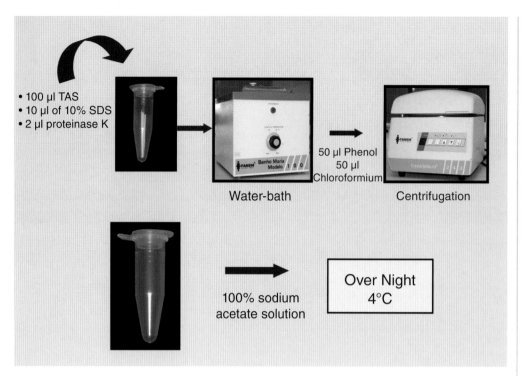

• 100 µl TAS
• 10 µl of 10% SDS
• 2 µl proteinase K

Water-bath

50 µl Phenol
50 µl
Chloroformium

Centrifugation

100% sodium
acetate solution

Over Night
4°C

3-4

Fig. 3-4. Precipitation of genomic DNA.

Fig. 3-5. Genomic DNA obtained.

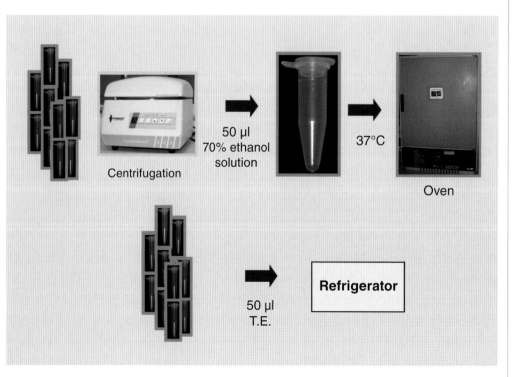

Centrifugation

50 µl
70% ethanol
solution

37°C

Oven

50 µl
T.E.

Refrigerator

3-5

Polimerase Chain Reaction (PCR)

Two new plastic cryotubes containing 2µL of genomic DNA, nucleotides (dATP, dTTP, and dGTP), DNA polymerase, oligonucleotides (primers) (Fig. 3-6), distilled water and PCR buffer solution (500mM KCl, 1.5mM MgCl$_2$, 100mM tris-HCl pH 9.0). This solution maintains pH and salinity necessary to synthesis (Fig. 3-7). The cryotubes are mounted on a termocycling device at 94°C for 5 minutes to break hydrogen bridges between DNA chains, causing them to denature (Fig. 3-7). After, temperature is decreased between 30 and 65°C for 30 seconds. This will promote biding of primers to their genomic DNA complementary sequences. Finally, temperature is increased to 72°C, for 2 to 5 minutes, to the synthesis of new DNA chains by DNA polymerase. These three steps denaturation, anneling and synthesis) are repeated 30 times, producing millions of copies of a double-strand DNA, exponentially increasing after each cycle (Fig. 3-8). Once the DNA amplification is finished, the samples are stored at -20°C for electrophoresis.

Fig. 3-6. Primers used in the reactions.

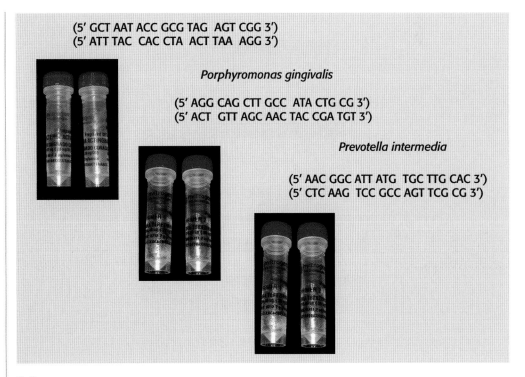

(5' GCT AAT ACC GCG TAG AGT CGG 3')
(5' ATT TAC CAC CTA ACT TAA AGG 3')

Porphyromonas gingivalis

(5' AGG CAG CTT GCC ATA CTG CG 3')
(5' ACT GTT AGC AAC TAC CGA TGT 3')

Prevotella intermedia

(5' AAC GGC ATT ATG TGC TTG CAC 3')
(5' CTC AAG TCC GCC AGT TCG CG 3')

3-6

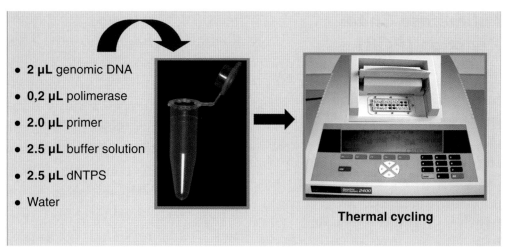

- **2 µL** genomic DNA
- **0,2 µL** polimerase
- **2.0 µL** primer
- **2.5 µL** buffer solution
- **2.5 µL** dNTPS
- Water

Thermal cycling

3-7

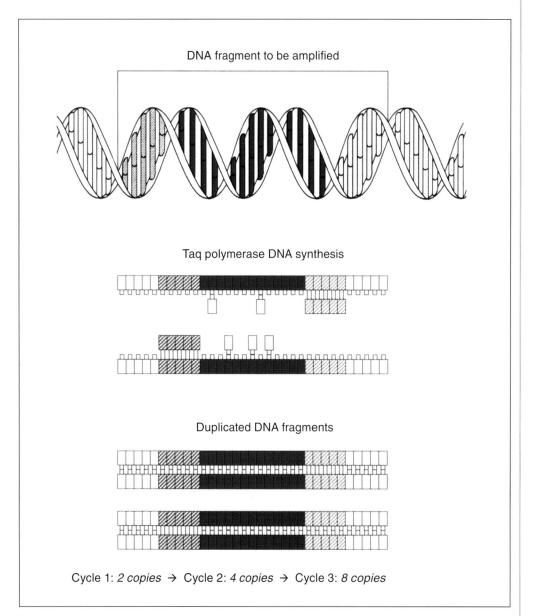

DNA fragment to be amplified

Taq polymerase DNA synthesis

Duplicated DNA fragments

Cycle 1: *2 copies* → Cycle 2: *4 copies* → Cycle 3: *8 copies*

3-8

Fig. 3-7. Polimerase chain reaction (PCR).

Fig. 3-8. Sequence of PCR and DNA amplification.

Electrophoresis

This procedure has the purpose to separate and visualize DNA fragments in agarosis gel. When submitted to an electric field in neutral pH, DNA molecules are attracted to the positive lead (anode). When de DNA migration occurs in a matrix with some frictional resistance, the small fragments can move easier than extensive fragments. A matrix made in agarose (Type II – Sigma), similar to purified gelatin, has a pore size that permits separation from 200bps to 50kbps, according to gel concentration. When gel concentration is less than 0.3%, frictional resistance to DNA migration will be mild, and extensive fragments can be quite separated. However, for complete separation of smaller fragments, it is necessary to increase gel concentration up to 2% or more.

The agarose gel for electrophoresis is prepared from TAE 1X dissociation, heating 0.8% agarose until its complete melting. Before pouring it onto the gel platform, a gel comb is inserted to form the wells, where DNA samples will be deposited.

After it solidifies, the gel is immersed on the electrophoresis tank with buffer solution (TAE 1X) at a neutral pH. A magnetic field is formed by means of electrical stimulation, leading to DNA migration on the mixture of electrophoresis gel and 6µL ethidium bromate (dye) which, under ultraviolet light, generate positive and negative bands for each microorganism analyzed. On each gel column, samples of DNA ladder are deposited too. It serves as reference for base pair identification and contamination control; the other column represents blank wells (where water is deposited instead of genomic DNA to evidence possible contamination).

As a result, the gel provides differential inverse fragment migration in relation to molecule size, where smaller fragments reach greater distances when compared to bigger ones (Fig. 3-9).

Finally, to observe marked bands after electrophoresis, the gel must be analyzed with an ultraviolet transluminator, where band signature is considered positive while its absence a negative result (Fig. 3-10).

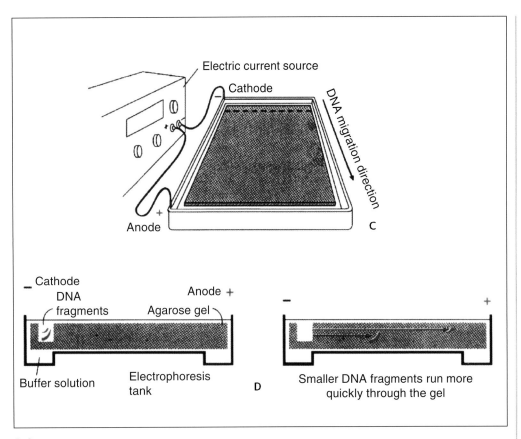

Electric current source

Cathode

DNA migration direction

Anode

C

Cathode
DNA fragments

Anode +

Agarose gel

Buffer solution

Electrophoresis tank

D

Smaller DNA fragments run more quickly through the gel

3-9

Fig. 3-9. Electrophoresis gel: separation and visualization of DNA fragments (according to Farah, 1997).

Fig. 3-10. Detection of presence or absence of *Actinobacillus actinomycetemcomitans, Porphyromonas gingivalis,* and *Prevotella intermedia* according to each individual.

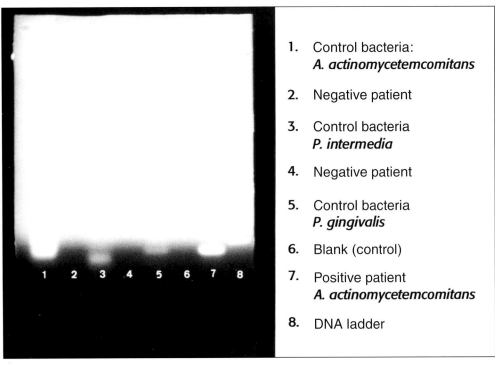

1. Control bacteria:
   A. actinomycetemcomitans

2. Negative patient

3. Control bacteria
   P. intermedia

4. Negative patient

5. Control bacteria
   P. gingivalis

6. Blank (control)

7. Positive patient
   A. actinomycetemcomitans

8. DNA ladder

3-10

Final considerations

Due to the interest and necessity of more knowledge on peri-implant tissues, along with the great development in molecular biology for studies on microbiology, Matos (2005) studied the possible role of implant-abutment junction of one and two stage implants on the quality of periimplant microflora. The microorganisms investigated were *Actinobacillus actinomycetemcomitans, Porphyromonas gingivalis* and *Prevotella intermedia*. According to the results, in spite of its high prevalence in both patient groups, there is no relation between the presence of *Actinobacillus actinomycetemcomitans* and its clinical parameters of evaluation (Graph 3-1). According to the literature, the presence of *Actinobacillus actinomycetemcomitans* does not implies on a pathologic condition, since the studies

of Buchmann et al. (2003) on the external surface of abutments showed highly pathogenic microorganisms, although in lower levels. In contrast, Mombelli et al. (1995) did not found these bacteria, even with the study being conducted on partially edentulous patients with a history of periodontal disease, factors that theoretically increase the likelihood of pathogenic species such as *Actinobacillus actinomycetemcomitans*. A possible explanation for this is the difficult to maintain anaerobic environment when utilizing culture technique, leading to false-negative results.

There is no significant difference regarding to *Porphyromonas gingivalis* colonization in groups with the classic two-stage approach and Novum (Graph 3-2). The influence of remaining teeth on the periimplant microflora generates great amounts of black-pigmented gram-nega-

Graph 3-1. Prevalence of *Actinobacillus actinomycetemcomitans* in the studied groups.

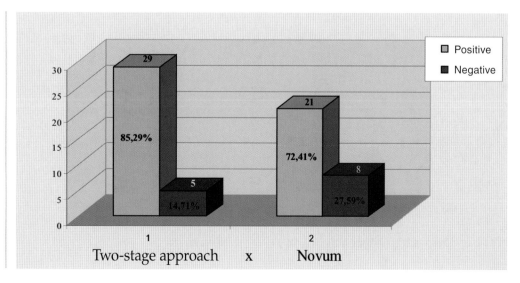

tive bacteria, while not found on completely edentulous patients. On the other hand, the prevalence of *Porphyromonas gingivalis* is also related to the history of previous periodontal or periimplant disease.[45]

In the same study, Matos (2005) observed mean pocket probing depths of 2.5mm for protocol group and of 1.5mm for Novum group. This possibly could justify the results obtained on the prevalence of *Porphyromona gingivalis* and *Prevotella intermedia* for two-stage approach and Novum groups, being (14.71%, 11.77%) and (17.25%, 24.14%), respectively (Graphs 3-2 and 3-3). These results are different from others,[6,48] which present a prevalence of 80% and 81.3% for *Porphyromonas gingivalis* and 53.3% for *Prevotella intermedia*. However, these studies investigated

partially edentulous patients, and according to the authors, there was pathogen transmission from periodontal to periimplant pockets.

According to the literature, *Porphyromonas gingivalis* and *Prevotella intermedia* have a strong symbiosis relationship, and since they present relation with sulcus probing depth, these findings could explain the results obtained by this author, although these values are not in accordance with adequate conditions for colonization of these periodontal pathogens.[27,49]

Although the Novum group had shown the least mean periimplant probing depths, it demonstrated the highest prevalence for these pathogens. These results do not agree with the literature.[38,48,49]

The pathogenesis of periim-

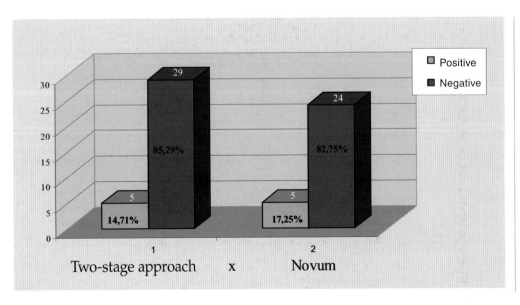

Graph 3-2. Prevalence of *Porphyromonas gingivalis* in the studied groups.

Graph 3-3. Prevalence of *Prevotella intermedia* in the studied groups.

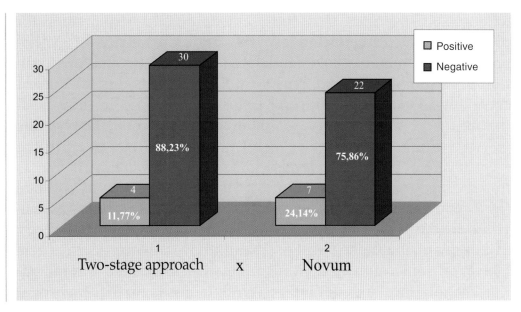

plant disease and its risk factors are not well known,[42] because even in the presence of occlusal overloading, there is loss of connective tissue insertion or epithelial adherence, with an increase on probing depth, providing an anaerobic environment and the development of pathogenic flora. These microflora can penetrate more rapidly on the periimplant sulcus due to plaque accumulation, resulting in biological breakdown because of the nature of connective tissue attachment on the implant surface, when compared to natural teeth. These facts also difficult to establish the main reasons of failure during treatment, in accordance to results observed by several authors,[19,20,21,33] once they do not verified significant differences between study groups,

leading to the belief in a possible mechanical cause responsible for differences on osseous marginal crest levels between two-stage approach and Novum.

The loss of osseointegration can occur either by infectious diseases, i.e., highly pathogenic microbiota, or through biomechanical causes, mainly due to occlusal overloading, with micromovement between abutment and implant, preventing the reestablishment of osseous modelling/remodelling. Such overload is not the only factor responsible for this, being the flexibility of metallic infra-structure, the marginal fit at implant-abutment interface, and the prosthesis design additional factors. Thus, it is very important to use prefabricated components to reduce marginal gaps. However,

Matos (2005) verified that the presence of such interface does not influence microbial colonization of periimplant region, only contributing to a pathologic condition.

According to the literature,[7,19,20,21,26] alveolar bone crest levels in one-stage systems depend on the location of superficial design, while in the two-stage systems of implant-abutment height. However, some authors believe that the interface does not influence the amount of periimplant osseous resorption.[23,50]

One possible explanation for the high prevalence of pathogenic species in shallow periimplant pockets and to the existence of deeper healthy sulci beyond 3mm could be the role of immunological system in the disease process.[42,52]

In this way, the hypothesis that etiological factors associated to periimplant pathology could have a more decisive role than that associated to oral microflora needs further investigation and requires new research strategies.

References

1. ABRAHAMSSON, I.; BERGLUNDH, T.; LINDHE, J. Soft tissue response to plaque formation at different implant systems. A comparative study in the dog. *Clinical Oral Implant Research*, v. 9, p.73-79, 1998.
2. ASHIMOTO, A. et al. Polymerase chain reaction detection of 8 putative periodontal pathogens in subgingival plaque of gingivitis and advanced periodontitis lesions. *Oral Microbiology and Immunology*, v. 11, n. 4, p.266-273, Aug. 1996.
3. AUGTHUN, M.; CONRADS, G. Microbial findings of deep peri-implant bone defects. *International Journal of Oral and Maxillofacial Implants*, v. 12, n. 1, p.106-112, Jan./Feb. 1997.
4. BAPOO-MOHAMED, K. Post-insertion peri-implant tissue assessment: a longitudinal study. *Journal of Oral Implantology*, v. 23, n. 3/4, p.225-231, 1996.
5. BRÅNEMARK, P-I. et al. Brånemark Novum: a new treatment concept for rehabilitation of the edentulous mandible. Preliminary results from a prospective clinical follow-up study. *Clinical Implant Dentistry and Related Research*, v. 1, n. 1, p.2-16, 1999.
6. BUCHMANN, R. et al. The microflora recovered from the outer-surfaces of the Frialit-2 implanto-prosthetic connector. *Clinical Oral Implant Research*, v. 14, n. 1, p.28-35, Feb. 2003.
7. COCHRAN, D.L. et al. Biologic width around titanium implants. A histometric analysis of the implanto-gingival junction around unloaded and loaded nonsubmerged implants in the canine mandible. *Journal of Periodontology*, v. 68, n. 2, p.186-198, Jan./Mar. 1997.
8. CHOW, J. et al. The Hong-Kong bridge protocol. immediate loading of mandibular Brånemark fixtures using a fixed provisional prosthesis: preliminary results. *Clinical Implant Dentistry and Related Research*, v. 3, n. 3, p.166-174, 2001.

9. DANSER, M.M. et al. Putative periodontal pathogens colonizing oral mucous membranes in denture-wearing subjects with a past history of periodontitis. *Journal of Clinical Periodontology*, v. 22, n. 11. p.854-859, Nov. 1995.

10. ELLEN, R. P. Microbial colonization of the peri-implant enviroment and its relevance to long-term success of osseointegrated implants. *International Journal of Prosthodontics*, v. 11, n. 5, p.433-441, Sept./Oct. 1998.

11. ENGQUIST, B. Simplified methods of implant treatment in the edentulous lower jaw. a controlled prospective study. Part I: One-stage versus two-stage surgery. *Clinical Implant Dentistry and Related Research*, v. 4, n. 2, p.93-103, 2002.

12. ENGSTRAND, P. et al. Brånemark Novum: Prosthodontic and dental laboratory procedures for fabrication of a fixed prosthesis on the day of surgery. *International Journal of Prosthodontics*, v. 14, n. 4, p.303-309, Jul./Aug. 2001.

13. ESPOSITO, M. et al. Differential diagnosis and treatment for biologic complications and failing oral implants: A review of literature. *The International Journal of Oral and Maxillofacial Implants*, v. 14, n. 4, p.473-490, Jul./Aug. 1999.

14. FARAH, S.B. DNA no diagnóstico das doenças humanas. In: ____. *DNA segredos & mistérios*. São Paulo: Sarvier, 1997. p.103-140. cap. 5.

15. GARG, A.K. The Brånemark Novum implant system: Rehabilitating the edentulous mandible. *Dental Implantology Update*, v. 13, n. 8, p.57-63, Aug. 2002.

16. GATEWOOD, R.R.; COBB, C.M.; KILLOY, W.J. Microbial colonization on natural tooth structure compared with smooth and plasma-sprayed dental implant surfaces. *Clinical of Oral Implant Research*, v. 4, p.53-64, 1993.

17. GOUVOUSSIS, J.; SINDHUSAKE, D.; YEUNG, S. Cross-infection from periodontitis sites to failing implant sites in the same mouth. *The International Journal of Oral and Maxillofacial Implants*, v. 12, n. 5, p.666-673, Sept./Oct. 1997.

18. HARTROTH, B.; SEYFAHRT, I.; CONRADS, G. Sampling of periodontal pathogens by paper points: evaluation of basic parameters. *Oral Microbiology Immunology*, v. 14, p.326-330, 1999.

19. HERMANN, J.S. et al. Crestal bone changes around titanium implants. A radiographic evaluation of unloaded non-submerged and submerged implants in the canine mandible. *Journal of Periodontology*, v. 68, n. 11, p.1117-1130, Oct./Dec. 1997.

20. _____. Crestal bone changes around titanium implants. A histometric evaluation of unloaded non-submerged and submerged implants in the canine mandible. *Journal of Periodontology*, v. 71, n. 9, p.1412-1424, Sept. 2000.

21. _____. Crestal Bone changes around titanium implants: A methodological study comparing linear radiographic with histometric measurements. *The International Journal of Oral and Maxillofacial Implants*, v. 16, n. 4, p.475-485, 2001.

22. HEYDENRIJK, K. et al. Microbiota around root-form endosseous implants: A review of the literature. *The International Journal of Oral and Maxillofacial Implants*, v. 17, n. 6, p.829-838, 2002.

23. _____. Clinical and radiologic evaluation of 2-stage imz implants placed in a single-stage procedure: 2 year results of a prospective comparative study. *The International Journal of Oral and Maxillofacial Implants*, v. 18, n. 3, p.424-432, 2003.

24. JANSEN, V.K.; CONRADS, G.; RICHTER, E. J. Microbial leakage and marginal fit of the implant-abutment interface. *The International Journal of Oral and Maxillofacial Im-*

plants, v. 12, n. 4, p.527-540, Jul./Aug. 1997.

25. KELLER, W.; BRÄGGER, U.; MOMBELLI, A. Peri-implant microflora of implants with cemented and screw retained suprastructures. *Clinical Oral Implant Research,* v. 9, p.209-217, Jan. 1998.

26. KING, G.N. et al. Influence of the size of the microgap on crestal bone levels in non-submerged dental implants: a radiographic study in the canine mandible. *Journal of Periodontology,* v. 73, n. 10, p.1111-1117, Oct. 2002.

27. KOJIMA, T.; YASUI, S.; ISHIKAWA, I. Distribution of Porphyromonas gingivalis in adult periodontitis patients. *Journal of Periodontology,* v. 64, n. 12, p.1231-1237, Dec. 1993.

28. KOKA, S. et al. Microbial colonization of dental implants in partially edentulous subjects. *Journal of Prosthetic Dentistry,* v. 70, n. 2, p.141-144, Aug. 1993.

29. KÖNÖNEN, E. et al. Are certain oral pathogens part of normal oral flora in denture-wearing edentulous subjects? *Oral Microbiology Immunology,* v. 6, n. 2, p.119-122, Apr. 1991.

30. LANG, N. P. et al. Histologic probe penetration in healthy and inflamed peri-implant tissues. *Clinical Oral Implant Research,* v. 5, p.191-201, 1994.

31. LEE, K.H. et al. Microbiota of successful osseointegrated dental implants. *Journal of Periodontology,* v. 70, p.131-138, Feb. 1999.

32. LYONS, S.R.; GRIFFEN, A.L.; LEYS, E.J. Quantitative Real-Time PCR for Porphyromonas gingivalis and total bacteria. *Journal of Clinical Microbiology,* v. 38, n. 6, p.2362-2365, Jun. 2000.

33. MATOS, D.A.D. *Análise comparativa da presença de patógenos bucais em dois esquemas de reabilitação oral sobre implantes.* 2005.101f. Dissertação (Mestrado em Odontologia) – Universidade do Sagrado Coração, Bauru, SP.

34. MOMBELLI, A. et al. The microbiota of osseointegrated implants in patients with a history of periodontal disease. *Journal of Clinical Periodontology,* v. 22, n. 2, p.124-130, Feb. 1995.

35. NAKAZATO, G. et al. In vivo plaque formation on implant materials. *The International Journal of Oral and Maxillofacial Implants,* v. 4, n. 4, p.321-326, 1989.

36. NISHIMURA, K. et al. Periodontal parameters of osseointegrated dental implants. *Clinical Oral Implant Research,* v. 8, p.272-278, 1997.

37. ÖKTE, E. et al. Bacterial adhesion of Actinobacillus actinomycetemcomitans serotypes to titanium implants: SEM evaluation. A Preliminary Report. *Journal of Periodontology,* v. 70, n. 11, p.1376-1382, Nov. 1999.

38. PAPAIOANNOU, W. et al. The effect of periodontal parameters on the subgengival microbiota around implants. *Clinical Oral Implant Research,* v. 6, n. 4, p.197-204, Dec. 1995.

39. PORTER, J. M. Same-day restoration of mandibular single-stage implants. *Journal of Indian Dental Association,* v. 81, n. 3, p.22-25, Fall. 2002.

40. QUIRYNEN, M. et al. An in vivo study of the influence of the surface roughness of implants on the microbiology of supra- and subgingival plaque. *Journal of Dental Research,* v. 72, n. 9, p.1304-1309, Sept. 1993.

41. QUIRYNEN, M. et al. The influence of titanium abutment surface roughness on plaque accumulation and gingivitis: Short-term observations. *The International Journal of Oral and Maxillofacial Implants,* v. 11, n. 2, p.169-178, Mar./Apr. 1996.

42. _____; DE SOETE, M.; VAN STEENBERGHE, D. Infectious risks for oral implants: Review of the literature. *Clinical Oral Implant Research,* v. 13, n. 1, p.1-19, 2002.

43. RAMS, T. E. et al. The subgingival microbial flora associated with human dental implants. *Journal of Prosthetics Dentistry,* v. 51, n. 4, p.529-534, Apr. 1984.

44. RIGGIO, M.P.; LENNON, A.; ROY, K.M. Detection of Prevotella intermedia in subgingival plaque of adult periodontitis patients by polymerase chain reaction. *Journal of Periodontal Research*, v. 33, n. 6, p.369-376, Aug. 1998.

45. RUTAR, A. et al. Retrospective assessment of clinical and microbiological factors affecting periimplant tissue conditions. *Clinical Oral Implant Research*, v. 12, p.189-195, 2001.

46. SHIBLI, J. A. et al. Microbiologic and radiographic analysis of ligature-induced peri-implantitis with different dental implant surfaces. *The International Journal of Oral and Maxillofacial Implants*, v. 18, n. 3, p.383-390, May/Jun. 2003.

47. SLOTS, J. et al. Detection of putative periodontal pathogens in subgingival specimens by 16S Ribosomal DNA amplification with the Polymerase Chain Reaction. *Clinical Infectious Diseases*, v. 20 (Suppl 2), p. 304-307, Jun. 1995.

48. SOCRANSKY, S.S, et al. Microbial complexes in subgengival plaque. Journal of Clinical Periodontology, v. 25, p.134-144, 1998.

49. SUMIDA, S. et al. Transmission of Periodontal Disease-Associated Bacteria from Teeth to Osseointegrated Implant Regions. *The International Journal of Oral and Maxillofacial Implants*, v. 17, n. 5, p.696-702, Sept./Oct. 2002.

50. TODESCAN, F.F. et al. Influence of the microgap in the peri-implant hard and soft tissues: A histomorphometric study in dogs. *The International Journal of Oral and Maxillofacial Implants*, v. 17, n. 4, p.467-472, 2002.

51. VAN WINKELHOFF, A.J.; WOLF, J.W.A. Actinobacillus actinomycetemcomitans-associated peri-implantitis in an edentulous patient. A case report. *Journal of Clinical Periodontology*, v. 27, p.531-535, Jul. 2000.

52. VAN WINKELHOFF, A.J. et al. Smoking affects the subgingival microflora in periodontitis. *Journal of Periodontology*, v. 72, n. 5, p.666-671, May. 2001.

53. WATANABE, K.; FROMMEL, T.O. Porphyromonas gingivalis, Actinobacillus actinomycetemcomitans and Treponema denticola detection in oral plaque samples using the polymerase chain reaction. *Journal of Clinical Periodontology*, v. 23, n. 3, p.212-219, Mar. 1996.

54. ZAMBON, J.J.; NISENGARD, R.J. Bactérias produtoras de pigmento negro. In:_____ . *Microbiologia e imunologia oral*. Rio de Janeiro: Guanabara Koogan, 1994. p.183-186.

55. ZITZMANN, N.U. et al. Soft tissue reactions to plaque formation at implant abutments with different surface topography. An experimental study in dogs. *Journal of Clinical Periodontology*, v. 29, n. 5, p.456-461, May. 2002.

4

SOFT TISSUE MANAGEMENT AND SMILE ESTHETICS

Glécio Vaz de Campos

Introduction

The esthetics of periimplant and periodontal soft tissues is a fundamental factor for success in dental treatment. This has demanded great efforts from professionals to optimizing surgical and restorative procedures. The harmonious interplay among dental specialties (Periodontics, Operative Dentistry, Prosthodontics, Orthodontics and Implantology) favors the esthetic diagnosis, planning, clinical treatment sequence, and outcome maintenance for each single case.

The periodontal plastic surgery involves techniques giving predictability for defects such as marginal tissue recession, loss of papilla, ridge alteration and marginal tissue asymmetry (Wennström, 1996). Based on the success obtained from periodontal defects, this procedures can be used to correct periimplant defects such as the lack of keratinized tissue, papillary alterations, loss of tissue thickness, and show through of prosthetic abutments. However, the biological characteristics of periimplant tissue must be respected, because although similar in nature to periodontal tissue, it has some peculiarities. (Berglundh et al., 1990) These techniques are delicate and very difficult, which implies therapeutic results varying according to surgeon's experience. Still, one has to consider the periodontal phenotype expression because it implies on different techniques for tissue manipulation (Baldi et al., 1999; Müller et al., 2000) and the quality of blood supply during surgery (Tinti et al., 1995; Hürzeler and Weng, 1999). The clinician has to bear in mind that continuous education is necessary to justify therapeutic procedures. This will reflects on treatment choice, outcomes, and long-term prognosis.

The periodontal phenotypes are evaluated on the next section, as well as its clinical and surgical implications, soft tissue esthetic defects, and the treatment planning for clinical cases.

Periodontal phenotype

Periodontal plastic surgery focuses on surgical techniques where the success is evaluated according to postoperative wound healing, formation of scars and predictability of treatment outcome. For this, methods to diagnose circumjacent tissues to periodontal defects and rigorous biological criteria are necessary (Müller and Eger, 2002).

A thorough periodontal examination must include quantitative and qualitative aspects as the following: pocket depth, tooth mobility, furcation involvement, the amount of keratinized tissue, gingival thickness, and alveolar bone type (Kao, Pasquinelli, 2002).

The quality of periodontal tissues can help the clinician to solve routine dilemmas such as: tissue recession after crown cementation, the severe atrophy of alveolar bone after tooth loss, patients with localized gingival recession, color changes in the periimplant tissues, and the level of tissue shrinkage in the postoperative period.

Ochsenbein and Ross (1969) have classified the periodontal soft tissue as thick-flat or thin-scalloped and suggested that underlying bone contour determines the gingival phenotype. Other studies (Eger et al., 1996; Müller and Eger, 1997; Müller et al., 2000) confirmed the presence of distinct periodontal phenotypes and their clinical implications.

The thick-flat type has a fibrous, dense appearance with a large band of keratinized tissue. Its flat topography suggests a thick osseous architecture. This pattern provides tissues more resistant to toothbrushing abrasion, cavity preparation, retraction cord insertion, and placement of margin restorations. The surgical procedures performed are more predictable, due to the less postoperative remodeling.

This is important during clinical crown lengthening, root coverage and removal of teeth before implant placement.

On the other hand, the thin-scalloped type has a friable, delicate appearance with a narrow band of keratinized tissue. Its scalloped topography suggests a thin osseous architecture, being subjected to dehiscence and fenestration areas (Fig. 4-1). The thinnest area can be found in the upper canine and lower premolar regions ranging from 0.7mm to 0.9mm (Eger, Muller and Heinecke, 1996). Taking into account that the epithelial layer has 0.3mm, these regions show a connective tissue thickness of 0.4 to 0.6mm. Those teeth have a high incidence of marginal tissue recession (Serino et al., 1994), being the surgical procedures less predictable. It is difficult to ascertain about final tissue position during clinical crown lengthening or flap surgery. Breakdown of thin cortical bone or tissue perforation in full thickness flap surgery is a common finding (Figs. 4-6 and 4-7). In this case, postoperative results largely depend on the thickness of keratinized tissue for coronal flap position (Baldi, Pini Prato, Pagliaro et al., 1999; Müller, Stahl and Eger, 2000) and minimal blood supply necessary to involved tissues (Tinti, Parma and Benfenati, 1995; Hürzeler and Weng, 1999). In areas of great esthetic demand, it is recommended to wait for at least 6 months until stabilization of marginal tissue before final restorative treatment (McGuire, 1998) (Box 4-1).

Individuals with healthy gingival tissues and thick phenotype have greater probing depths than that with thin phenotype (Olsson et al., 1993; Eger et al., 1996; Muller et al., 2000). Different probing depths associated to several gingival thicknesses generate individualized structures of biologic width. It is well established that the biological width must be considered during restorative in teeth and implants. Gargiulo, Wentz and Orban (1961) observed that the connective tissue attachment plus junctional epithelium measure 1mm and the gingival sulcus has 0.7mm. Overall, it is recommended that distance between osseous crest and restoration margin must be 3mm (Brägger, Lauchernauer and Lang; 2002). A thorough analysis of data showed by Gargiulo et al. (1961) reveals a considerable individual variation of these distances. Thus, the biological width depends on the periodontal phenotype (Portoriero and Carnevale, 2001; Müller and Eger, 2002) (Fig. 4-2). In individuals with thin gingiva and narrow band of keratinized tissue, the sum of mean values (3mm) is too large, while the biological width is violated

Box 4-1. Clinical characteristics of periodontal phenotypes*

Thick phenotype	Thin phenotype
Bone/soft tissue flat architecture	Bone/soft tissueScalloped architecture
Fibrous and dense soft tissue	Friable and delicate soft tissue
Broad band of attached gingival	Narrow band of attached gingival
Thick underlying tissue	Thin underlying tissue
Can withstand mechanical trauma	Fenestration and dehiscence
Reacts to periodontal disease showing pocket and infra-osseous defect	Reacts to periodontal disease and traumatism showing marginal tissue recession
Square dental form	Triangular dental form

*Adapted from Kao RT, Pasquinelli K. CDA 2002;30:521-6

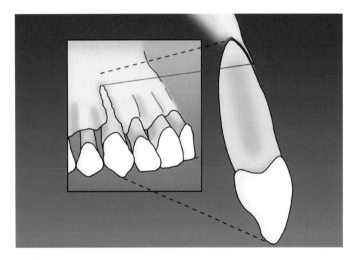

4-1A

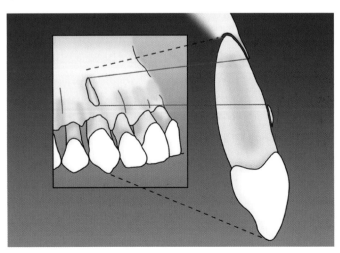

4-1B

Fig. 4-1A and B. Dehiscence and osseous fenestration. In patients with thin phenotype or types III and IV (Maynard; Wilson, 1980), dehiscence (A) or fenestration (B) areas are common during full thickness flap surgery.

in individuals with thick gingiva and a large band of keratinized tissue (Figs. 4-2 and 4-3).

Clinical practice has shown that these two phenotype cat-egories are not sufficient to clas-sify all variations found in peri-odontal patients.

The classification proposed by Maynard and Wilson (1980),

Fig. 4-2. Clinical crown lengthening for esthetic purposes in patients with thin bone.

4-2A. Periodontal probes positioned at the height of gingival contour (zenith) according to treatment planning.

4-2B. Initial incision in the region of central incisors with a round microblade (no. 6961 – G Hartzell & Son, Concord, CA, USA).

4-2C. Partial thickness el-evated flap with the same microblade. Observe the apical position of osseous crest: osteotomies are not necessary.

4-2D. Area after surgical debridement.

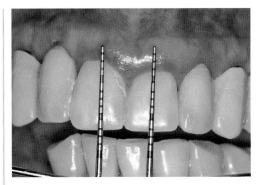

4-2A

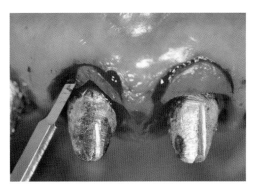

4-2B

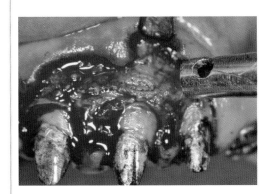

4-2C

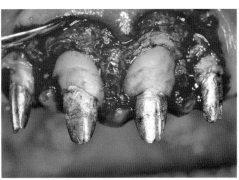

4-2D

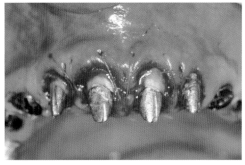

4-2E

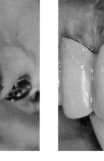

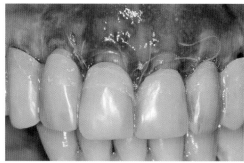

4-2F

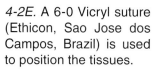

4-2E. A 6-0 Vicryl suture (Ethicon, Sao Jose dos Campos, Brazil) is used to position the tissues.

4-2F. Five days postoperative view showing maintenance of gingival levels established on surgery.

4.2G. Postoperative view showing final healing process.

4.2H. Final crowns cemented on prepared teeth. Observe high quality, excellent gengival tissue contour.

4-2G

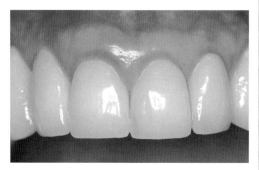

4-2H

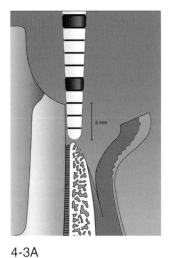

3 mm

4-3A

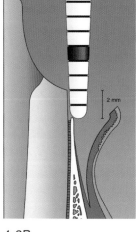

2 mm

4-3B

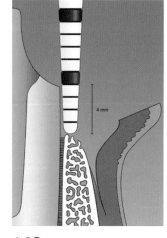

4 mm

4-3C

Fig. 4-3. Diversity of biological width according to the preparation margin:

4-3A. Mean biological width observed in most cases (3mm).

4-3B. In patients with thin phenotype, the biological width is less than 3mm.

4-3C. In patients with thick phenotype, the biological width is more than 3mm.

seems to be the most suitable to categorize periodontal/bone thickness and the band of keratinized tissue.

Based on this system, the advantages and disadvantages of each case can be assessed, giving more safety and predictability to the surgical outcomes (Figs. 4-4 and Fig.4-5).

Periodontal Tissue – Type I

This type is found on 40% of patients. The band of keratinized tissue and the bucco-lingual thickness of alveolar bone are considered normal or "ideal" (Maynard and Wilson, 1980) (Fig. 4-4A).

Fig. 4-4. Periodontal phenotypes (Maynard and Wilson, 1980).

4-4A and A'. Type I, normal bone an keratinized tissues.

4-4B and B'. Type II, normal bone and narrow band of keratinized tissue.

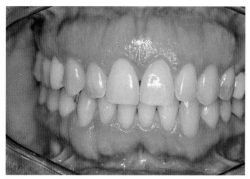

4-4A

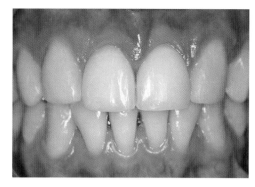

4-4B

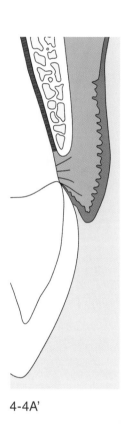

4-4A'

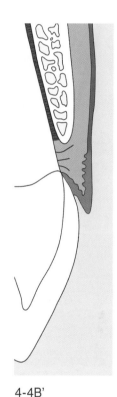

4-4B'

CLINICAL ASPECT

❑ The height of keratinized tissue ranges from 3 to 5mm, revealing a thick aspect on palpation.
❑ The flat topography suggests thick bone architecture.

SURGICAL IMPLICATIONS

❑ **Full thickness flap:** abundant bone is visualized overlying roots without dehiscence and fenestrations; the bone crest is near to the cementoenamel junction.
❑ **Partial thickness flap:** sufficient thickness to divide the soft tissue without damaging the periosteum and perforate the flap.
❑ **Suture:** soft tissue resistant

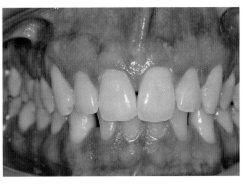

4-5A

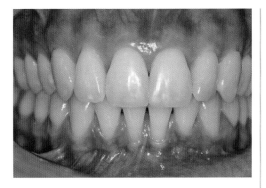

4-5B

Fig. 4-5. Periodontal phenotypes (Maynard and Wilson, 1980).

4-5A and A'. Type III, thin bone and normal keratinized tissue.

4-5B and B'. Type IV, thin bone and narrow keratinized tissue.

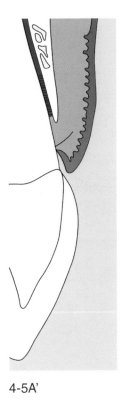

4-5A'

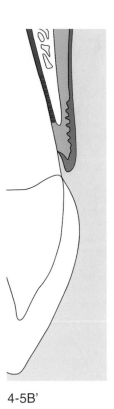

4-5B'

to tension. Less chance of flap or circumjacent tissue dilaceration.

❑ **Blood supply:** a thick flap and abundant bone favor the blood supply to involved tissues.

CLINICAL CROWN LENGHTENING

❑ **Advantages**: (1) surgical access to osteotomy or osteoplasty can be gained by means of full or partial thickness flap; (2) flaps hardly are perforated or nutrition deficient, (3) in the instance of inadequate tissue cooptation at interproximal region, the height of the papilla is still preserved due to osseous characteristics.

❑ **Clinical note:** the biological width should be more than 3mm, to accommodate thicker tissues.

CONNECTIVE TISSUE GRAFT

❑ **Advantages:** (1) partial thickness flap is easy to obtain, (2) thick bone and gingival tissues adjacent to the defect provide adequate graft nutrition.

❑ **Clinical note:** (1) verify coronal flap reflection: in case of inadequate mobility, incise remaining fibers, (2) thicker repositioned flaps over too thick grafts lead to excess volume in the grafted sites.

Periodontal Tissue – Type II

The type II occurs in 10% of patients. The band of keratinized tissue is narrow and the buccolingual thickness of alveolar bone is normal (Maynard and Wilson, 1980) (Fig. 4-4B).

CLINICAL ASPECT

❑ The keratinized tissue on labial surface is less than 2mm in height.

❑ The subjacent bone appears to be thick on palpation.

SURGICAL IMPLICATIONS

❑ **Full thickness flap:** normal bone is visualized with complete coverage of dental roots;

the bone crest is near the cementoenamel junction; careful flap reflection does not damage osseous cortical.

❑ **Partial thickness flap:** delicate tissue thickness requires great attention from its initial course to mucogingival junction (Fig. 4-6A). From this point, is more easy to divide flap.

❑ **Suture:** delicate soft tissue that requires great care on needle insertion and surgical closure (Fig. 4-7C).

❑ **Blood supply:** adequate bone favors flap nutrition; however, the narrow band of keratinized tissue requires slight manipulation to avoid perforations and dilacerations.

CLINICAL CROWN LENGHTENING

❑ **Advantages:** bone covering roots minimizes complications from soft tissue manipulation (perforation, dilaceration, and grasping) (Figs. 4-6 and 4-7). This favors flap healing on desired position.

❑ **Clinical note:** (1) the use of a periosteal elevator in full thickness flaps does not affect alveolar bone; however, one has to be extremely careful to avoid soft tissue damage (Fig. 4-6C), (2) tissue thickness can be controlled with a scalpel in partial thickness design; however, it is necessary to avoid internal beveled incision because the amount of keratinized tissue removed will aggravate the compromised gingival condition.

CONNECTIVE TISSUE GRAFT

❑ **Advantages:** (1) in the areas adjacent to the defect where edge-to-edge suturing is not possible, normal bone offers sufficient protection until reepithelization; (2) either vertical or horizontal releasing incisions can be placed.

❑ **Clinical note:** great care must be exercised to obtain an uniform partial thickness flap containing connective and epithelial tissue layer. Otherwise, flap necrosis and lack of blood supply will occur.

Periodontal Tissue – Type III

This type occurs in 20% of patients. The keratinized tissue is normal or "ideal" and the bucco-lingual thickness of alveolar bone is thin, with less than adequate trabecular bone (Fig. 4-5A).

CLINICAL ASPECT

❑ Although having adequate tissue thickness, roots are palpable in the mucogingival line.

SURGICAL IMPLICATIONS

❑ **Full thickness flap:** there is a thin cortical plate overlying roots, or even the presence of dehiscence and fenestrations (Fig. 4-1). The osseous crest can be found away from cementoenamel junction.

❑ **Partial thickness flap:** adequate thickness to divide soft tissue, leaving an intact periosteum; less chance of flap perforation.

❑ **Suture:** resistant to tension. Less chance of flap dilaceration (Fig. 4-7) during surgical closure.

❑ **Blood supply:** a thick flap and a thin bone determine that nutrition be provided at the expenses of soft tissue.

CLINICAL CROWN LENGHTENING

❑ **Advantages:** (1) easy to divide flap, providing its repositioning on the desired position; (2) no need for osteotomy or osteoplasty.

❑ **Clinical note:** the surgical periosteal elevator can remove delicate parts of cortical plate (Fig. 4-7A). In this sense, a partial thickness flap is recommended. The scalpel blade can easy divides the gingival tissues and maintains the integrity of cortical plate. In areas with great fenestrations and dehiscence (Fig. 4-1), this approach conserves collagen fibers attached to roots, facilitating nutrition and flap closure.

CONNECTIVE TISSUE GRAFT

❑ **Advantages:** a partial uniform thickness flap favors graft coverage and nutrition.

❑ **Clinical note:** mal-positioned incisions in areas adjacent to defects can create additional complications. This is a common finding in sites without sufficient bone. Horizontal rather than vertical releasing incisions must be made.

Periodontal Tissue – Type IV

This type occurs in 30% of patients. The keratinized tissue height is less than 2mm and the bucco-lingual thickness of alveolar bone is thin (Maynard and Wilson, 1980) (Fig. 4-5B).

CLINICAL ASPECT

❑ The topography of labial surface is well scalloped due to root convexity. In these instances, there is an increasing likelihood of marginal tissue recession in the presence of etiological factors.

CLINICAL IMPLICATIONS

❑ **Full thickness flap:** there is a thin cortical plate covering dental roots, or even the presence of dehiscence and fenestration (Fig. 4-1); the osseous crest can be found distant away from cementoenamel junction;

❑ **Partial thickness flap:** critical condition to divide soft tissue (usually, the surgical blade reaches the bone, removing periosteum fragments; more chance of flap perforation (Fig. 4-6A).

❑ **Suture:** less resistant to tension. Great chance of flap dilaceration during surgical closure (Fig. 4-7C)

❑ **Blood supply:** thin flap and bone preventing nutrition.

CLINICAL CROWN LENGHTENING

❑ **Advantages:** no need for osteotomy or osteoplasty.

❑ **Clinical note:** (1) the use of a surgical elevator can dilacerate or perforate the full thickness flap (Fig. 4-6C) and thus remove more delicate portions of cortical plate (Fig. 4-7A). Perforations are common due to loss of surgical elevator control. Thus, a partial thickness flap is strong recommended; although difficult to obtain, tissue stability is verified during surgery, (2) the biological width on bone healthy areas must be less than 3mm; (3) in the absence of edge-to-edge cooptation, interproximal necrosis can occur; (4) the repositioned flap must be in close contact with labial bone to avoid a dense clot. Otherwise, a healing pattern by second intention is established, generating irregular gingival margins and necrotic sites.

CONNECTIVE TISSUE GRAFT SURGERY

☐ **Advantages**: none.
☐ **Clinical note**: (1) perforation and dilaceration are common findings during flap design (Figs. 4-6 and 4-7), even with complete removal of connective tissue, increasing the risk for necrosis; (2) when thicker gingival grafts are used (>1.0mm) its adaptation and coverage with the flap are difficult; (3) a decision for a full thickness flap may be the best option; however, there is a great risk for flap perforation (Fig. 4-6C) and detachment of underlying thin cortical bone (Fig. 4-7A); (4) surgery on these periodontal phenotype

appears to be beyond the visual acuity of the operator and instruments used.

According to the stated above, it is important to evaluate whether the patient has a thin or thick bone/periodontal phenotype, and the absence or presence of keratinized tissue. The knowledge of periodontal and periimplant phenotype helps to understand how the different tissue types respond to surgical approaches and restorative treatment.

Currently, periodontal surgery techniques have evolved to change the risk of clinical complications found on high risk periodontal phenotypes to more predictable clinical procedures and esthetic results (Müller and Eger 2002; Kao and Pasquinelli, 2002).

Fig. 4-6. Common accidents during soft tissue surgery.

4-6A. Perforation with a scalpel blade is a common finding in patients with thin periodontal phenotype.

4-6B. Traumatic releasing due to gross instrument and excessive force.

4-6C. Flap perforation due to unnecessary movements and loss of instrument control.

Fig. 4-7. Common accidents during soft tissue surgery.

4-7A. Thin cortical plate detachment during full thickness flap design in patients with periodontal phenotypes III and IV (Maynard and Wilson, 1980).

4-7B. Grasping of the flap with the forceps is due to excessive pressure applied over a delicate tissue.

4-7C. Flap dilaceration can occurs due to inadequate needle and suture, incorrect technique, and unnecessary movements during flap closure.

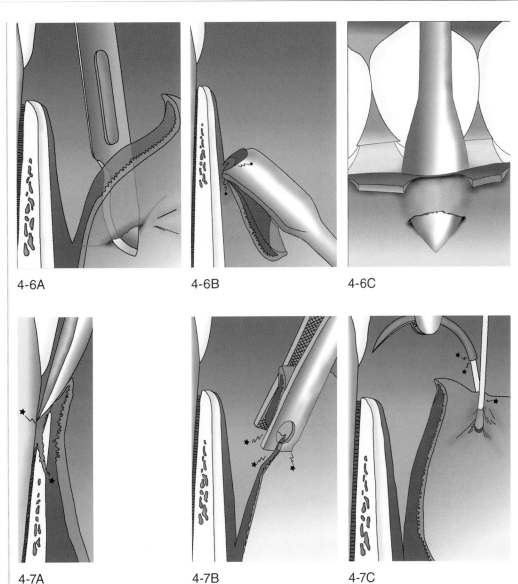

4-6A 4-6B 4-6C

4-7A 4-7B 4-7C

Periodontal Microsurgery

The periodontal microsurgery is a minimum invasive procedure done under the surgical microscope (Fig. 4-8) and with micro-instruments (Fig. 4-9) providing smaller incisions, avoiding vertical releasing incisions, resulting in an better edge-to-edge flap closure (Fig. 4-10). Avoidance of tissue trauma during surgery and the healing pattern result in a more comfortable postoperative situation and faster wound healing without scarring (Shanelec, 1991; Shanelec and Tibbetts, 1996; Tibbetts and Shanelec, 1998). This contributes to a better patient acceptance and to a more favorable and predictable esthetic result (Box 4-2).

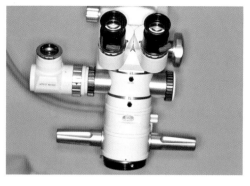

4-8A

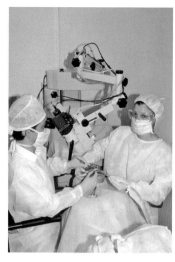

4-8B

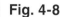

Fig. 4-8

4-8A. The surgical microscope has a wide range of magnification (3 to 20X), excellent illumination, and image capture concomitant to surgical procedure.

4-8B. The dental assistance can follow the surgical step on the monitor screen.

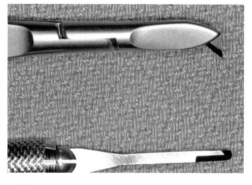

4-9A

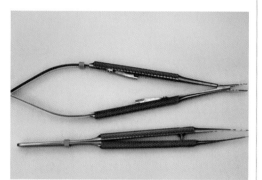

4-9B

Fig. 4-9. The microinstruments have robust handles and delicate and precise active points.

4-9A. Castroviejo blade-breaker and holder and round point microblade.

4-9B. Microneedle holder and forceps.

Box 4-2. Periodontal Microsurgery characteristics

Advantages	Development of new techniques Less traumatic tissue manipulation Less intraoperative bleeding Accurate wound closure Less healing time Primary wound healing Scarring reduction More postoperative comfort Improves patient acceptance to surgical procedures
Disadvantages	Elevated surgical time Previous laboratorial training Manual dexterity in both hands Extensive learning curve Initial cost

Box 4-3. Surgical Microscope characteristics

Advantages	Improved visual acuity Ergonomic work position Light intensity beyond 100.000 lux Control of light intensity Attenuation of visual fatigue Change of magnification according to clinical situation Simultaneous treatment documentation
Disadvantages	Previous laboratorial training Limited surgical field Training of auxiliary staff Initial cost

Fig. 4-10. Ideal microssuture.

4-10A. Incomplete coaptation of wound margins: a loose suture does not approximate wound margins.

4-10B. Invaginated flaps: excessive knot tension and incorrect position of needle angle of entry and exit.

4-10C. Overlap flaps: observe different bite sizes on both sizes of the wound.

4-10D. Adequate edge-to-edge wound closure due to microssuture technique. Primary wound healing will occur.

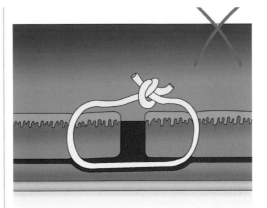

4-10A

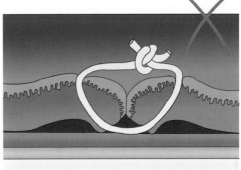

4-10B

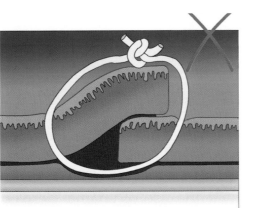

4-10C

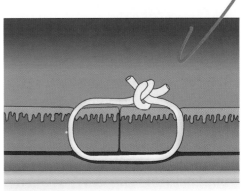

4-10D

The surgical microscope (Box 4-3) can be used in all phases: root preparation, incision and suturing. The operator selects the magnification according to the situation. The basic rule is to use maximum magnification on each surgical step to visualize the field of interest. For example, for root preparation with finishing burs, it is necessary to use a 13X magnification; to the horizontal incision at the papilla base from mesial to distal portions, an 8X magnification is enough.

One of the principles of microsurgery is to accomplish well defined and accurate incisions with a Castroviejo blade-breaker and holder (Shanelec and Tibbetts, 1996; Tibbetts and Shanelec, 1998). This instrument "breaks" a small fragment of a shaving blade (carbide). The blade is held on the active point of the instrument in an angle that favors the incision. The handgrip and cutting instrument precision provides a 90 degree initial incision (Fig. 4-11). This is the first rule of microsurgery because it will favors microssuture, which is the final surgical step.

The flap dissection with uniform thickness is facilitated through round point microblades (Fig. 4-9A) even in thin and delicate tissues.

Another favorable aspect is microssuture, which can be divided in two steps: (1) approximation and (2) coaptation (Fig. 4-12). On the first phase, the ob-jective is to stabilize the connective tissue graft and approximate wound margins with a 6-0 suture and a 15mm-length needle. On the second phase, the surgeon has to accurately approximate wound edges with an 8-0 suture and a 5mm-length needle. Thus, adequate coaptation of wound margins and primary wound healing are achieved.

The microsurgery learning requires dexterity on hands, eyes and mind. As the depth of field is limited, ranging from 66mm (3X) to 110mm (20X), only the active instrument point is visible. This requires proper training for handgrip and accurate movement of microinstruments (Michaelides, 1996; Shanelec and Tibbetts, 1996; Burkhardt and Hürzeler, 2000; Vaz de Campos and Tumenas, 2002).

Cortellini and Tonetti (2001) evaluated the use of microsurgical techniques associated to guided periodontal regeneration for interproximal and deep infra-osseous defects. It was concluded that microsurgery provides primary wound healing on interproximal regions, assures a low level of bacterial contamination, and offers optimal stability for flap margins. The gain on clinical attachment level and mild tissue recession are considerable.

Wachtel et al. (2003) evaluated the use of enamel derived matrix (Emdogain, Biora AB, Malmö Sweden) associated to

Fig. 4-11. Vertical and horizontal releasing microincisions. They are made with a Castroviejo blade-breaker and holder slight less than 90 degrees. This favors a well-defined incision and control of blade penetration.

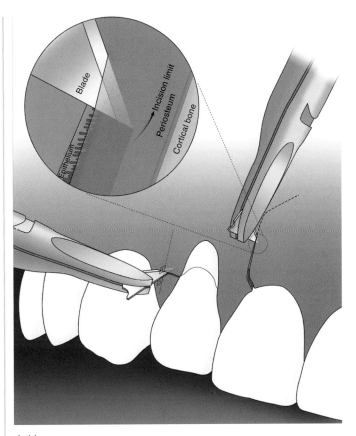

4-11

Fig. 4-12. Microsuture steps:

4-12A. Apposition with a 6-0 suture (needle 15mm). This primary wound apposition serves to eliminate gaps and stabilize wound edges (yellow).

4-12B. Coaptation is responsible for a close contact (8-0 suture, needle 5mm) of wound margins, known as "edge-to-edge coaptation".

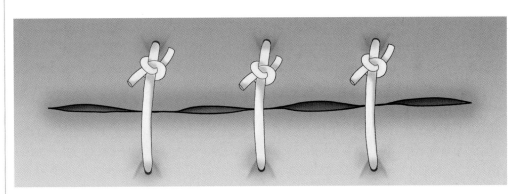

4-12A

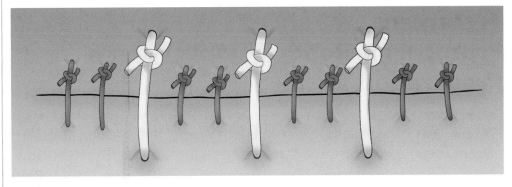

4-12B

microsurgery. It was observed that primary wound healing was important to prevent contamination and decrease postoperative marginal tissue recession. However, this study was not conclusive about Emdogain and microsurgery.

The precision of microinstruments and the versatility of surgical microscopy have improved and creating new techniques (Box 4-4) impossible to the naked eye (Vaz de Campos and Tumenas, 1998; Vaz de Campos and Tumenas, 1999; Cortellini and Tonetti, 2001; Vaz de Campos e Vaz de Campos 2002; Vaz de Campos et al., 2003; Vaz de Campos et al., 2004).

Although clinical evidence shows a direct relationship between periodontal microsurgery and more esthetic and predictable results, research studies are necessary to demonstrate the technical benefits of periodontal microsurgery compared to conventional techniques (Burkhardt and Hürzeler, 2000; Belcher, 2001, Cortellini and Tonetti, 2001; Wachtel et al., 2003).

Treatment Protocol for Root Preparation

Patient (Chief) Complaint: the patient feels uncomfortable during smile due to marginal tissue recession in both upper ca-

nines and conoid lateral incisors (Figs. 4-13A and B). The patient was submitted to an orthodontic treatment with partial outcomes.

Clinical examination: the patient has good health condition, with controlled risk factors for caries and periodontal disease. On the right canine, marginal recession is 4mm; on the left canine, marginal recession is 5mm. The height of keratinized tissue is 2mm on the upper central incisors, 3mm on the upper lateral incisors, 2mm on the right canine, and 1mm on the left canine. A type III periodontal phenotype can be identified. The roots of teeth 14 and 24 have a palatal inclination; the root of tooth 23 has a distal angulation. Cervical enamel hypoplasic defects can be seen on teeth 13, 11, 23 and on the incisal border of tooth 12. Radiographic analysis of teeth 13, 12, 11, 21 and 22 shows adequate osseous crest levels. On the region of teeth 23 and 24, the osseous crest is well-defined, but more apical to cementoenamel junction (Fig. 4-13C).

Esthetic diagnosis

The smile esthetics involves the harmonious integration between dental and periodontal (periimplant) tissues to the face components (Rufenacht, 2000). One can say that the fundamentals of

Fig. 4-13. Initial view – clinical case:

4-13A. 4mm marginal tissue recession on tooth 13 and of 5mm on tooth 23, conoid clinical crown of teeth 12 and 22.

4-13B. Unpleasant smile due to extensive radicular exposition on teeth 13 and 23 and lateral incisors 12 and 22.

4-13C. Periapical radiographs of upper anterior teeth. Observe an intact osseous crest on teeth 13, 12, 11, 21, and 22. Teeth 23 and 24 have a well defined crest but more apical to cementoenamel junction.

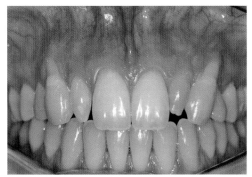
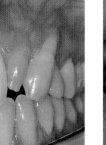
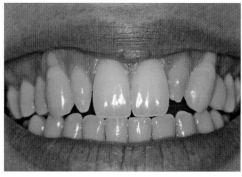

4-13A

4-13B

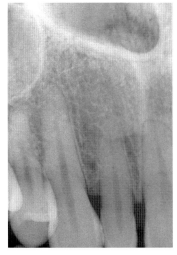
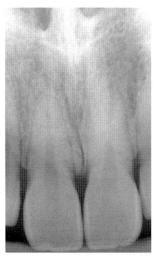
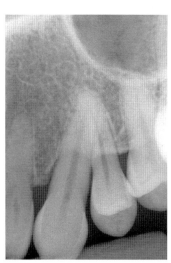

4-13C1

4-13C2

4-13C3

Esthetic Dentistry are: (1) create teeth with a pleasant proportion, (2) create a tooth arrangement in harmony with lips, gingival tissue and face (Figs. 4-14 to 4-16). These objectives are established through intra and extra-oral reference points and reinforced by perspective and illusion effects (Chiche and Pinault, 1994).

Box 4-4. Predictability of root coverage technique (Wennström, 1996)

Surgical technique	Predictability
Free gingival graft associated to coronally positioned flap	63%
Laterally positioned flap and double papilla technique	64%
Free gingival graft	72%
Guided tissue regeneration	74%
Coronally positioned flap	83%
Subepithelial connective tissue graft	91%

Esthetic reference lines

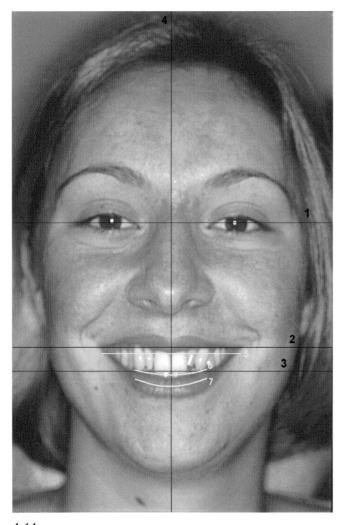

Fig. 4-14. Esthetic reference lines:

(1) Pupillary line: evaluate incisal plane and gingival margins.

(2) Comissure line: evaluate incisal length at rest and during smile; gingival zenith position during smile.

(3) Occlusal plane: evaluate parallelism with comissure and papillary lines.

(4) Facial midline: evaluate midposition of central incisors and mediolateral discrepancies.

(5) Smile line: only shows incisive papilla.

(6) Incisal border line.

(7) Lower lip line: the parallelism between incisal border and lower lip line gives a pleasant smile.

4-14

Initial clinical status

Fig. 4-15. Initial clinical status:

(1) Marginal tissue recession on 13 and 23;

(2) Reduced height of keratinized tissue on 13 and 23;

(3) Scalloped periodontal phenotype showing root convexity;

(4) Unfavorable dental axis on teeth 23 and 24;

(5) Inadequate crown shape on teeth 13, 12, 23 and 24;

(6) Enamel hiploplasic defect on teeth 13, 12, 11 and 23;

(7) Undercontoured crown on tooth 24;

(8) Altered left buccal corridor.

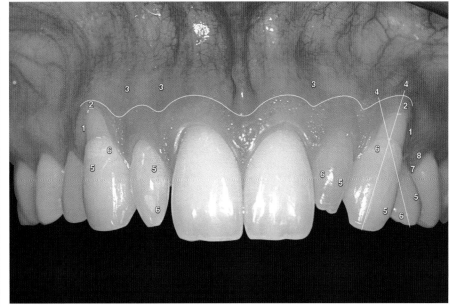

4-15

Esthetic planning

Fig. 4-16. Esthetic planning:

(1) Root coverage on teeth 13 and 23;

(2) Cervical restorations on teeth 13 and 23;

(3) Restoration of crown contour on teeth 12 and 22;

(4) Resin restorations to improve dental axes of teeth 23 and 24;

(5) Enameloplasty of teeth 23 and 24.

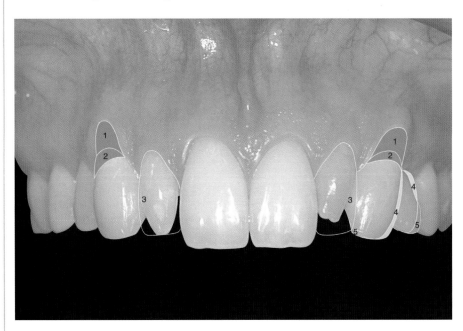

4-16

Treatment sequence

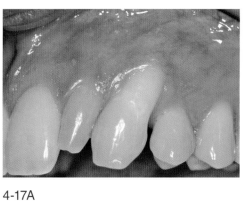

4-17A

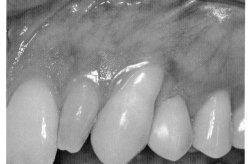

4-17B

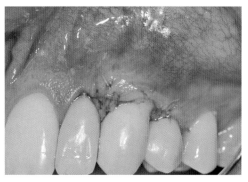

4-17C

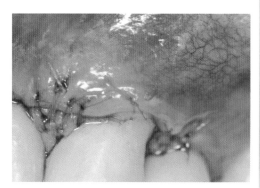

4-17D

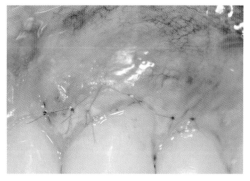

4-17E

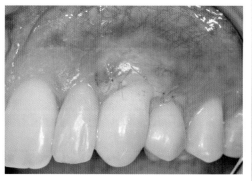

4-17F

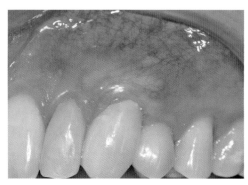

4-17G

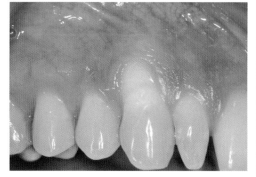

4-17H

Fig. 4-17

4-17A. Clinical pre-operative aspect of left canine. Marginal tissue recession of 5mm with a 1mm of keratinized tissue. Too thin gingival tissue, suggesting dehiscence and fenestration. Observe diastema between canine and first premolar as well as the altered dental axis of these teeth.

4-17B. After direct restoration to reestablish contact point and improve dental axis of teeth 23 and 24.

4-17C. Immediate postoperative view of periodontal microsurgery with subephitelial connective tissue graft for root coverage.

4-17D. Immediate postoperative situation (13X magnification). Observe approximation (6-0) and coaptation (8-0) microssuture of wound margins. Graft was positioned more apical to cementoenamel junction. Resin composite material will be added to cervical margin.

4-17E. Fifth days postoperative view (13X). Tissues kept the desired position during wound healing.

4-17F. Fifth day postoperative view showing less trauma to adjacent tissues.

4-1G. Thirty days after microsurgery. Note direct restorations on teeth 22, 23 and 24.

4-17H. Clinical pre-operative view of right canine. Observe marginal tissue recession of 4mm with 2mm of keratinized tissue.

4-17I. Immediate postoperative view of periodontal microsurgery with subephitelial connective tissue graft.

4-17J. Immediate postoperative view (13X). Observe approximation (6-0) and coaptation (8-0) microssuture. Graft was positioned more apical to cementoenamel junction.

4-17K. After 5 days, observe the fast reephitelization and stability of wound margin position.

4-17L. After 5 days, before suture removal. Less trauma is observed in adjacent tissue.

4-17M. Thirty days after microsurgery. Resin composite was added to teeth 13 and 12.

4-17N and O. Postoperative view of two donor sites. Continuous sutures (6-0) providing good approximation of wound margins.

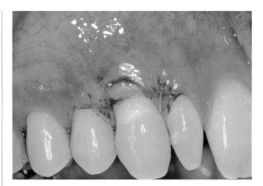

4-17I

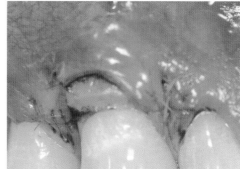

4-17J

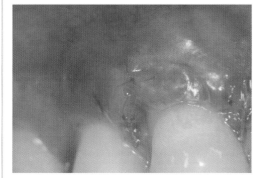

4-17K

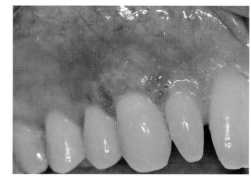

4-17L

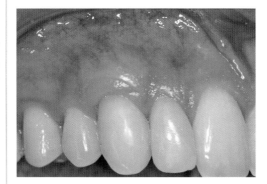

4-17M

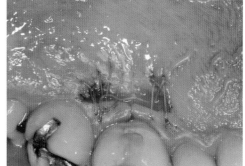

4-17N

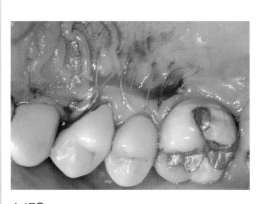

4-17O

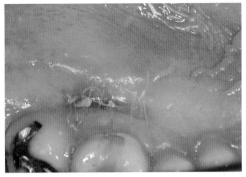

4-17P

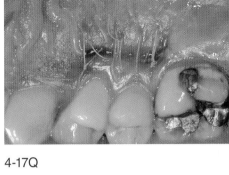

4-17Q

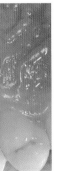
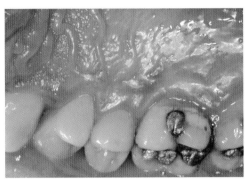

4-17R

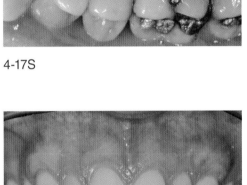

4-17S

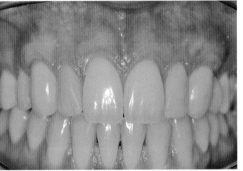

4-17P and Q. Postoperative view after 5 days – suture removal. Observed reduced trauma to donor sites.

4-17R and S. Postoperative view after 21 days. Observe complete ephitelialization and few signs of graft harvest.

4-17T. Pre-operative clinical aspect.

4-17U. The surgical and restorative treatments provided excellent gingival aspect and pleasant clinical crowns.

4-17V. Pre-operative smile.

4-17W. An esthetic smile showing integration between teeth, lips and gingival tissue.

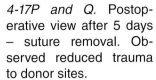

4-17T

4-17U

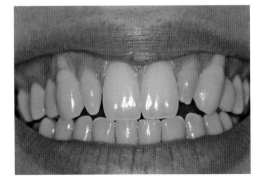

4-17V

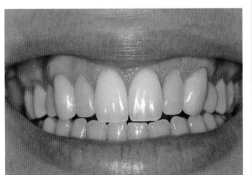

4-17W

Control and follow-up

❑ An occlusal splint was made just after restorative treatment.

❑ Support periodontal therapy was established in 4-month intervals.

❑ Restorations are examined annually to maintain their ideal characteristics.

❑ The case presented above has 4 years of follow-up without gingival tissue alterations, which demonstrates predictability of this technique.

Periimplant soft tissue

The use of dental implants in esthetic regions is a complex and sensitive procedure (Hürzeler and Weng, 1996; Salama et al., 1997; Sadoun et al., 1999). To achieve success in implant dental prosthetics, factors such as esthetics, function and biological principles must be balanced. This idea generated the concept that the implant must be "prosthetically driven" (Garber and Belser, 1995). Thus, the prosthetic planning determines the implant position rather than the osseous availability. Most cases require bone grafts previous to implant placement, as well as soft tissue to give harmonious transition between crown and implant. Several surgical procedures have been used to reestablish lost bone and create adequate sites to implant placement (Adell et al., 1990; Nevins and Mellonig, 1992; Isakssan, 1994; Buser et al., 1996).

Other surgical techniques try to improve periimplant soft tissue quantity and quality by palatal (Hertel et al., 1994; Tinti and Parma-Benfenati, 1995; Han, 1996; Tinti and Parma-Benfenati, 2002), or connective tissue grafts (Raplay et al., 1992; Han et al., 1995; Azzi et al., 2002). The increasing esthetic demand has driven implantodontists and periodontists to create periimplant soft tissue with a more natural esthetics. Microsurgery has optimized plastic periodontal techniques. It offers more safety and the possibility of wound healing by primary intention. Thus, observed results are faster, predictable, and esthetical. The periimplant microsurgeries can be made in four different moments:

I. Before implant installation

Substituting a tooth for an implant: a less traumatic removal can be through delicate soft tissue manipulation (periotomes and surgical elevators). This avoids cortical plate fracture and necrosis, as well as less postoperative tissue shrinkage (Fig. 4-18).

Extraction alveolar socket: the use of autogenous block grafts requires palatal positioning of labial flap to provide adequate closure and blood supply to wound healing. Usually, the keratinized tissue disappears on the labial aspect leaving a thin mucosa. In this sense, subephitelial connective tissue grafts can augment soft tissue thickness and create a band of keratinized tissue (Fig. 4-19).

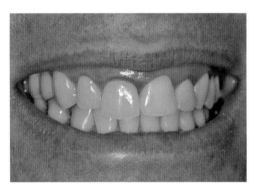

4-18A

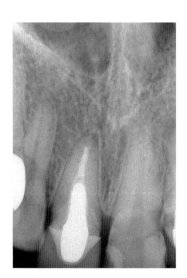

4-18B

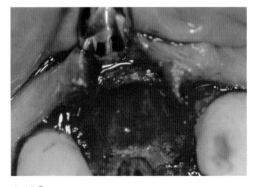

4-18C

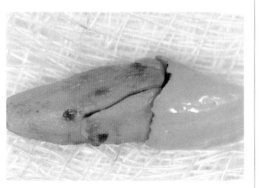

4-18D

Fig. 4-18. Plastic periimplant microsurgery before implant placement. The tooth was not removed yet.

4-18A. The patient smile shows marginal tissue inflammation, suppuration and slight mobility on tooth 11.

4-18B. Periapical radiographic image suggestive of middle third root fracture.

4-18C. Removal of tooth 11. Intrasucular incisions are made on teeth 12, 11 and 21. After flap dissection, fractured root was removed with periotomes and delicate elevators to preserve the labial plate.

4-18D. Image of fracture line and crown aspect.

4-18E. A 5-0 horizontal mattress suture (Poliglactin 910) is made before interrupted sutures.

4-18F. Occlusal aspect 5 days after. Suture was not removed.

4-18G. Frontal aspect 5 days after. Suture was not removed. Observe postoperative tissue quality due to a less traumatic procedure.

4-18H. Thirty days after surgery. Observe less tissue shrinkage.

4-18I. After suture removal, tissue conditioning was attempted with a provisional prosthesis.

4-18J. Occlusal aspect. Observe adequate soft tissue on labial site.

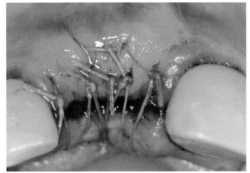
4-18E

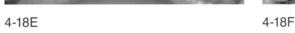
4-18F

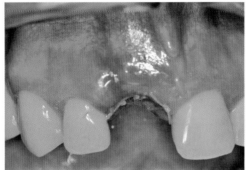
4-18G

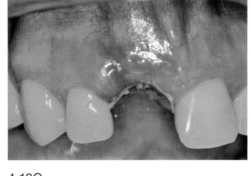
4-18H

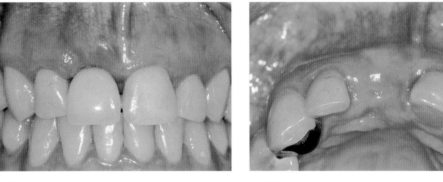
4-18I

4-18J

Fig. 4-19. Plastic periodontal microsurgery after tooth removal.

4-19A. Temporary crown on the anterior region showing lack of keratinized tissue.

4-19B. Radiographic image showing bone graft performed.

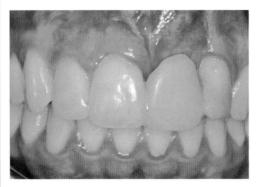
4-19A

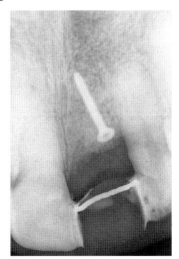
4-19B

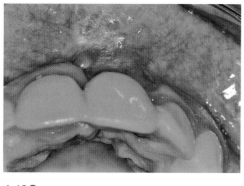

4-19C

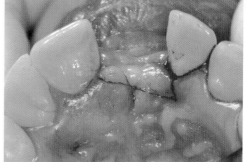

4-19D

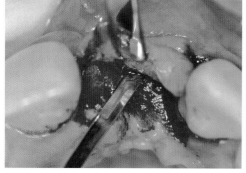

4-19E

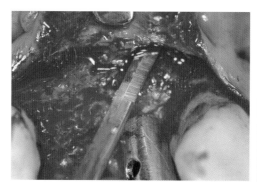

4-19F

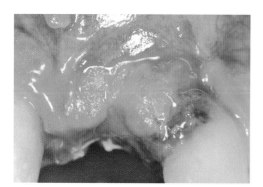

4-19G

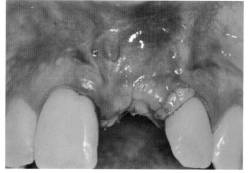

4-19H

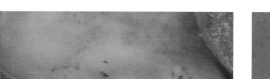

4-19I

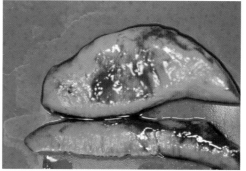

4-19J

4-19C. Occlusal view. Observe the loss of soft tissue.

4-19D. Initial incision palatal to the alveolar ridge.

4-19E. Initial flap dissection with microblade.

4-19F. Flap coronal releasing is achieved.

4-19G. Inicisons made on the donor site. Note the absence of vertical releasing incisions.

4-19H. Epithelial graft layer removal.

4-19I. Placement of connective tissue graft on the receptor area.

4-19J. Microsuturing finished.

4-19K. A 8-0 (Poliglactin 910) microsuture view (13X magnification). The graft and flap are approximated.

4-19L. Post-operative view, 5 days after: observe the complete graft integration to the soft tissue.

4-19M. Immediate post-operative occlusal view.

4-19N. Post-operative view: approximation suture (white 6-0) and coaptation suture (blue 8-0).

4-19O. Continuous 6-0 suture on the donor site.

4-19P. Fifth day post-operative view.

4-19Q. Preoperative view.

4-19R. Post-operative view, 30 days after; note the increased thickness on the region of 21. Mesial papilla on tooth 22 has improved considerably.

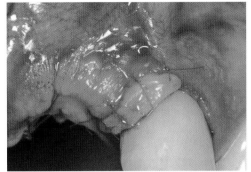

4-19K

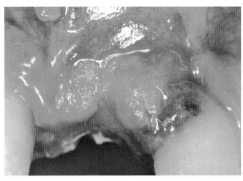

4-19L

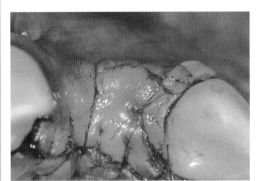

4-19M

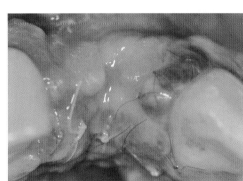

4-19N

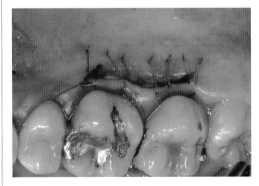

4-19O

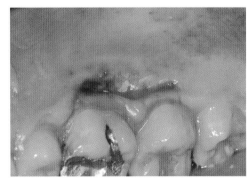

4-19P

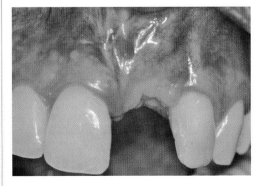

4-19Q

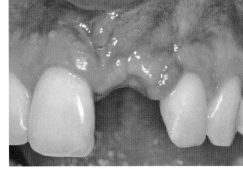

4-19R

2. Second surgical phase

During healing abutment connection, two different procedures can be made depending on tissue characteristics and defect configuration:

Without connective tissue graft: the masticatory palatal mucosa is rotated to the labial site. Usually, this is enough to create soft tissue volume lost due anterior surgical procedures (Fig. 4-20).

With connective tissue graft: for more accentuated soft tissue absence on labial or occlusal aspects. The palatal donor sites give an adequate amount of connective tissue, which can be shaped according to the situation of the receptor area. The graft length depends on the donor site thickness. Thus, thicker areas provide smaller grafts; otherwise, the mesiodistal graft dimension is augmented. The graft can be folded or rolled according to the size of the defect. The correct positioning of periimplant soft tissue around the healing abutment determines its initial configuration. The tissue is further defined by crown emergency profile (Fig. 4-21).

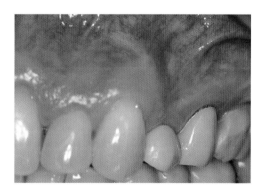

4-20A

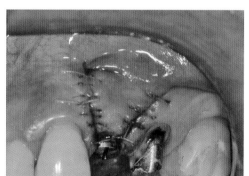

4-20B

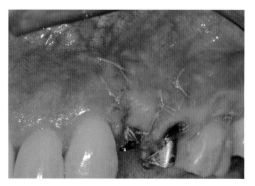

4-20C

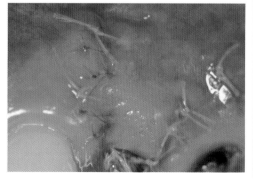

4-20D

Fig. 4-20. Plastic periimplant microsurgery. Vertical releasing microincisions.

4-20A. Observe the region of tooth 24. Note thin soft coverage and the lack of keratinized tissue.

4-20B. Immediate postoperative view, microssutures of approximation and coaptation. The palatal tissue was adapted to the labial aspect of the implant.

4-20C. Fifth day postoperative view. Observe the absence of trauma to adjacent areas and fast wound healing.

4-20D. Fifth day post-opertative view (13X magnification). In this phase, it is difficult to identify incision sites.

4-20E. Customized abutment installation (Procera, NobelBiocare, Göteborg, Sweden).

4-20F. Definitive restoration. Observe the soft tissue augmentation and the periimplant natural contour.

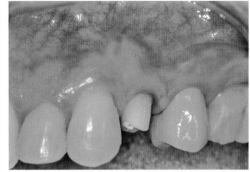
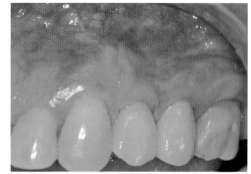

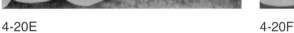

4-20E   4-20F

Fig. 4-21. Plastic periodontal microsurgery with connective tissue graft augmentation.

4-21A. Frontal view 6 months after implant placement. Observe loss of mesial papilla on tooth 21 and of keratinized tissue on the implant site.

4-21B. Radiographic image showing more apical implant position.

4-21C. Flap microssuture over the connective tissue graft adapted around healing abutment.

4-21D. Palatal donor site after continuous suture.

4-21E. Frontal view five days after showing wound healing on the mesial of 21.

4-21F. Occlusal view five days after showing labial tissue augmentation.

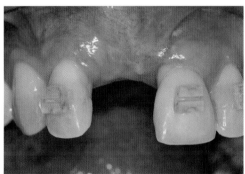
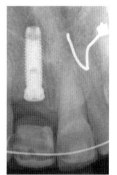

4-21A   4-21B

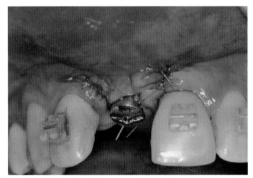
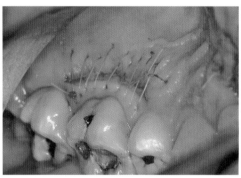

4-21C   4-21D

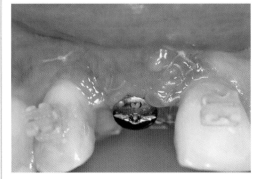
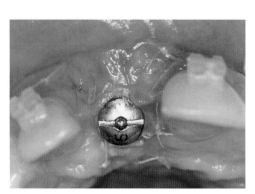

4-21E   4-21F

3. Provisional crown phase

When the patient presents with crown and prosthetic abutment installed, it is necessary to augment soft tissue height and thickness, or to recreate unsatisfactory papilla. Flap dissec-

tion and the use of subepithelial connective tissue grafts between flap and the prosthetic component can bring natural esthetics to soft periimplant tissues (Figs. 4-22 and 4-23). The provisional crown will guide soft tissue healing to a more natural looking appearance (Touati, 1995).

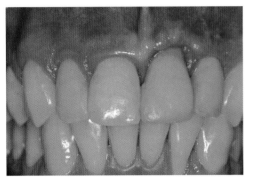
4-22A

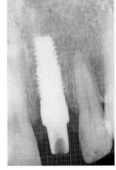
4-22B

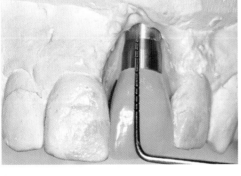
4-22C

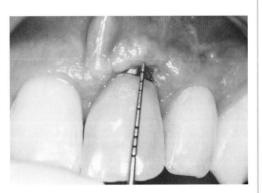
4-22D

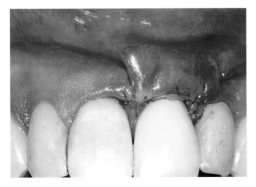
4-22E

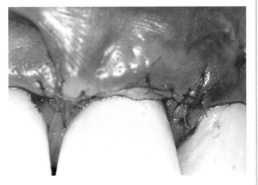
4-22F

Fig. 4-22. Plastic periodontal microsurgery during provisional restoration.

4-22A. Frontal view showing zenith unbalance between teeth 11 and 21.

4-22B. Radiographic image, new abutment installed (GengiHue – 3I).

4-22C. Master cast after determining the level of finish line configuration and the provisional crown.

4-22D. Abutment and provisional crown installation. Periodontal probe showing the amount of soft tissue to be covered.

4-22E. Periimplant microsurgery augmented by connective tissue graft. Immediate post-operative view.

4-22F. Immediate post-operative view (13X magnification). Observe approximation and coaptation microsutures.

4-22G. Initial view.

4-22H. Definitive restoration in position.

4-22I. Initial view: observe gingival discrepancy on tooth 21.

4-22J. Definitive restoration: observe balance between gingival and peri-implant marginal tissues.

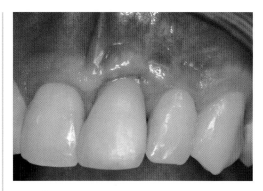

4-22G

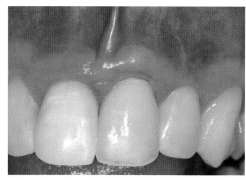

4-22H

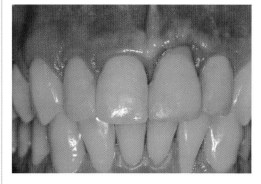

4-22I

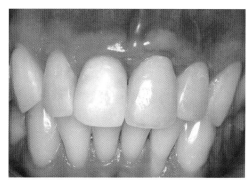

4-22J

Fig. 4-23. Plastic peri-implant microsurgery during provisional restoration phase.

4-23A. The patient complaints of prosthetic abutment on region 11.

4-23B. Radiographic image showing implant satisfactory conditions (IntraLock, Boca Raton, FL, USA).

4-23C. Frontal view. Prosthetic abutment showing through gingival tissue is evident.

4-23D. Connective tissue graft microsurgery on the immediate postoperative period. A new provisional crown was fabricated one week before surgery.

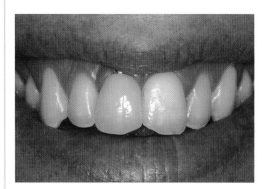

4-23A

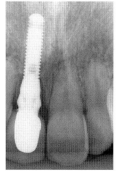

4-23B

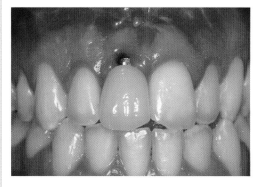

4-23C

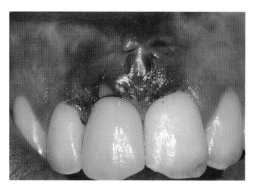

4-23D

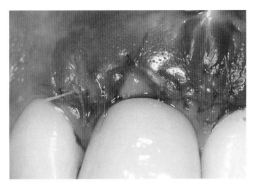

4-23E

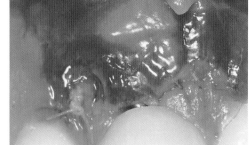

4-23F

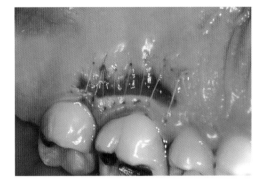

4-23G

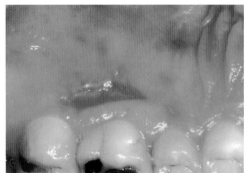

4-23H

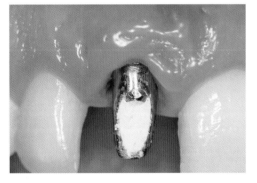

4-23I

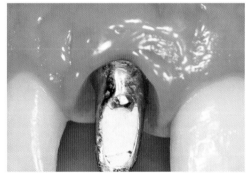

4-23J

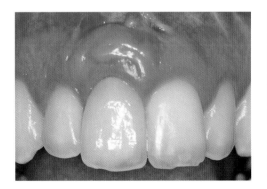

4-23K

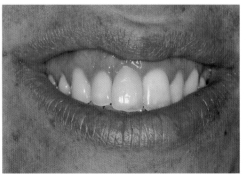

4-23L

4-23E. Immediate post-operative view (13X magnification). Observe that 6-0 (white) and 8-0 (blue) microssutures provide edge-to-edge coaptation of wound margins and adequate graft position on the desired area.

4-23F. Post-operative view 5 days after.

4-23G. Continuous suture in the donor site.

4-23H. Five day post-operative view after 6-0 suture removal.

4-23I. Ten day post-operative view (13X magnification). Acrylic resin has been added to the provisional crown.

4-23J. Thirty day post-operative view. Observe tissue remodeling on interproximal papilla.

4-23K. Definitive ceramic crown on implant 11. Change of resin restoration on tooth 21.

4-23L. The patient smile shows the reestablishment of periimplant soft tissue contours.

4. Maintenance phase

Once the definitive prosthesis has been made, it is difficult to perform plastic periimplant surgery. However, satisfactory results can be obtained in especial conditions, through connective tissue graft insertion between flap and prosthetic abutment already installed (Fig. 4-24). The achievement of predictable and esthetics results during soft tissue management depends on biological differences between tooth and implant insertion apparatus. Collagen fibers of periimplant mucosa run parallel to the implant surface, having its origin on osseous crest. The junctional epithelium is almost as twice long as compared to the healthy periodontium (Berglundh, 1991). Another important surgical aspect is the lack of blood supply to periimplant tissues due to absence of periodontal ligament (Berlundh et al., 1994).

These drawbacks are critical during plastic periodontal conventional surgery, especially on patients with thin phenotype. Manipulation of delicate soft tissue gives rise to mal-nutrition and prevents graft revascularization.

However, microsurgery techniques provide adequate precision during edge-to-edge approximation and coaptation, favoring primary wound healing intention. Thus, it increases predictability on technique-sensitive areas with great esthetic demands. The clinical cases on Figs. 4-18 to 4-24 illustrate several applications of periodontal microsurgery on the different phases of esthetic implant rehabilitation.

Conclusion

❑ The great esthetic appeal requires adequate technical and scientific knowledge to provide correct diagnosis and treatment planning of clinical cases.

❑ The identification of periodontal phenotype is important before soft tissue manipulation. Individual histological and anatomic characteristics dictate appropriate care and limitations of each case.

❑ Plastic periodontal microsurgery has the objective to minimize tissue trauma and provide wound healing by first intention. This treatment philosophy has broadened new perspectives on more safe, fast, predictable, and esthetic solutions.

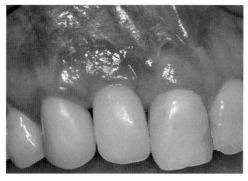

4-24A

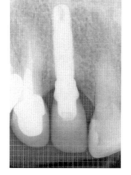

4-24B

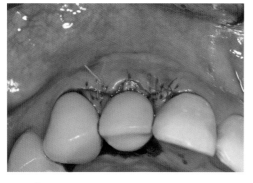

4-24C

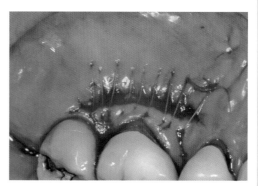

4-24D

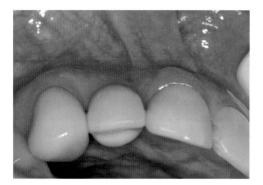

4-24E

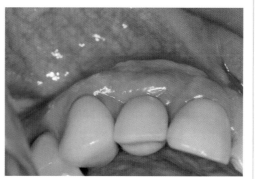

4-24F

Fig. 4-24. Plastic periodontal microsurgery during phase maintenance.

4-24A. Implant and crown on the region of tooth 12 made 15 years ago, showing loss of labial tissue thickness.

4-24B. Radiographic image showing osseous crest integrity.

4-24C. Immediate postoperative view after microsurgery augmented by subepithelial connective graft.

4-24D. Donor site after continuous 6-0 suture.

4-24E. Occlusal view. Observe the loss of labial soft tissue on the region of 12.

4-24F. Wound healing after 30 days and the new labial thickness.

References

1. ADELL, R.; LEKHOLM, V.; GRON-DAHL, K.; BRANEMARK, P-I.; LINDSTRÖM, J.; JACOBSSON, M. Reconstruction of severely resorbed edentulous maxillae using osseointegrated fixtures in immediate autogenous bone grafts. *Int J Oral Maxillofac Implants* 1990; 5:233-46.

2. AZZI, R.; ETIENNE, D.; TAKEI, H.; FENECH, P. Surgical thickening of the existing gingival and reconstruction of interdental papillae around implant supported restorations. *J Periodontics Restorative Dent* 2002; 22:71-77.

3. BALDI, C.; PINI-PRATO, G.; PAGLIARO, U. et al. Coronally advances flan procedure for root coverage. Is flap thickness a relevant predictor to achieve root coverage? A 19 – case series. *J Periodontol* 1999; 70:1077-84.

4. BELCHER, J.M. A perspective on periodontal microsurgery. *Int J Periodont Restorative Dent* 2001; 21:191-6.

5. BERGLUNDH, T.; LINDHE, J.; ERICSSON, I.; MARINELLO, C.P.; LILJENBERG, B.; THOMSEN, P. The soft tissue barrier at implants and teeth. *Clin Oral Implants Res* 1991; 2:81-90.

6. BERGLUNDH, T.; LINDHE, J.; JONSSON, K.; ERICSSON, I. The topography of the vascular systems in the periodontal and peri-implant tissues in the dog. *J Clin Periodontol* 1994; 21:189-193.

7. BRÄGGER, U.; LAUCHENAUER, D.; LANG, H.P. The surgical lengthening of the clinical crown. *J Clin Periodontol* 1992; 19:58-63.

8. BURKHARDT, R.; HÜRZELER, M.B. Utilization of the surgical microscope for advance plastic periodontal surgery. *Pract Periodont Aesthet Dent* 2000; 12:171-80.

9. BUSER, D.; DULA, K.; HIRT, H.P.; SCHENK, R.K. Lateral ridge augmentation using autografts and barrier membranes: A clinical study with 40 partially edentulous patients. *J Oral Maxillofac Surg* 1996; 54:420-32.

10. CHICHE, G.J.; PINAULT, A. *Esthetic of anterior fixed prosthodontics.* Chicago: Ed Quintessence 1994.

11. CORTELLINI, P.; TONETTI, M.S. Microsurgical approach to periodontal regeneration. Initial evaluation in a case cohort. *J Periodontal* 2001; 72:559-69.

12. EGER, T.; MÜLLER, H.P.; HEINECKE, A. Ultrasonic determination of gingival thickness. Subject variation and influence of tooth type and clinical features. *J Clin Periodontol* 1996; 23:839-45.

13. GARBER, D.A.; BELSER, U.C. Restoration-driven implant placement with restoration-generated site development. *Compend Cont Educ Dent* 1995; 16:796-804.

14. GARGIULO, A.W.; WENTZ, F.M.; ORBAN, B. Dimensions and relations of the dentogingival junction in humans. *J Periodontol* 1961; 32:261-67.

15. HAN, T.J.; KLOKKEVOLD, P.A.; TAKEI, H.H. Strip gingival autograft used to correct mucogingival problems around implants. *Int J Periodontics Restorative Dent* 1995; 15:405-11.

16. HAN, T.J. Surgical aspects of dental implants. In: CARRANZA JR., F.A.; NEWMAN, M.G. (eds). *Clinical Periodontology,* 8.ed. Philadelphia: WB Saunders, 1996.

17. HERTEL, R.C.; BUDJOR, P.A.; KALK, W.; BAKER, D.L. Stage 2 surgical techniques in endosseous implantation. *Int J Oral Maxillofac Implants* 1994; 9:273-78.

18. HOUAISS, A.; VILLAR, M.S.; FRANCO, F.M.M. *Dicionário da língua portuguesa.* Rio de Janeiro: Ed. Objetiva, 2001.

19. HÜRZELER, M.B.; WENG, D. Peri-implant tissue management: Optimal timing for an aesthetic result. *Pract Periodont Aesthet Dent* 1996; 8(9):857-68.

20. HÜRZELER, M.B.; WENG, D. Func-

tional and esthetic outcome enhancement of periodontal surgery by application of plastic surgery principles. *Int Periodontics Restorative Dent* 1999; 19:36-43.

21. ISAKSSAN, S. Evaluation of three bone grafting techniques for severely resorbed maxillae in conjunction with immediate endosseous implants. *Int J oral Maxillofac Implants* 1994; 9:679-88.

22. KAO, R.T.; PASQUINELLI, K. Thick vs. thin gingival tissue: a key determinant in tissue response do disease and restorative treatment. *CDA*, 2002; 30:521-26.

23. MCGUIRE, M.K. Periodontal plastic surgery. *Dent Clin North Am* 1998; 42:441-64.

24. MICHAELIDES, P.L. Use of the operating microscope in dentistry. *J Calif Dent Assoc* 1996; 24:45-50.

25. MÜLLER, H.P.; EGER, T. Gingival phenotypes in young male adults. *J Clin Periodontol* 1997; 24:65-71.

26. MÜLLER, H.P.; HEINECKE, A.; SCHALLER, N.; EGER, T. Masti-gatory mucosa in subjects with different periodontal phenotypes. *J Clin Periodontol* 2000; 27:621-26.

27. MÜLLER, H.P.; STAHL, M.; EGER, T. Dynamics of mucosal dimensions after root coverage with a bioresorbable membrane. *J Clin Periodontol* 2000; 27:1-8.

28. MÜLLER, H.P.; EGER, T. Mastigatory mucosa and periodontal phenotype: a review. *Int J Periodontics Restorative Dent,* 2002; 22:172-183.

29. NEVINS, M.; MELLONIG, J.T. Enhancement of the damaged edentulous ridge to receive dental implants: a combination of allograft and the Gore-Tex membrane. *Int J Periodontics Restorative Dent* 1992; 12:97-111.

30. OCHSENBEIN, C.; ROSS, S. A reavaluation of osseous surgery. *Dent Clin North Am* 1969; 13:87-102.

31. OLSSON, M.; LINDHE, J.; MARI-NELLO, C.P. On the relationship between crown form and features of the gingival in adolescents. *J Clin Periodontol* 1993; 20:570-77.

32. PONTORIERO, R.; CARNEVALE, G. Surgical crown lengthening: a 12-month clinical wound healing study. *J Periodontol* 2001; 72:841-48.

33. RAPLEY, J.W.; MILLS, P.M.; WY-LAM, J. Soft tissue management during implant maintenance. *Int J Periodontics Restorative Dent* 1992; 12:373-81.

34. RUFENACHT, C.R. *Principles of esthetics integration.* Berlim: Quintessence, 2000.

35. SAADOUN, A.P.; LEGALL, M.; TOUATI, B. Selection and ideal tri-dimensional implant position for soft tissue aesthetics. *Pract Periodont Aesthet Dent* 1999; 11(9): 1063-72.

36. SALAMA, H.; SALAMA, M.; LI, T.G.; ADAR, P. Treatment planning 2000 – an esthetically oriented revision of the original implant protocol. *J Esthet Dent* 1997; 9(2):55-67.

37. SHANELEC, D.A. Current trends in soft tissue. *Calif Dent Assoc J* 1991; 19(12):57-60.

38. SHANELEC, D.A.; TIBBETTS, S. Recent advances in surgical technology. In: CARRANZA, F.A.; NEWMAN, M.G (eds). *Clinical Periodontology.* Philadelphia: Saunders 1996; 677-84.

39. SERINO, F.; WENNESTRÖN, J.L.; LINDHE, J.; ENERTH, L. The prevalence and distribution of gingival recession in subjects with a high standard of oral hygiene. *J Clin Periodontol* 1994; 21:57-63.

40. TIBBETTS, L.S.; SHANELEC, D.A. Periodontal microsurgery. *Dent Clin North Am* 1998; 42:339-59.

41. TINTI, C.; PARMA-BENFENATI, S. Coronally positioned palatal sliding flap. *Int J Periodontics Restorative Dent* 1995; 15:298-310.

42. TINTI, C.; PARMA-BENFENATI, S. The ramp mattress suture: a new suturing technique combined with a surgical procedure to obtain papillae between implants in the buc-

cal area. *Int J Periodontics Restorative Dent* 2002; 22:63-9.

43. TOUATI, B. Custom-guided tissue healing for improved aesthetics in implant supported restoration. *Int J Dent Symp* 1995; 3:36-9.

44. VAZ DE CAMPOS, G.; TUMENAS, I. Microcirurgia plástica periodontal: uma alternativa biológica e estética no recobrimento de raízes. *Rev Assoc Paul Cir Dent*, 1998, 52:319-23.

45. VAZ DE CAMPOS, G.; TUMENAS, I. Microcirurgia plástica periodontal com matriz dérmica acelular. *Rev Assoc Paul Cir Dent*, 1999, 53:487-91.

46. VAZ DE CAMPOS, G.; VAZ DE CAMPOS, F.T. Microcirurgia plástica periodontal. In: CARDOSO, R.J.A.; GONÇALVES, E.A.N. *Estética*, v.3, São Paulo: Ed. Artes Médicas, 2002; cap. 14, p. 283-316.

47. VAZ DE CAMPOS, G.; TUMENAS, I. Microcirurgia plástica periodontal. In: Opinion makers. *Tecnologia e informática*. São Paulo: Ed. VM Comunicações, 2002, p.66-73.

48. VAZ DE CAMPOS, G.; LOPES, C.J.; CHINEN, M.C.; AUDA, S.M.; TOZZI, C. Microcirurgia plástica periodontal na reconstrução de papila interdental. In: LIMBERTE, M.S.; MONTENEGRO, J.R. *Estética do sorriso – arte e ciência*. São Paulo: Ed. Santos, 2003, cap. 14, p.183-92.

49. VAZ DE CAMPOS, G.; LOPES, C.J.; LACERDA NETO, A. Tratamento estético e expectativa do paciente. Microcirurgia plástica periodontal e dentística restauradora. In: MIYASHITA, E.; FONSECA, A.S. *Odontologia estética – o estado da arte*. São Paulo: Ed. Artes Médicas, 2004, cap, 21. p.507-30.

50. WACHTEL, H.; SCHENK, G.; BÖHM, S.; WENG, D.; ZUHR, O.; HÜRZELER MB. Microsurgical access flap and enamel matrix derivative for the treatment of periodontal intrabony defects: a controlled clinical study. *J Clin Periodontol* 2003; 30:496-504.

51. WENNSTRÖM, J.L. Mucogingival therapy. *Ann Periodontol* 1996; 1:671-701.

5

WHEN TO REPLACE TEETH BY IMPLANTS

Reinaldo Janson
Ziad Jaboult
Euloir Passanezzi
Adriana Campos Passanezzi Sant'Ana

Introduction

Every clinical situation is different. Every patient is different. Every clinician is different.

For a long time, every attempt to preserve compromised teeth was valid: teeth with periodontal disease were heroically treated and, in many cases, had a long-term survival.[4-8,11,13,14,19,22,24,25,28]

The introduction of osseointegrated dental implants by Prof. Per-Ingvar Brånemark in 1982 has brought a new alternative for oral rehabilitation of teeth with uncertain prognosis,[1,3,7,10,12,18,20] where the same could be replaced with implants with long term predictability.

The decision of whether to replace teeth with implants is not always a simple question.[7,11,21,34]

However, during explanation of the most simple to the most complex treatment planning, the clinician will be able to decide the best and most predictable treatment for each single case.

In this chapter, we will discuss the several factors that influence whether to maintain or replace teeth with implants.

Variables

Three different variables are important to achieve adequate treatment whether to extract a tooth (or teeth) or not.

The first corresponds to the dental status. The evaluation is based on treatment type to eliminate its cause and to predict the necessary restorations.[4,5,8,13,14,22] Although by itself it indicates tooth removal, it does not determines the type of rehabilitation to be fabricated.[5,9,12,18,21,24]

The second variable regards to the patients. Their judgment and correct analysis will help clinicians on the treatment options, indicating the least and the most likely for each patient.

The third variable represents the implant itself. During tooth removal, one has to decide whether the implant is the best option or a conventional dental prosthesis would achieve satisfactory results.[1,3,10,12,18,34]

The great challenge is not to decide on cases where the clinician had already identified hopeless teeth[11,28] (Figs. 5-1 to 5-4), where any prosthesis type is adequate (fixed, removable or implant-supported), but in cases with a questionable prognosis. In these situations, the clinician must consider whether to maintain and treat or to remove and replace teeth with implants.[11,21,35,39]

This evaluation must be done on factors such as long-term function and the best treatment option.

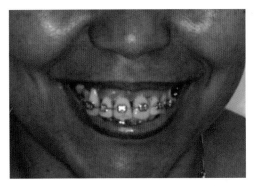

5-1

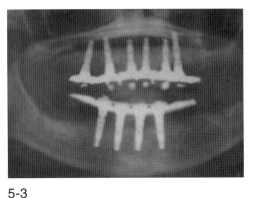

5-2

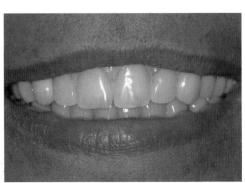

5-3

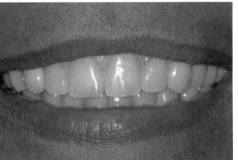

5-4

Fig. 5-1. Patient frontal view showing pathological labial tooth migration of upper anterior teeth.

Fig. 5-2. Radiographic image showing extensive alveolar bone loss.

Fig. 5-3. Radiographic image of implants installed.

Fig. 5-4. Frontal view after treatment with implant prostheses.

Tooth variables

This is the key factor in the decision making process. It will determine the necessary treatment to remove disease and restore teeth. When the tooth is hopeless (as in the case of vertical fractures) it must be removed. The two other variables will determine the rehabilitation type to be executed.

Within tooth variables, endodontic,[6,19,22] periodontal,[2,4,13,19,23,25,26,36] restorative,[13,14,24,33] and orthodontic treatment must be considered for each dental situation. They must consider the tooth role in the treatment planning.

Endodontic treatment. A judicious evaluation of pulp health is paramount for a long-term success. Although endodontic treatment has been shown a high success index, certain situations prevent an adequate endodontic therapy. The presence and size of periapical pathologies represents a new endodontic variable that must be thorough evaluated. Root canal retreatment requires special attention in cases of periapical lesions and intraradicular posts.

Periodontal treatment. The decision depends on individual susceptibility to infectious marginal periodontal disease (periodontitis) and the available periodontal support to neutralize occlusal forces.

The patient susceptibility is related to the periodontal immunologic profile, determined by HLA haplotypes, characterizing the risk to periodontitis, being classified in classes A or DR HLA antigens.[2,15,32,36,37]

However, being the relation between haplotype and periodontitis not confirmed, the individual susceptibility can be screened with the Periodontal Susceptibility Test (PST) proposed by Kornman[17] and Kornman, Crane, Wang, diGovane, Newman, Pirk, Wilson, Higginbottom and Duff. A blood sample is sent to the laboratory. DNA analysis will show whether the individual is genotype-positive or negative to the interleukin-1 (IL-1).

The actual evidence sustains that, when bacterial disease affects genotype-positive individuals, the likelihood of severe generalized periodontitis is six-fold increased. Thus, compromised individuals must be monitored carefully to maintain dentobacterial plaque levels under control.

Besides, genotype-positive heavy smoker individuals composed 86% of severe periodontitis cases in a student population. The genotype-negative smokers can have more clinical benefits on reduction or interruption of smoking, at least about the risk reduction on severe periodontal disease.

The PST is a susceptibility

test which informs whether the patient will be further subject to severe periodontitis. Clinical longitudinal studies must explore its use to make it more accessible, being this worthwhile to decide whether to replace teeth with implants.

The available periodontal support to neutralize occlusal forces must be considered regarding individual tooth and the number of abutments for splinting and stabilization.

The periodontal support is defined as the number of inserted periodontal ligament fibers divided by the root volume unit. It is uniform along cylindrical and diminishes progressively on tapered roots (Figs. 5-5A and B).

Thus, while the loss of periodontal support in cylindrical roots is proportional to the loss of alveolar bone, the same one-third loss in tapered roots represents half the periodontal support (Figs. 5-6A and B).

Besides, lateral forces manifest themselves along coronoapical extension, even during axial forces (Fig. 5-6C). In this situation, a wider periodontal ligament space must be provided, increasing the physiological mobility limits of those teeth.

Perhaps, that is the reason why tapered roots are not considered adequate abutments for prosthesis fabrication (Shillingburg, Hobo, Whitsett, Jacobi, Bracket[33]).

The implications of root configuration and alveolar bone level on periodontal support and occlusal force distribution can be investigated by photoelastic analysis (Figs. 5-5 and 5-6).

Bearing in mind that each tooth can withstand twice the load applied, the loss of half of periodontal support can generate secondary occlusal trauma, requiring tooth splinting or replacing with implant. In this sense, it is important to remember that the loss of periodontal support begins at the osseous crest and follows an apical direction, compromising areas of more fiber insertion. Thus, teeth with tapered roots will be severely affected. A 2mm bone loss can be extremely significant since the involved areas provide most periodontal ligament fibers by root volume unit, jeopardizing tooth prognosis (Passanezi, Sant'Ana, Rezende, Greghi, Janson[30], Passanezi, Sant'Ana, Rezende, Greghi[31]).

Besides, occlusal force neutralization still depends on the cantilever generated between clinical crown (load arm) and its root alveolar insertion (resistance arm). The ideal stated crown-to-root ratio is less than or equal to 1. Otherwise, it can jeopardize periodontal ligament homeostasis as the load arm becomes greater than the resistance arm.

Regarding to tooth substitution, not only the number of teeth to be extracted must be

Fig. 5-5. Photoelastic analysis of occlusal force distribution on dental prototypes mounted in the semi-adjustable articulator simulating normal and reduced periodontal support.

5-5A. Occlusal axial force distribution on posterior teeth with normal periodontal support. The first photoelastic fringe was produced with a load of 10kgf. Observe force concentration on apical root portion.

5-5B. Occlusal axial force distribution on posterior teeth with one third reduced periodontal support. The first photoelastic fringe was produced with a load of 5kgf. Based on these findings, a 50% loss in periodontal support can be deducted.

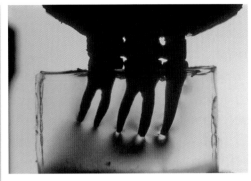

5-5A

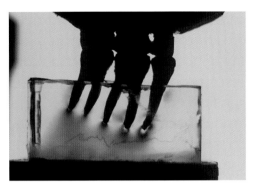
5-5B

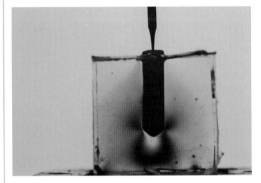
5-6A

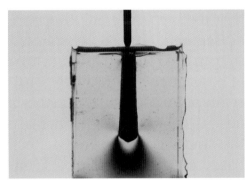
5-6B

Fig. 5-6. Photoelastic analysis of occlusal force distribution on dental prototypes mounted in the semi-adjustable articulator.

5-6A and B. First photoelastic fringe distribution on cylindrical and tapered roots. In these situations, apical portions are wider than coronal portions. Force concentrates on apical portions, illustrating that axial forces result in tooth intrusion without lateral force reactions.

5-6C. First photoelastic fringe distribution on cylindrical and tapered roots. In this situation, apical portion is narrower than coronal portion. Contrary to the situation in figures 5-6A and B, force now concentrates on apical and lateral root portions. The same effects could be observed in dental implants. However, the existence of periodontal ligament contributes to the axial distribution of forces. On the other hand, these force distribution mechanisms on dental implants probably depends on bone resilience and its ultra-structural characteristics. Thus, the evidence of connective tissue on bone-implant interface can be regarded as a biological adaptation and not the failure of osseointegration

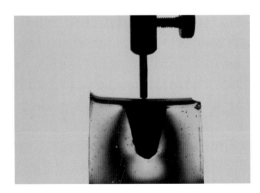
5-6C

considered, but also the number of abutments to provide adequate occlusal force distribution. Two important aspects must be considered: (1) when the total amount of remaining periodontal support is not equal or less than that of removed abutments and, (2) when teeth distribution is not adequate for conventional dental prosthesis fabrication.

In the first scenario, implant indication is immediate, while in the second the design of the reconstruction depends on the principles of tooth stabilization suggested by Roy (Grant, Stern and Listgarten[9]). According to this, teeth on different directional segments must be splinted into an arch to increase root area of resistance and provide a fulcrum point inside the prosthesis design. Also, this will increase the mesiodistal ferule effect. Based on these principles, Lindhe and Nyman[24] obtained excellent results during treatment of advanced periodontal disease.

Thus, individual susceptibility to periodontal disease, risk factors, and mechanisms of force neutralization constitute the main factors during decision making process of tooth splinting or replacement. The clinical crown lengthening must be considered after bone height evaluation and before visualization of landmark structures (mandibular canal, maxillary sinus), adjacent teeth and endodontic therapy.[6,8,13]

Restorations:[5,6,7,8,19,22] endodontically treated teeth must receive post and core restoration to avoid root fracture. Teeth with crown fracture and biologic width violation must undergone clinical crown lengthening through periodontal surgery or orthodontic forced eruption.

Orthodontic treatment:[21] drifted teeth must be evaluated whether orthodontic movement will be sufficient to improve prognosis. Severely tilted molars, crossbite and extrusion problems are some issues considered in the treatment planning. The need of root canal therapy and periodontal surgery in cases of posterior bite collapse is a clinical dilemma.

Overall treatment planning: the importance of a tooth within the overall planning must be considered: is the tooth considered a fixed or removable prosthesis abutment? The implant treatment is been considered within the same or to adjacent quadrant? If the tooth must serve as an abutment, additional stresses will be generated. Thus, tooth replacement must be considered when implant therapy is planned for the same quadrant.

Patient variables

This includes social history, medical conditions, economic factors, motivation, chief complaint, caries and periodontal disease susceptibility, as well as esthetic desires.[11,15,34]

Smoking is a risk factor for periodontitis. It decreases the success level of implant therapy, leading to bone loss over time. Although smoking does not contra-indicate implant treatment, patients must be informed on this outcome. Also, uncontrolled diabetes, patient medication related to xerostomic conditions and high caries prevalence index are important issues that deserve attention before establishing a treatment strategy, in addition to the patient motivation. Table 5-1 summarizes some risk factors that must be taken into account.

The esthetic desire, especially in the anterior region, along with patient's age, high lip line and periodontal phenotype are decisive and must be thoroughly evaluated to achieve success in implant dentistry. Table 5-2 summarizes indications for tooth maintenance or implant installation.

Implant variables

The implant treatment must be considered simple with a low level of complexity and complex level.[1,3,12,20]

Simple treatment

In those instances, tooth removal, implant placement and prosthetic reconstruction must be done in a casual way. For this, complications such as bone loss or anatomic involvement during surgery must not be observed. Immediate implant installation can be considered in the absence of pathologies, loss of cortical plate or labial recession. A flapless surgery can help to prevent loss of osseous crest. Also, bone graft techniques can be used in conjunction with implant placement for difficult cases.

Low level of complexity

It involves cases with few anatomic or patient related limitations. However, is still possible to perform treatment without major surgery. Bone loss in height and can be considered an anatomic limitation, because it implies the need of shorter implants and/or bone grafts. This situation can occur during tooth removal (loss of cortical plate) or bone resorption due to periodontal disease.

Patient limitations: any medical condition in which pharmacological therapy needs to be altered before implant surgery, i.e., the use of anticoagulants or uncontrolled diabetes. Also, patients must be reminded of postoperative complications due to smoking habits.

Complex treatment

Additional surgeries must be done before implant installation, such as maxillary sinus and alveolar bone crest augmentation. Also, medically compromised patients must have a more conservative treatment.

Assessment method

A simple method can be proposed to help the decision making process of tooth maintenance or replace it with implant. Each variable was divided into different procedures. After, a score was attributed to each procedure.

Table 5-1. Factors related to tooth preservation or implant placement

Tooth preservation	Implant placement
Smoker	Medication causing xerostomy
Uncontrolled diabetes	
Medically compromised patients	
Low level of caries susceptibility	High level of caries susceptibility
Low predisposition to periodontal disease	High predisposition to periodontal disease
Patient apprehensive regarding implant treatment	Patient motivated regarding implant treatment
Great esthetic demand	

Table 5-2. Esthetic factors related to tooth preservation or implant placement

Tooth preservation	Implant placement
High lip line	Low lip line
Two adjacent implants	Single implant, pontic related
Loss of adjacent periodontal ligament	Adjacent teeth without loss of periodontal ligament
Thin-scalloped gingival phenotype	Thick-flat gingival phenotype
Intact dentition	Recession, black triangle
Great esthetic demand	Low esthetic demand

The highest score level (10) indicates tooth removal and implant placement. The lowest score level (1) indicates tooth maintenance and treatment. A score between 3 to 5 represents the *grey zone*, where the clinicians' knowledge and skills are fundamental to tooth prognosis, on the basis of factors previously discussed.[38,39]

Table 5-3 summarizes the score levels.

Evaluation scale

❑ Tooth preservation = sum of scores between 1 to 3.
❑ Grey zone = scores between 3 to 5.
❑ Implant therapy = scores between 5 to 10.

Table 5-3. Evaluation scale in the decision making process

Numerical values	Endodontic procedures
1	Root canal therapy
2	Retreatment
3	Complicated cases: – Retreatment with periapical pathology – Retreatment with post removal – Root canal treatment with extensive periapical pathology
	Periodontics
1	Clinical crown lengthening
1	Bone loss >3mm
1	Mobility grade III or above
1	Furcation lesion (grade II or III)
	Restorative
1	Prosthetic crown
1	Post and core restoration
2	Fixed or removable dental abutment prosthesis
	Implant therapy
1	Implants on the same quadrant
1	Simple treatment
0	Low level of complexity
-1	Complex treatment

Clinical case presentations

Case 1

The patient had a root fracture on tooth 11. Adequate root canal therapy and bone levels were seen on this radiograph. However, poor crown-to-root ratio impedes orthodontic extrusion or clinical lengthening to rees- tablish its biologic width (Figs. 5-7 and 5-8).

Taken into account these factors, replacement of the remaining root with implant followed by screwed retained prosthesis was the best option (Figs. 5-9 to 5-11).

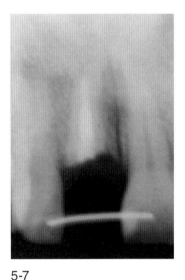 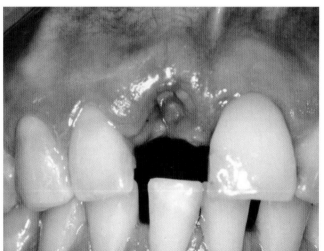

5-7   5-8

Fig. 5-7. Periapical radiograph showing remaining root with endodontic treatment and preservation of adjacent bone crest.

Fig. 5-8. Clinical view showing good gingival condition and adequate edentulous space.

Fig. 5-9. Implant installation after tooth extraction. A small fenestration can be seen in the apical portion.

Fig. 5-10. Periapical radiograph showing implant and the fixation screw securing membrane during bone regeneration.

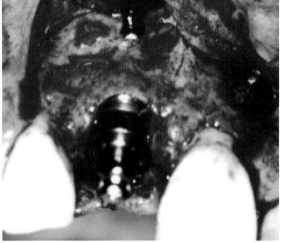 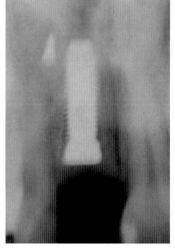

5-9   5-10

Fig. 5-11. Final view. Observe adequate gingival levels due to the preservation of adjacent osseous crest.

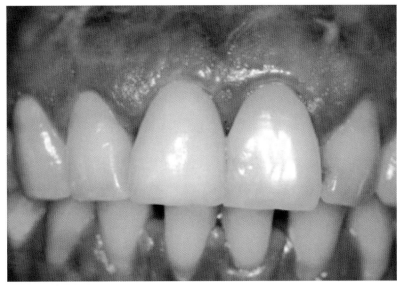

5-11

Case 2

This patient presented with a three unit fixed prosthesis with abutment teeth 46 and 48. Periapical radiograph demonstrated cervical carious lesion on tooth 46 jeopardizing its long term prognosis (Fig. 5-12). In case of conventional treatment, prosthesis removal, clinical crown lengthening, endodontic therapy, post and core restoration, and a new fixed prosthesis would be fabricated. The local bone condition was good in height and width. Teeth 46 and 47 were replaced with two implants. Crown on tooth 48 remained in position (Fig. 5-13).

Fig. 5-12. Periapical radiograph showing the extent of carious lesion compromising long-term prognosis of fixed dental prosthesis.

Fig. 5-13. Periapical radiograph showing substitution of teeth 46 and 47 for two dental implants. Crown on tooth 48 remains in position.

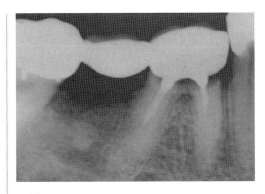

5-12

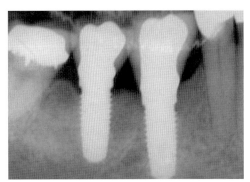

5-13

Case 3

The tooth 24 had a distal angular bone defect and mobility caused by periodontal problems and occlusal trauma (Figs. 5-14 and 5-15).

Treatment option was tooth removal, immediate implant installation and fabrication of a implant retained prosthesis (Figs. 5-16 to 5-19).

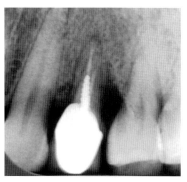

5-14

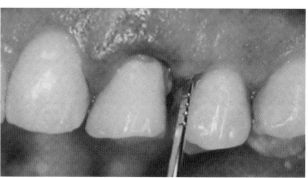

5-15

Fig. 5-14. Radiographic image showing distal angular bone defect and poor crown-to-root ratio.

Fig. 5-15. Distal probing on tooth 24 confirming bone loss.

Figs. 5-16 and 5-17. Careful tooth removal preserving adjacent osseous structures and immediate implant installation.

Figs. 5-18 and 5-19. Periapical radiograph and final clinical view, showing bone and soft tissue recovering around dental implant.

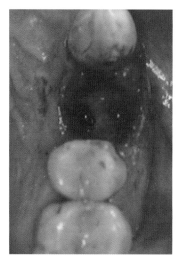

5-16

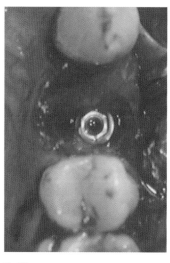

5-17

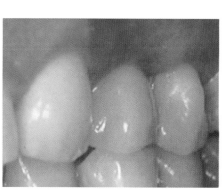

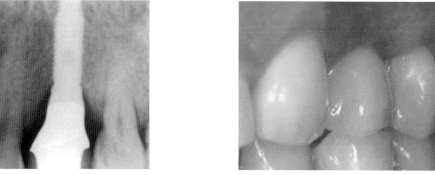

5-18

5-19

Case 4

The patient's chief complaint was his inferior teeth. A periodontal maintenance program had been institutionalized without long-term success. The teeth presented with generalized mild to severe bone loss. Without adequate periodontal response, the treatment option was complete inferior teeth removal, implant placement and a fixed prosthesis installation.

Fig. 5-20. Panoramic radiograph showing periodontal involvement of inferior teeth.

Fig. 5-21. Open surgical field showing generalized bone loss of involved teeth.

Figs. 5-22 and 5-23. Final radiographic and clinical views. Five implants and a fixed prosthesis were placed in the mandible. Observe good gingival response.

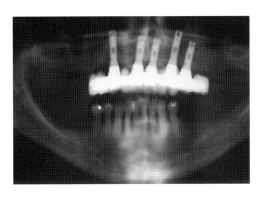

5-20

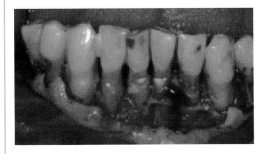

5-21

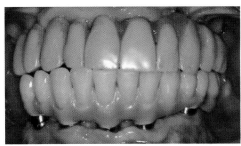

5-22

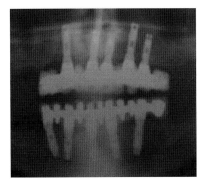

5-23

Conclusion

Nowadays, Implantology is a time-honored procedure in dentistry. It can be incorporated and help to treat simple or complex cases, providing patients with successful long-term oral rehabilitations.

References

1. ADELL, R.; LEKHOLM, U.; ROCKLER, B.; BRÅNEMARK, P-I. A 15-years study of osseointegrated implants in the treatment of edentulous jaws. *Int J Oral Surg* 1981; 10: 387-416.
2. AMER, A. et al. Association between HLA antigens and periodontal disease. *Tissue antigens*, 31:53-8, 1988.
3. ARNOUX, J.P. The use of Brånemark implants in the treatment of severe periodontitis. *Real Clin* 1992; 3: 359-369.
4. BECKER, W.; BERG, L.; BECKER, B.E. The long term evaluation of periodontal treatment and maintenance in 95 patients. *Int J Periodontics Rest Dent* 1984, 2:55-62.
5. CARNEVALE, G.; GIANFRANCO, D.F.; TONELLI, M.P.; MARIN, C.; FUZZI, M.A. A retrospective analysis of the periodontal-prosthetic treatment of molars with interradicular lesions. *Int. J Periodontics Restorative Dent* 1991; 11: 188-205.
6. COHEN, A.; MACHTOU, P. Endo-periodontal lesions: Biologic and mechanical considerations. *J Parodontol* 1996; 15: 235-250.
7. DAVANPARNAH, M. et al. To conserve or implant: which choice of therapy? *The Int. J. Period. Rest. Dent.* 2000; 20: 413-421

8. FUGAZZOTTO, P.A.; PARMA-BEN-FENATTI, S. Preprosthetic periodontal consideration: crown length and biologic width. *Quintessence Int* 1984; 15: 1247-1256
9. GRANT, D.A.; STERN, I.B. & LISTGARTEN, M.A. *Periodontics* 6th ed., S. Louis, Mosby, 1988 pp. 479-526, 1056-74.
10. HASS, R.; MENSDORFF-POUILLY, N.; MAILATH, G.; WATZEK, G. Brånemark single-tooth implants. *J Prosthetic Dent* 1995; 7: 4-9.
11. HARRISON, J.W.; SVEC, T.A. The hopeless tooth: When is treatment futile? *Quintessence International* 1999, v30; 12:846-850.
12. JEMT, T.; LEKHOLM, U.; ADELL, R. Osseintegraded implants in the treatment of partially edentulous patients. *Int J Oral Maxillofac Implants* 1989; 4: 211-217.
13. KALDAHL, W.B.; BECKER, C.M.; WENTS, F.M. Periodontal surgical preparation for specific problems in restorative dentistry. *Prosthet Dent* 1984; 51: 36-41
14. KARLSSON, S. Failures and length of service in fixed prosthodontics after long-term function. *Swed Dent J* 1989; 13: 185-192.
15. KASLICK, R.S.; WEST, T.L.; CHASENS, A.L. Association between ABO blood groups, HL-A antigens and periodontal diseases in young adults: a follow-up study. *J. Periodontal.*, 51: 339-42,1980
16. KORNMAN, K.S. Conference on PST. International Meeting of Periodontics and restorative Dentistry. Boston 1997.
17. KORNMAN, K.S.; CRANE, A.; WANG, H.Y.; DI GIOVANE, F.S.; NEWMAN, A. Interleukin-1 genotype as a severity factor in adult periodontal disease. *J Clin Periodontol.* 1997; 24(1): 72-7.
18. LANGER, B.; SULLIVAN, D.Y. Osseointegration: Its impact on the in-

terrelatioship of periodontics and restorative dentistry. Part 3. Peridontal prosthesis redefined. *Int J Perodontics Restorative Dent* 1989; 9: 241-261.

19. LANGER, B.; STEIN, S.D.; WAGENBERG, B. An evaluation of root resections. Aten year study. *J. Periodontol* 1981; 52: 719- 722.

20. LEKHOLM, U.; VAN STEENBERGHE, D.; HERMANN, I.; BOLENDER, C.; FOLMER, T.; GUNNE, J. et al. Osseointegrated implants in the treatment of partially edentulous jaws: A prospective 5-year multicenter study. *Int. J oral Maxillofac Implants* 1994; 9: 627-635.

21. LEWIS, S. Teratment planning: Teeth versus implants. *Int J Periodontics Restorative Dent,* 1996; 46: 367-377.

22. LINDHE, J. Treatment of furcation-involved teeth. *Textbook of Clinical Periodontology.* Copenhagen: Munksgaard, 1989; 512-532.

23. LINDHE, J. Pathogenesis of plaque associated periodontal disease.In: Textbook of Clinical Periodontology. Copenhagen: Munkgaard, 1989:153-190.

24. LINDHE, J. & NYMAN, S. The role of occlusion in periodontal disease and the biological rationale for splinting in the treatment of periodontitis. *Oral Sci. Rev.,* 10: 11- 43, 1977.

25. LINDHE, J.; WESTFELT, E.; NYMAN, S.; SOCRANSKY, S.S.; HEIJI, L.; BRATTHALL, G. Healing following surgical/nonsurgical treatment of periodontal disease. A clinical study. *J. Clin Periodontol* 1982; 9: 115-128.

26. MCFALL, W.T. Tooth loss in 100 treated patients with periodontal disease. Along –term study. *J Periodontol* 1982; 53: 539-549.

27. NAERT, I.; KOUTSIKAKIS, G.; DUYCK, J.; QUIRYNEN, M.; JACOBS, R.; VAN STEENBERGHE, D. Biologic outcome of single-implant restoration as tooth replacements: A long term follow-up study. *Clin Impl Dent and related research,* v.2, 4, 2000.

28. NYMAN, S.; LINDHE, J. A longitudinal study of combined periodontal and prosthetic treatment of patients with advanced periodontal disease. *J. Clin Periodontol* 1979; 4: 163-169.

29. NYMAN, S.R.; LANG, N.P. Tooth mobility and the biological rationale for splinting teeth. *Periodontol 2000* 1994; 4: 15-22.

30. PASSANEZI, E.; SANT' ANA, A.C.P.; REZENDE, M.L.R.; GREGHI, S.L.A.; JANSON, W.A. Occlusión traumatogênica em Periodoncia y Implantologia. In: PANTALÉON, D.S.; PASSANEZI, E. Odontologia clínica. Prática contemporânea. v.2. São Paulo: Artes Médicas, 2004, cap. 7, pp.205-50.

31. PASSANEZI, E.; SANT' ANA, A.C.P.; REZENDE, M.L.R.; GREGHI, S.L.A. Epidemiologia da Doença Periodontal In: PAIVA, J.S.; ALMEIDA, R.V. Periodontia Baseada em Evidência. São Paulo: Artes Médicas, 2005.

32. REINHOLDT, J.; BAY, I.; SVEJGAARD, A. Association between HLA - antigens and periodontal disease. *J. Dent. Res,* 56: 1261-3, 1977.

33. SHILLINGBURG, H.T.; HOBO, S.; WHITSETT, L.D.; JACOBI, T. & BRACKETT, S.E. *Fundamentals of Fixed Prosthodontics.* 3rd ed., Chicago: Quintessence, 1997, pp. 90-91.

34. SIMON, J.F. Retain or extract: The decision process. *Quintessence International,* 1999, v30; 12: 851-854.

35. SPEAR, F. When to restore, when to remove: the single debilitated tooth. Compendium/April 1999, 316-328.

36. TERASAKI, P.I. et al. Low HL-A2 frequency and periodontitis. *Tissue Antigens,* 5: 286-8, 1975.

37. VAN DYKE et al. Reactor paper: risk factors involving host defense mechanisms. *Risk Assessment in Dentistry:* 105-108, 1989.

38. WANG, H.L.; BURGETT, F.G.; SHYR, Y.; RAMFJORD, S. The influence of molar furcation involvement and mobility on future clinical periodontal attachment loss. *J Periodontol* 1994; 65: 25-29.

39. WARREN, J.J.; HAND, J.S.; LEVY, S.M.; KIRCHNER, H.L. Factors related to decisions to extract or retain at – risk teeth. *J Public Health Dent* 2000; 60(1): 39-42.

6

TREATMENT PLANNING AND PROCEDURES TO ADEQUATE IMPLANT POSITIONING TOWARD ESTHETICS AND FUNCTION

Luis Guillermo Peredo-Paz

Marcos dos Reis Pereira Janson

Introduction

Nowadays, osseointegration can rehabilitate single, partial and completely edentulous patients. In addition to adequate comfort and function, esthetics is a fundamental factor on treatment planning. In totally edentulous patients, the residual alveolar ridge atrophy poses a major problem to adequate implant positioning. Thus, surgical reconstructive procedures are recommended. On the other hand, when implants rehabilitate partial segments or a single tooth, a "tooth-implant contiguous interface" will be created. To adequately positioning those implants and still maintains in-tact the gingival architecture for functional and esthetic reasons, some parameters have to be considered:

❏ **Residual alveolar ridge height on edentulous area**: bone height and the gingival level will influence the length of final clinical crown. It is well known that corono-apical implant positioning must be 3mm below the cementoenamel junction of adjacent teeth to provide a more adequate emergency profile and natural crown contour.[54] Also, it is very important to avoid thread exposition above bone level because there is a great risk for contamination and implant failure.[2] Thus, without adequate bone level, the implant will be more apically positioned, increasing crown length and compromising final esthetic results.

❑ **Adequate bone width**: an inadequate bone height and width can contra-indicate implant rehabilitation because there is no sufficient buccolingual bone to stabilize the implant. In some cases, the lack of labial cortical plate will drive implants to a more palatally position. This will create an overcontoured crown in an attempt to produce alignment with adjacent teeth. Also, dental hygiene and esthetic deficiencies will result.

❑ **Adequate room for prosthesis fabrication:** the prosthetic crown must have compatible shape, contour, color and soft tissue relationships. Thus, adequate balance between crown and adjacent teeth must be achieved.[3] This is the first question to be answered during treatment planning to guide the next procedures.

❑ **Apical room between adjacent roots:** the adjacent root tips must provide at least 1mm between root and implant to avoid perforation. At this moment, it is important to establish implant diameter,

although this choice must take into account the following parameter.

❑ **Enough room for implant platform and adjacent roots at osseous crest level:** the distance between bone crest and the proximal contact point determines the presence or absence of interdental papilla.[61] Bone around osseointegrated implants suffers mild vertical and horizontal resorption at abutment connection. Thus, a continuity is established between implant surface and oral environment.[60] As the papilla at tooth-implant interface is supported by adjacent osseous crest, the horizontal distance between implant platform and adjacent root will determine its presence or absence. This is a very important factor depending on the cervical tooth width to be restored.

According to the five cited factors above, the first two presents with surgical and/or orthodontic approaches, while the last three are directly related to orthodontic movement. In this chapter, we will explore the importance of these factors, how they change in the absence of teeth, and the therapeutic approaches indicated to restore function and esthetics.

Determining factors for esthetic planning

Influence of bone resorption patterns on the final implant positioning

All organ tissues underwent substantial changes during aging. The bone tissue is one with most metabolic transformations. Some of these will be highlighted here to comprehend the resorption patterns that govern the final shape of the jaws and thus, what the clinician needs to know before three-dimensional implant positioning.

The osseous tissue supports the human body and the skeletal muscles. Although facial esthetics is the product of measures and proportions, the soft tissue (skin, connective tissue, subcutaneous fat, and face musculature) lies on the maxillary structures. Its arrangement is primarily influenced by bone face volume and height, mimic and masticatory muscles tone, and gravity force.[16] On aging, the quantity and quality of collagen and elastin found on connective tissue diminishes, the skin gets more laxity, and the expression lines more apparent. These changes are more pronounced on totally edentulous individuals. Premature teeth extraction has a profound impact on the lower third of the face (distance from chin to nose), breaking smile esthetics.

Although bone sustains soft tissues and musculature, tooth arrangement in maxillary arches provides most of the labial support. Before understanding phenomena related to tooth extraction, it is important to have in mind that in the first stages of tooth development, the alveolus is just created after the formation of Hertwig epithelial root's sheath.[8,47] This means that alveolar bone cannot exist without teeth. Thus, in the absence of masticatory stimuli transmission and bone support for fiber insertion, the alveolus does not retain its configuration. Initially, the alveolus will be filled by blood clot. This blood clot will be removed in a few days and biochemistry signals sent to the formation of an immature, non-organized (woven) bone. After 90 days, a new mineralized bone matrix can be found on the post-extraction socket.

However, the entire process of bone resorption is not precisely known.[14] Thus, one cannot drive its pattern to reestablish the initial maxillary contours. Without adjacent dental support, the interproximal osseous crest becomes flat to mimic the labial aspect of residual bone.[11,60,63] The new architectural pattern leads to the resorption of strategic (esthetic) areas for implant positioning (Figs. 6-1 and 6-2).

In this way, the final success of dental prosthesis depends on treatment response provided by hard (bone) and soft (skin and musculature) tissues. Today, such treatment is defined by implant placement with or without graft adjunctive techniques, orthodontic movements and integrated clinical procedures.

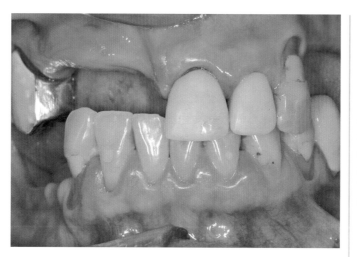

6-1

Fig. 6-1. Frontal view of premature tooth and extensive alveolar bone loss.

Fig. 6-2. The importance of tooth and lip support can be evidenced during smile esthetics. In the past, the only solution for this patient was a removable appliance.

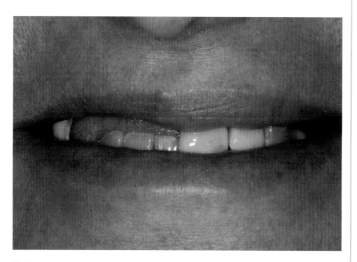

6-2

Fig. 6-3. Observe marginal tissue inflammation on tooth 22 and gingival discrepancy on tooth 24 (pontic).

Fig. 6-4. Extraction of tooth 22. Observe extreme bone loss on the region of tooth 24.

Fig. 6-5. Implant placement and guided bone regeneration with membrane barrier.

Fig. 6-6. Final aspect showing gingival tissues and prosthetic crowns. Observe excellent esthetics. Compare with figure 6-3.

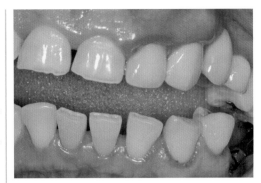

6-3

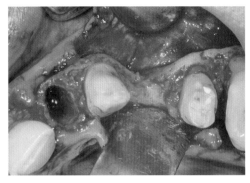

6-4

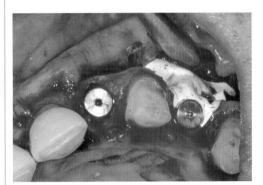

6-5

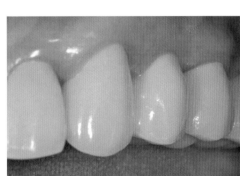

6-6

Fundamental aspects to achieve esthetic results on implant rehabilitation

A detailed clinical examination of the proposed area and the pre-surgical planning are fundamental aspects to achieve desired esthetic results. The following factors must be considered and studied thoroughly before implant placement:

❑ Osseous crest – height and volume.
❑ Soft tissue – quantity, quality and spatial position.
❑ Periodontal phenotype (biotype).
❑ Esthetics - smile line.
❑ Implant – size, form and position.
❑ Surgical procedure.
❑ Provisional restorations and emergence profile.
❑ Type of final restoration.

Osseous crest – height and volume

The residual ridge reduction is a continuous and slow process[5] varying from individual to individual,[2-4] accelerated by the wearing of total or removable prostheses without osseointegrated implants.[69] During the first year after tooth extraction, maxillary arch height reduces 2 to 3mm, being this of 4 to 5mm in the mandibular arch.[68] The reduction in the anterior residual ridge height in mandible is four times the rate of the loss in the maxilla.[14,58] In the maxilla, a centripetal or horizontal resorption occurs,[32,35] being the horizontal resorption rate twice of the vertical rate.[28] The vertical resorption of maxillary bone in the anterior region can occurs to the level of nasal spine. In some cases, fusion of internal and external cortical plates leads to an extremely thin alveolar ridge. In the posterior maxilla, vertical and horizontal atrophies occur almost at the same time. Bone can be resorbed to the level of maxillary sinus.[13] In addition; the decrease in density and number of osseous trabeculae is seen on aging. In the mandible, a centrifugal resorption occurs.[58] The resorp-

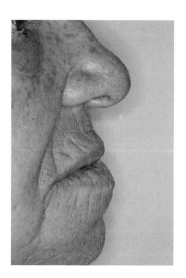

6-7

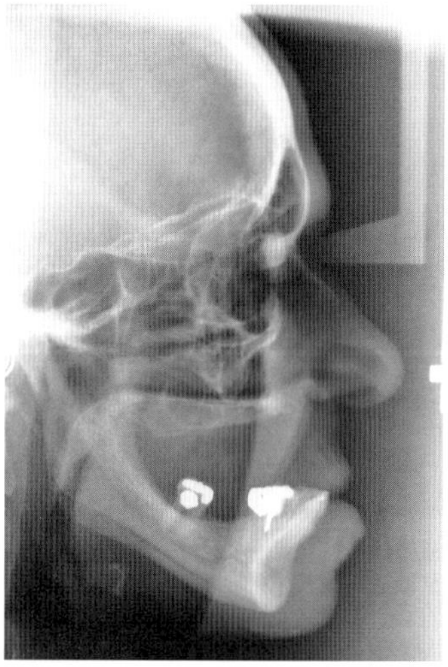

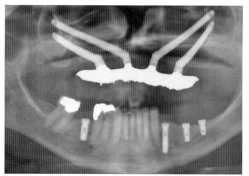

6-8

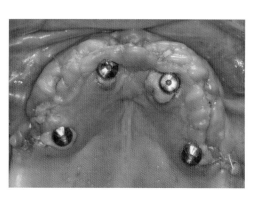

6-9

6-10

Fig. 6-7. Patient lateral view. Observe the loss of tissue support.

Fig. 6-8. Cephalometric view showing severely resorbed maxilla and mandibular protrusion.

Fig. 6-9. Installation of four zygomatic fixtures and a fixed prosthesis.

Fig. 6-10. Final radiographic aspect. Now, progressive bone changes can be minimized with the use of osseointegrated implants.

Fig. 6-11. Frontal view of the same patient showing the reestablishment of lip support. Observe patient's high lip line.

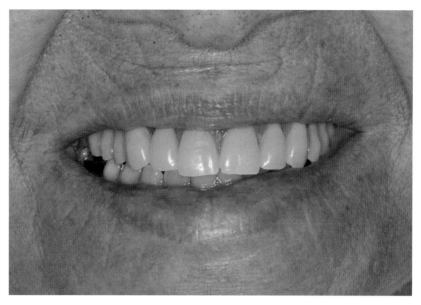

6-11

tion is more pronounced in the posterior mandible than the anterior mandibular region. Also, the resorption on the mandible occurs in the lingual premolar and bucal molar areas. Another important aspect is that due to the resorption pattern and to changes in the intermaxillary relationships, the maxilla will appears smaller than mandible over time[55] (Figs. 6-7 to 6-11).

Soft tissue – quantity, quality and spatial position

The soft tissue evaluation can detect the need for augmentation procedures. Periimplant mucosa is rich in collagen fibers that run parallel to the implant surface. The "biological width" around dental implants is comparable to that on dental apparatus.[20] The literature has still not established whether the presence of a keratinized mucosa is essential to implant placement.[57] However, the presence of a 3mm fibrous periimplant tissue leads to marginal stability, manipulation during surgical procedures, improves esthetics, favors the emergence profile, acts like a barrier against contamination and inflammation, facilitate impression making, and masks the prosthetic abutment connection (Figs. 6-12 to 6-20).[8]

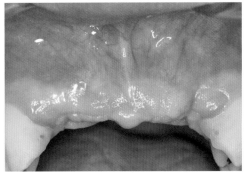
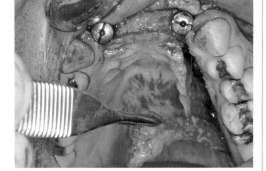

6-12

6-13

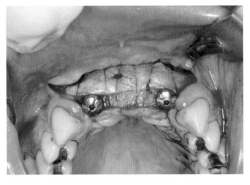
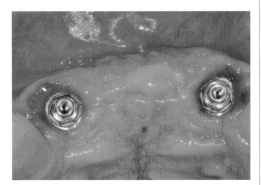

6-14

6-15

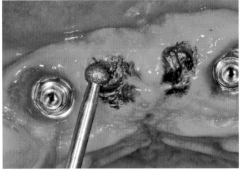
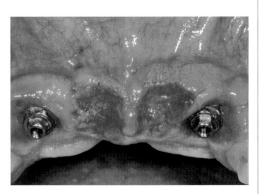

6-16

6-17

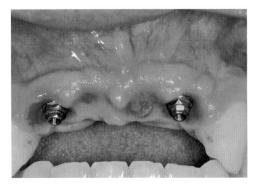
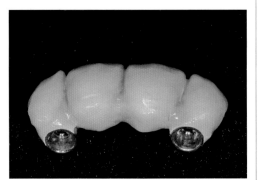

6-18

6-19

Fig. 6-12. Anterior alveolar ridge aspect before implant surgery.

Fig. 6-13. Subepithelial connective soft tissue graft removed from palate.

Fig. 6-14. Graft sutured in position.

Fig. 6-15. Observe tissue volume obtained after complete wound healing.

Fig. 6-16. Gingival conditioning with a round diamond bur.

Fig. 6-17. Pontic area delineated on soft tissue.

Fig. 6-18. Soft tissue contouring with provisional crowns.

Fig. 6-19. Intaglio surface of the definitive prosthesis. Observe adequate space for soft tissue papilla.

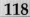

Fig. 6-20. Final aspect of implant-supported prosthesis. Observe the interaction between ceramic crowns, gingival tissue and implants.

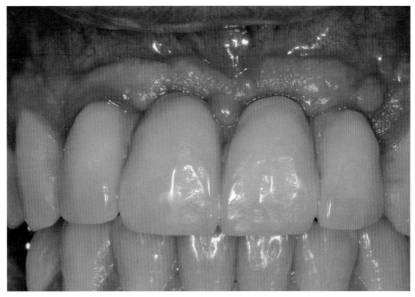

6-20

Periodontal phenotype (biotype)

Basically, there are two periodontal biotypes, thin-scalloped and thick-flat, accounting for 15% and 85% of the population, respectively. According to Kois,[38] the thicker the tissue, the more it can withstands trauma and recession; on the other hand, pocket formation and junction epithelium migration are facilitated. Thinner tissues are more prone to tearing and recession; thus, papillae are lost after surgical procedure.

The tooth shape determines the height and width of interproximal gingival tissues. Square teeth have a broader contact area and black triangles rarely occur. Tapered tooth forms show more incisal contact points. Thus, soft tissue that fulfills embrasure area is considerable. There is a great chance of black triangles after flap surgery. Usually, triangular teeth show more amplitude for interdental bone crest. However, the difference between labial contours and interdental bone crest drives the implant more apically.[60] In these cases, implant designs with anatomic platforms must be used.

Esthetics – smile line

The analysis of the height of the smile line is very important. A high lip line (exposing teeth cervical areas and significant gingival tissue) (Fig. 6-11) can be seen on 15% of cases. Patients with medium lip line (68.4% of cases) show two-thirds of clinical crown and gingival papilla (Fig. 6-29). The lowest percentage (20.48%) is attributed to patients with a low lip line, exposing one-third of clinical crown. Besides, the lip line can be classified in straight, curve or inverted. This factor determines whether the implant abutment–prosthetic cylinder interface will be exposed during smile,[27] the adequate crown length, and the relation of implant and gingival tissues.

Implant size, form, and position

SURGICAL GUIDE: INVALUABLE TOOL

Every "attempt" of three-dimensional implant positioning begins with a diagnostic wax-up and the fabrication of a surgical guide. Accurate implant placement is paramount to satisfy function, esthetics, phonetics, and oral hygiene procedures.[15]

The clinician must bear in mind that the three-dimensional positioning is always driven by the dental prosthesis, wax-up or surgical guide.[17,27,29,41,70] Implant surgery without previous prosthetic planning simply is nonsense. Thus, after the casts being related in a semi-adjustable articulator, the dental technician shapes the final contours of the desired prosthesis, transferring all necessary information to a clear acrylic guide. This template must be adapted to teeth and/or soft tissue. After, three aspects must be considered:

- The three-dimensional implant and prosthesis positioning (bucco-lingual, corono-apical, and mesiodistal);
- The need for bone/soft tissue augmentation to improve final esthetics;
- The patient expectations (prosthesis type, esthetics, function, cost-benefit ratio).

The clinician has a wide array of materials and techniques to construct surgical guides: they can be made from duplicated dental wax-up, existing total or removable prosthesis. For single-tooth implant restorations, acrylic rests on adjacent teeth are sufficient. Also, metallic balls, gutta-percha or several radiopaque products can be included in the final design. Recently, the use of computerized tomography and stereolithographic techniques have improved their quality.[12,67]

Francischone, Vasconcelos and Brånemark (2000)[35] denominated "reverse treatment planning" the preoperative technical procedures that aim to provide safety and predictability for correct implant position, especially in cases of great esthetic demand.

Fig. 6-21. Frontal view depicting vertical and horizontal bone loss. Observe thin alveolar bone crest, jeopardizing final implant position.

Fig. 6-22. Diagnostic wax-up to determine the soft tissue lost volume, crown length, and surgical guide configuration.

Fig. 6-23. Bone graft positioned for horizontal augmentation.

Fig. 6-24. Surgical guide during implant positioning.

Fig. 6-25. Observe harmonious interaction between dental implants and grafted/local bone.

Fig. 6-26. Second surgical stage; healing abutments installed and flap sutured.

Fig. 6-27. Try-in of metallic infra-structure.

Fig. 6-28. Final screwed prosthesis in position. Observe the volume and quality of gingival tissue obtained. This would not be possible without "reverse treatment planning".

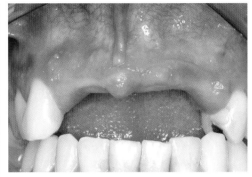
6-21

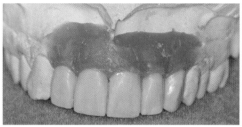
6-22

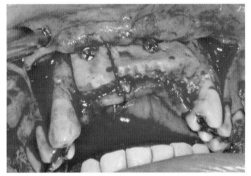
6-23

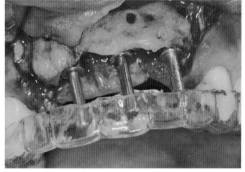
6-24

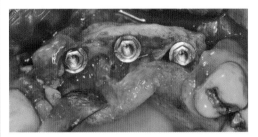
6-25

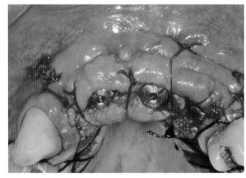
6-26

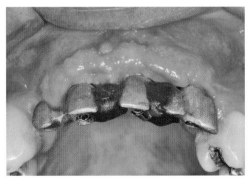
6-27

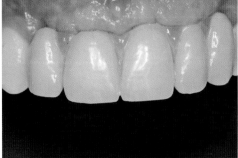
6-28

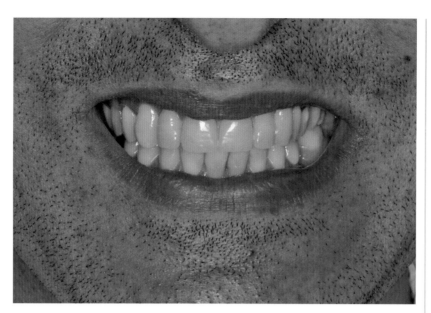

6-29

Fig. 6-29. The patient has a medium lip line. However, smile esthetics was achieved with great success.

IMPLANT DESIGN

The first implant launched in the market had a 3.75mm diameter cylindrical-threaded body. This design still is the most widely used. Today, most implant systems have a 3.75mm diameter body and 4.1mm diameter platform. With the success of partial and single-tooth implant restorations, new concepts were incorporated to the initial design and used in different clinical situations.[71] Implants with anatomical platform contours can be placed between adjacent teeth to preserve surrounding bone architecture. Thus, dental papilla can be maintained. Possible indications for tooth replacement are central incisors and premolars due to their round cross-sectional format.

The implant diameter is most related to root diameter at the emergence bone level, and not always with the cementoenamel junction. Available versions include implants ranging from 3.3 to 6.0mm diameter. A correct choice can improve the emergence profile and final esthetics.[53] Differences between tooth and implant diameter must be minimized with soft tissue conditioning by provisional restorations.[26,44,72]

CORONO-APICAL POSITIONING

In patients with adequate periodontal support, the implant must be positioned at level of the cementoenamel junction. The implant cervical level must be more apically positioned when adjacent teeth show differences on CEJ levels (teeth with reduced periodontal support).[6,19,59] Other options include implant placement 2 to 3mm above a line connecting zenith of adjacent teeth.[48] Wider-diameter implants requires less apical positioning for adequate emergence profile than standard-diameter implants (Fig. 6-30).

BUCCO-LINGUAL POSITIONING

First, clinicians must decide whether final reconstruction will be a screwed or cemented-type (Figs. 6-31 and 6-32). Implants for cemented restorations can have emergence profiles similar to natural teeth. For screwed prostheses on posterior regions, implants must follow the same orientation of cemented crowns. Also, in the anterior region, implants must be lingually positioned to avoid esthetic compromising of labial surfaces.

According to Potashnick,[51] for each millimeter toward palatal surface, the implant must be positioned 1mm more apical to maintain natural emergence profile.[49] Deviations from sagital axis orientation (10 degrees or more) can compromise final esthetic results.[19] On the one hand, too palatal implant positioning results in a soft tissue overcontoured margin. On the other hand, too labial placement leads to gingival recession and long clinical crowns.

For implants positioned between adjacent teeth, a rule of thumb consists of drawing an imaginary line across their cusp tips and place the fixture slightly to lingual direction. For the lower anterior region, implants must be inclined from labial to lingual avoiding natural mandibular bony concavities,[52] i.e., to follow jaw anatomy.

In relation to the posterior maxillary region, cemented or screw-retained restorations have shown favorable results. In the first case, implant must be placed in a buccal position, parallel to the alveolar bone ridge. In the second case, implants must be inserted in the central fossa region to provide screw access. Fixtures installed in the posterior mandibular region must be tipped toward the lingual as one progresses distally in the arch.[55] Thus, perforation or lingual fenestrations can be avoided.

MESIODISTAL POSITIONING

Incorrect mesiodistal positioning can prevents development of tooth-implant papilla, affects blood supply and leads to bone crest resorption and loss of mar-

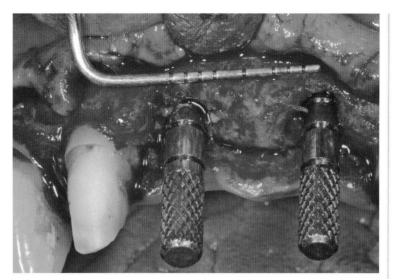

6-30

Fig. 6-30. Clinical case showing mesio-distal parameters: 2mm from tooth to implant and 3mm between adjacent implants.

Fig. 6-31. Occlusal view: parallelism and adequate space for papillae.

Fig. 6-32. Final positioning. Observe implant platform level.

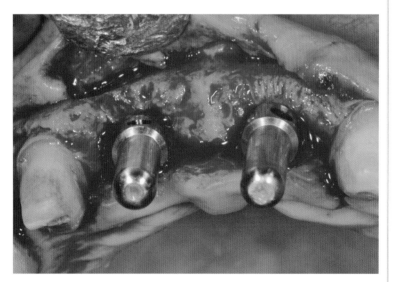

6-31

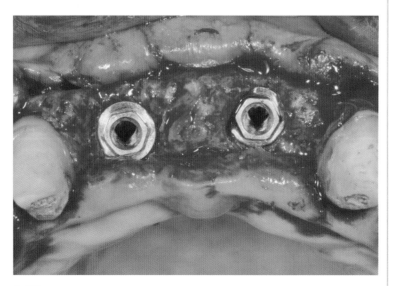

6-32

ginal soft tissue. After tooth extraction, papilla undergoes mesiodistal flattening and loss of labio-palatal architecture.[36] Clinicians have to bear in mind that, when the distance from tooth contact point to the interproximal bone crest is 5mm or less, papilla fills the space almost 100% of time.[43] The ideal horizontal distance between tooth and implant must be of 2mm. Similar, a minimum of 3mm is recommended between adjacent implants.[18] One study[59] has shown that the mean height of papillary tissue between two adjacent implants can reach up to 3.4mm with a range of 1 to 7mm (Fig. 6-33). Thus, judicious manipulation of soft tissues is recommended during surgery to avoid esthetic complications. When two adjacent teeth need to be replaced, interproximal bone crest levels can be maintained if implants were inserted one following the osseointegration of the other.[37] Besides, an alternative is to insert one implant and fabricate a cantilevered dental prosthesis. For totally edentulous patients, the minimum distance between the centers of two adjacent implants is 7mm. In cases where the anterior maxillary region is too resorbed, fewer implants must be inserted in the mesiodistal position.

In the posterior region, when the mesiodistal space for the first lower molar is 13 to 14mm, is possible to insert two implants with 3.75mm or 4.1mm diameter, following the same root angulation.[21] However, the available space is 11 to 12mm. In these cases, a wide-diameter platform implant can be used. It is interesting to center the implant in order to better distribute occlusal forces on dental prosthesis.[5] A seven-year follow up study on 60 unitary crowns joining two 3.75mm diameter implants showed high success rates, being the most important parameter the mesiodistal value (12mm) between two adjacent implants at bone crest level.[5]

THREE-UNIT FIXED IMPLANT PROSTHESIS

The same rules applicable to single-tooth restorations can be used. However, as the space required for dental prosthesis increases, the influence of anatomic and occlusal becomes more decisive.

Usually, a tripod configuration is recommended for a three-unit fixed prosthesis: the middle implant is buccal or lingually offset (Figs. 6-24 to 6-26), counteracting torque generated by lateral chewing forces.[45,64] One FEA study[52] showed that buccal or lingual displacement of 1mm not always decrease tension forces applied on prosthetic screws. However, implants placed in a straight line can lead to screw loosening and, in some cases, implant fracture.[66] When inadequate thickness is

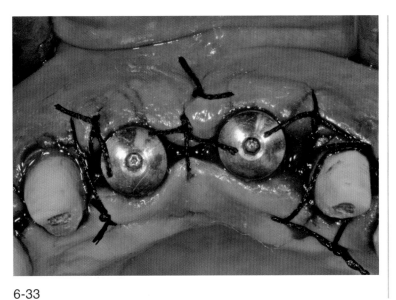

Fig. 6-33. Healing abutments and flap closure.

6-33

found on buccolingual direction, a slight inclination on implant platform is sufficient.

Timing of surgical procedures

There exist several types of clinical and protocol approaches in osseointegration surgery: immediate placement after tooth extraction, delayed-immediate, and delayed implant placement.

The use of immediate loading in any of these three alternatives depends on separate clinical situations and correct "reverse planning",[35] with restoration-generated site development.[28] The documented success rate of immediate loading is high; however; it must be carefully planned and executed in the esthetic zone. Any complications during pre, intra, and postoperative periods can cause irreversible damage to the esthetic appearance. Poor surgical design, osseous concavities found in the anterior maxilla, fenestrations, and the incorrect corono-apical implant positioning lead to undesirable esthetic effects (Figs. 6-34 to 6-49).[17]

Provisional restorations and emergence profile

The emergence profile is that portion of axial tooth contour extending from the base of the gingival sulcus past the free gengival margin into the oral environment. (Figs. 6-41 to 6-43; 6-48). The maintenance of an adequate emergence profile has immediate long-term effects. The final objective is to establish a biomimetic effect, avoiding re-

tentive contours that favor plaque accumulation and prevent oral hygiene procedures. The peri-implant soft tissue configuration depends on its volume and the three-dimensional implant positioning during surgery (Figs. 6-50 to 6-52).

Marginal tissue stability is fundamental to finalize restorative treatment. However, it can be a long task. According to Bennani and Baudoin,[8] 0.9mm of gingival recession can be observed until de third postoperative month.

From the cited above, one can comprehend that provisional restorations are paramount and must be present in all phases of gingival conditioning and soft tissue maintenance. This will help to visualize final esthetic results.[35]

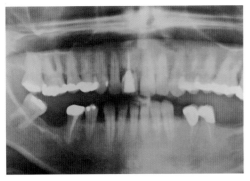

6-34

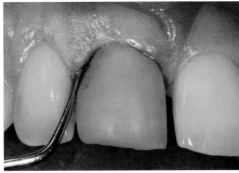

6-35

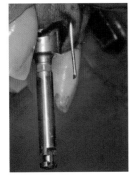

6-36

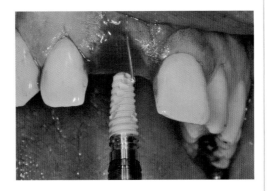

6-37

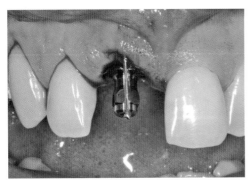

6-38

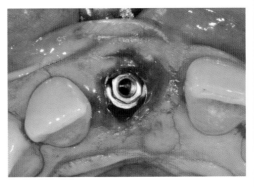

6-39

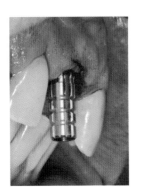

6-40

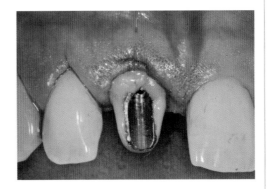

6-41

Fig. 6-34. Panoramic radiograph showing bone loss on tooth 11.

Fig. 6-35. Frontal view. Observe probing depth on mesial aspect of central incisor.

Fig. 6-36. Surgical preparation after tooth extraction.

Fig. 6-37. In this case, a conical implant design was chosen to avoid buccal fenestrations.

Fig. 6-38. Final corono-apical implant position related to the needle.

Fig. 6-39. occlusal view showing adequate implant placement.

Fig. 6-40. Temporary abutment for provisional restoration.

Fig. 6-41. Light-cure composite resin to obtain gingival emergence profile.

Fig. 6-42. Provisional screw-retained crown.

Fig. 6-43. Periapical radiograph. Observe that the implant design matches the alveolar socket configuration.

Fig. 6-44. Connective tissue graft removed.

Fig. 6-45. Connective tissue graft and provisional crown in position.

Fig. 6-46. Customized coping to capture emergence profile and transfer impression.

Fig. 6-47. Procera abutment in position.

Fig. 6-48. Procera crown luted with a resin-modified glass-ionomer cement.

Fig. 6-49. Final esthetic aspect. This patient has a medium lip line.

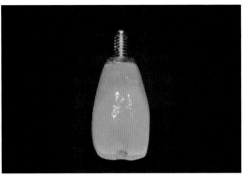

6-42

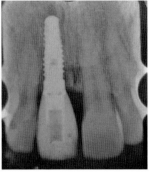

6-43

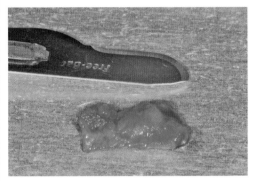

6-44

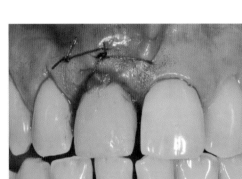

6-45

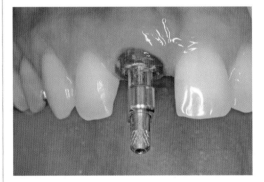

6-46

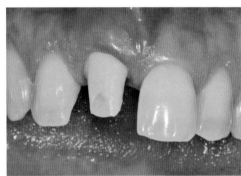

6-47

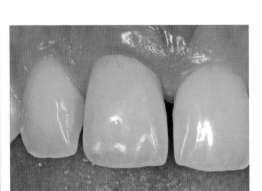

6-48

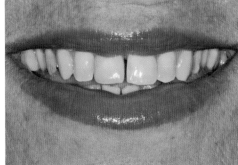

6-49

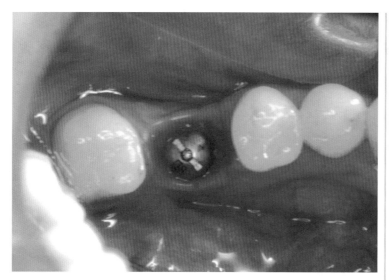

6-50

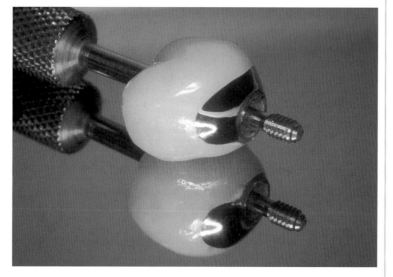

6-51

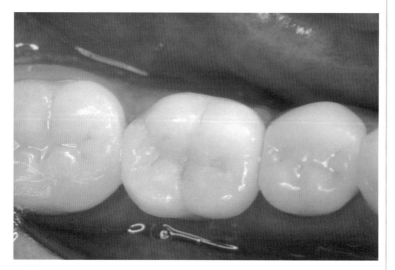

6-52

Fig. 6-50. Emergence profile obtained with acrylic resin build-up.

Fig. 6-51. Final restoration. Observe high polished surface to be in contact with gingival tissue.

Fig. 6-52. Final restoration in position. Screw access hole was restored with light-cure composite resin.

Type of final restoration

The type of the final restoration (screw or cemented) must be defined before surgical planning. Many authors state that retrievability is an important aspect, while some argue that definitive restorations must not be cemented over the top of the implant. With the introduction of STR (Single Tooth Restoration) and the CeraOne abutments, cemented prostheses have gained popularity on Dental Implantology. Nowadays, most single crowns are cemented because the screw access hole compromises tooth contact and esthetics. Besides, built-in customized abutments can correct implant inclination and provide more natural cervical contours (Figs. 6-47 and 6-48).[1]

The initial Brånemark protocol presented in 1977 has several advantages such as retrievability and the screw acting as a "security system" (Figs. 6-10, 6-11, 6-20 and 6-28). It means that screw loosening is indicative of occlusal overloading.[10] In situations of reduced occlusal space, the screwed type is considerably more predictable.

However, the choice of the restoration is related to multifactorial analysis and final decisions depend on important factors discussed between patient and clinician.

Orthodontic therapy previous to implant placement

Patients seeking treatment with osseointegrated implants show absence of one or more teeth. Usually, the edentulous space is not adequate due to adjacent tooth migration. This not only prevents correct contouring of ceramic crowns but also adequate implant placement. Orthodontic movements provide enough room for prosthetic crowns and help during alveolar ridge/soft tissue augmentation procedures, being less invasive and more predictable than surgical procedures. In addition, some of these patients have generalized malocclusion that can be treated according to patient desires. These possibilities must be taken into consideration during treatment planning and not after implant placement, because the chance to manage occlusal alterations is greatly reduced. One distinguished situation is the presence of fixtures in anterior upper region limiting the amount of horizontal trespass. Thus, effective communication between orthodontist and implantodontist is crucial to establish adequate chronological treatment sequence.

In order to create a positive symbiosis between these professionals, the five keys to implant positioning in orthodontics are discussed below.

Prosthetic room for dental restoration

In this scenario, two distinct situations can be visualized:

a) *the occlusal relationship is stable and there is no need for extensive orthodontic treatment to correct localized malocclusions:* in this case, the antero-posterior relationship between upper and lower teeth does not change. Minor alterations will be made to improve the edentulous space. However, it is necessary to know mesio-distal dimensions of teeth to be replaced. Homologous teeth on the opposite side of the arch are a good starting point. Also, the reader is encouraged to further reading[23,42] on dental proportions that adds interesting information. Regarding to the orthodontic movement, two types of movement can be done: mesialization or distalization with an open coil spring when there are spaces between adjacent teeth(Figs. 6-53A to C), or elongation of the arch by anterior tooth movement (Figs. 6-54A to M). This must be carefully assessed, because it will increase the

arch perimeter, with further implications to the anterior guidance.

b) *The patient has generalized malocclusion and need extensive orthodontic treatment:* in this case, the treatment planning involves the teeth dimensions and also the orthodontic criteria to resolve the malocclusion. The best way to give an accurate prognosis is through a diagnostic wax-up with the final tooth positions. This gives the orthodontist the perspective for planning tooth movements and also the anchorage. Two situations are possible:

b1) *implants are placed after orthodontic treatment:* when edentulous spaces are located in the anterior region, vertical occlusal dimension is stable and posterior teeth adequate for orthodontic anchorage (Figs. 6-55A to I);

b2) *some implants are installed in the beginning or during treatment to help orthodontic movements:* in this case, implants will serve as anchorage and help maintain the vertical dimension. However, it is necessary to have all final tooth positions in the diagnostic wax-up to avoid occlusal compromise (Figs. 6-56A to H).

Fig. 6-53

6-53A. This patient has compromised space to accommodate a fixed prosthesis. Observe the diastema between upper canine and first premolar.

6-53B. An open coil-spring provides space for two premolar teeth.

6-53C. The first premolar was mesialized and the first molar slightly distalized providing enough space for two premolars.

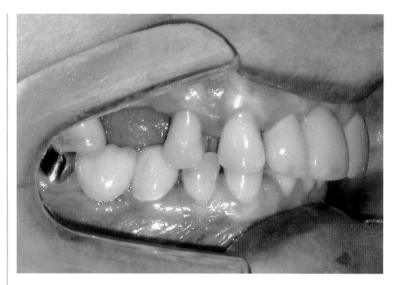

6-53A

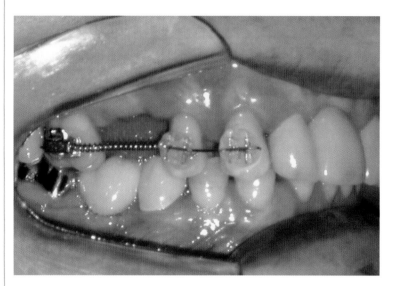

6-53B

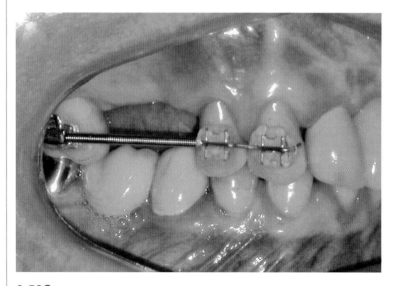

6-53C

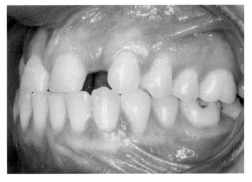

6-54A

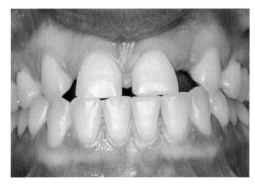

6-54B

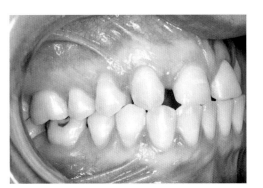

6-54C

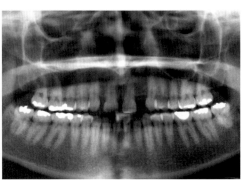

6-54D

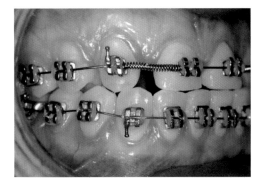

6-54E

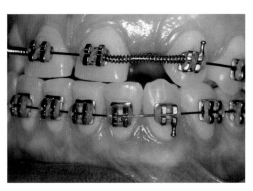

6-54F

Fig. 6-54

Fig. 6-54A, B and C. This 20-year old patient has an Angle Class I occlusion. Observe that the congenital absence of upper lateral incisors diminished the arch perimeter causing edge-to-edge anterior position.

6-54D. Panoramic radiograph showing lack of space for dental implants. The diastema between upper central incisors favors labial inclination.

6-54E, F. Initial orthodontics with open coil spring protruding the incisors.

6-54G, H. Final result of orthodontic treatment. Now it is possible to restore dental esthetics.

6-54I. Panoramic view showing the adequate spaces for the implants and aesthetics restorations.

6-54J, K and L. Frontal view showing good horizontal trespass of anterior teeth (J). Observe that Angle Class I occlusion was maintained (K, L) and a satisfactory esthetic result was obtained.

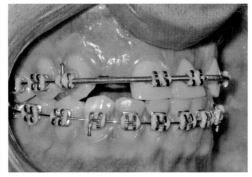

6-54G

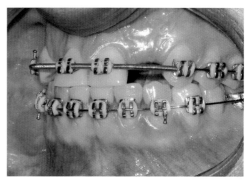

6-54H

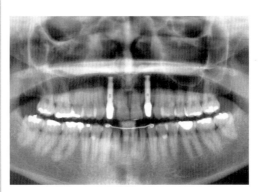

6-54I

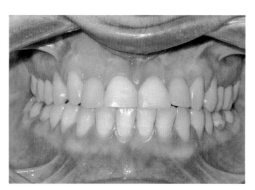

6-54J

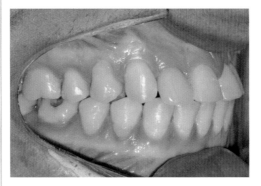

6-54K

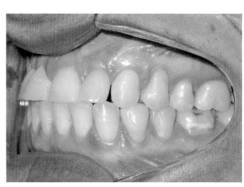

6-54L

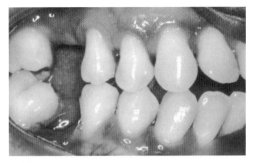

6-55A

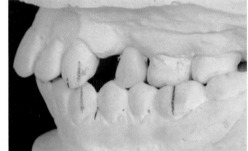

6-55B

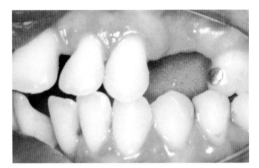

6-55C

6-55D

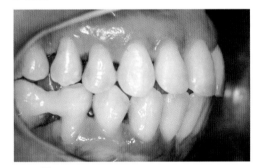

6-55E

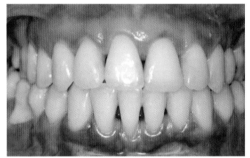

6-55F

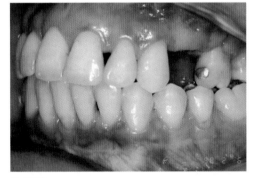

6-55G

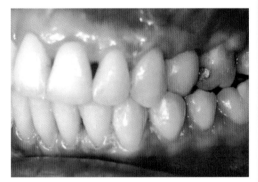

6-55H

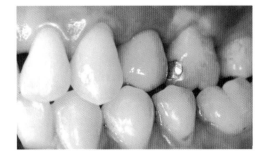

6-55I

Fig. 6-55

6-55A, B and C. This 36-year old patient has an Angle malloclusion class II, bone loss, diastemata between lower central incisors, and left posterior crossbite. Corrective orthodontic was done in both arches. Final outcome would be a canine Class I relationship, closing the upper right space and providing the proper space to restore the left space with a premolar implant. Thus, special concern on tooth anchorage was evident. In a Class I relationship, the upper first premolar must occlude between the lower first and second premolar. A diagnostic wax-up was necessary to visualize final tooth position (D), and maximal molar anchorage obtained. The final results are observed: a good canine Class I relationship was achieved, as well as adequate space for implant positioning (E, F and G). The implants were installed on the region of 24 (H). The crossbite was maintained due to its skeletal nature and because the patient refused to go through surgical expansion. Nevertheless, this inverted occlusal relationship is not harmful because upper canines provide guidance during lateral excursive mandibular movements.

Fig. 6-56

6-56A, B and C. This 44-year old patient has several lost teeth, canine Angle Class II relationship, and deep horizontal and vertical trespass. The deep overbite is the main obstacle to a satisfactory esthetic result. It is difficult to correct overbite through intrusion of anterior teeth, due to their great distance from posterior anchorage elements. Thus, it is necessary to insert some implants before orthodontic therapy in order to facilitate anchorage.

6-56D. A diagnostic wax-up was done to better evaluate orthodontic movements. In this case, the anterior reference was the upper canines positioning. Observe in the inferior arch that the canine will have an anterior movement to open space for the first premolar.

6-56E. One implant was placed in the region of 14 and a cantilever was created on the region of 13. After six months of osseointegration, the orthodontic treatment was initiated. The sinuous curve presented on the initial leveling wire supported by the implant anchorage helps to visualize the amount of vertical teeth movement necessary for this patient.

6-56F. After 18 months of treatment, there was adequate space in the region of 13 and 34 to place

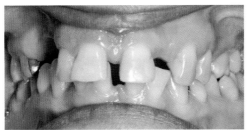

6-56A

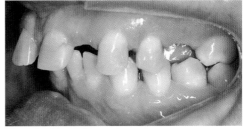

6-56B

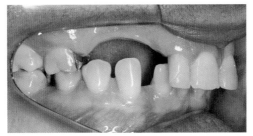

6-56C

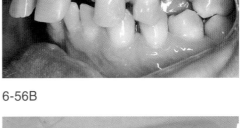

6-56D

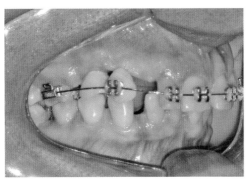

6-56E

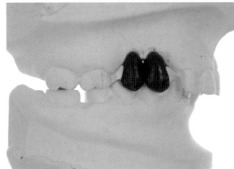

6-56F

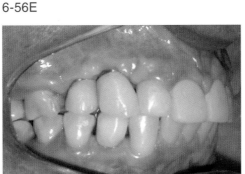

6-56G

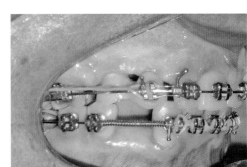

6-56H

dental implants. The upper and lower canines have a Class I relationship. Horizontal and vertical trespasses were correct.

6-56G and H. Lateral view at the end of orthodontic treatment with provisional restorations, showing good antero-posterior relationship. Final panoramic radiograph, where can be noted the adequate spaces for implants at right and left sides.

Apical space between adjacent roots

This section, the previous one and the next are intrinsically related, because when the root positioning must be included in the implant treatment planning. The space between the apical portion of the root is related to the implant diameter. The ideal situation occurs when there is 1mm between root and implant in both sides. Logically, dental ankylosis prevents tooth movement (Fig. 6-57C and D).

Root space at the level of osseous crest

This topic is related to the papilla preservation at the proximal level. According to Tarnow, Cho and Wallace,[5] after the implant-abutment connection, bone resorption around most coronal implant part ranges from 1.36mm to 1.40mm. In the vertical direction, values range from 1.5mm to 2.0mm.[31] This healing reaction occurs to establish a "biologic width". It is important to remember that the bone crest is responsible for maintenance of periimplant papilla. Thus, horizontal distance between implant and adjacent roots must be of 1.5mm. Theoretically, this will lead at least 0.2mm for the osseous crest. In this context, the implant platform diameter is crucial. Thus, not only adequate space is provided for coronal and apical dimensions, but also at the bone crest level. For example, upper central incisors and canines have mesio-distal dimensions from 8 to 10mm. When is necessary to replace a central incisor (8mm), one must subtract 1.5mm on each proximal area, leaving 5mm for implant platform. However, upper lateral incisors have a mesio-distal dimension of 5.5mm to 6.6mm.[39] In this situation, the implant platform must have a minimum of 3.0mm at most to preserve papilla, and this diameter is not so common. To resolve this situation the orthodontist is challenged with three possible alternatives: to increase mesio-distal space between adjacent roots, increase crown width (been aware that this also changes the anterior oclusal relationship) or reshape adjacent teeth without altering occlusion (Fig. 6-57A-G).

Height of alveolar ridge on the edentulous site

The alveolar bone, gingiva and restoration are the key elements of esthetic dentistry. Any deficiencies in these three parameters constitute the rationale for implant site conditioning. Some rules must be strictly follow to obtain good natural looking esthetics: the implant platform must be 1 to 3mm apical to the cementoenamel junction of adjacent teet,[1] and the implant threads have to be completely submerged.

For this, the proposed site must have enough bone and attached gingival tissue. In this scenario, the substitution of a periodontally compromised tooth for an implant is a difficult task, because several bone and gingival levels can be found. The number of remaining osseous walls is proportional to the severity of the defect.[50] In these situations, there is an irregular osseous topography with few or inexistent bone next to the crown contours. Several types of bone defects can be found as one reaches a more apical position during surgery: the fewer the walls the worse is the prognosis (Fig. 6-58B).

The orthodontic treatment in this situation is the forced tooth eruption. This procedure provides coronal bone growth through extrusion of dentogingival apparatus. Also, the band of keratinized gingiva is increased. However, it is necessary to have at least apical attachment representing one-third to one-fourth of root length and no inflammation signs.[1] This procedure have been denominated Orthodontically-guided Bone and Soft Tissue Regeneration (OGBSR)[34] (Fig. 6-58A-H). The alveolar bone height can also be modified with horizontal movements, described in the next section.

Appropriate thickness of the alveolar bone ridge

The alveolar bone ridge dictates indication for dental implants, its bucco-lingual position and the emergence profile.[7] Atrophied ridges will necessitate augmentation procedures. A good prognosis can be achieved with block or particulate bone grafts. Sometimes, orthodontic treatment can further prevent surgical invasive procedures. In this sense, two important aspects have to be mentioned: first, the teeth can be moved to atrophic areas without loss of stability. Some authors[33,56] have demonstrated in young adults the closure of spaces in the mandibular first molar area. During closure of spaces up to 10mm, the alveolar ridge follows the mesialization of the lower second molar. In adults there could be 2mm of bone loss at the crestal levels; however, these authors did not investigate alterations in the dentogingival insertion. According to Fontenelle,[22] teeth can be moved with or without bone. Nevertheless, direct resorption must occur during movement. On the other hand, indirect resorption is observed when the tooth is moved through the bone, without osseous apposition in the leading edge. This process can be seen when forces are exaggerated causing periodontal ligament hyalinization. The tooth movement can be done since adequate forces have been employed[46] (Figs. 6-59A to F).

The second aspect is the tissue response observed when teeth are moved to areas with less

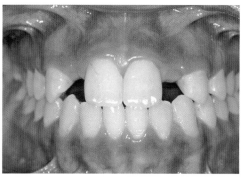

6-57A

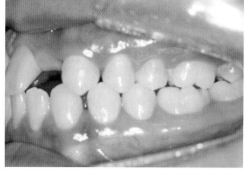

6-57B

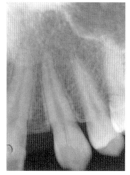

6-57C

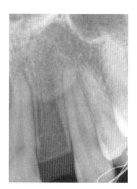

6-57D

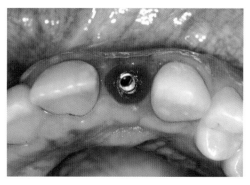

6-57E

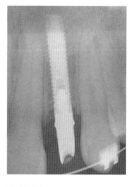

6-57F

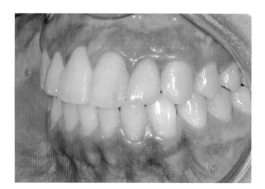

6-57G

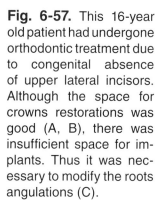

Fig. 6-57. This 16-year old patient had undergone orthodontic treatment due to congenital absence of upper lateral incisors. Although the space for crowns restorations was good (A, B), there was insufficient space for implants. Thus it was necessary to modify the roots angulations (C).

6-57D. Final space between adjacent roots after orthodontic treatment.

6-57E. Note adequate space for crown contours on the region of 22.

6-57F. Periapical radiograph showing that the implant does not interfere with bone crest levels.

6-57G. Excellent esthetics. Observe the harmony between crown contours and soft tissue levels.

Fig. 6-58. This 50-year old patient was presented with a great recession on left upper canine (A) and vertical bone loss (B). The tooth has a Grade II mobility.

6-58C. Forced eruption was planned to increase bone levels. The device was activated 1mm on each 15 day intervals, being sometimes this period superior to 30 days.

6-58D. Periapical radiograph showing the appliance bone level related to the adjacent teeth. The tooth was maintained in position for 4 months. Observe soft tissue quantity and quality on cervical canine area (Fig. 6-58C).

6-58E and F. The canine was substituted for an implant. Exposed implant threads on labial side were covered with autogenous bone graft harvested from the mesial aspect, which had height excess.

6-58G and H. Periapical radiograph showing adequate implant positioning. Excellent esthetics was achieved. This case demonstrates how to obtain adequate bone height through forced eruption of periodontally compromised teeth with less surgical invasive procedures.

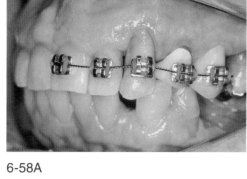

6-58A

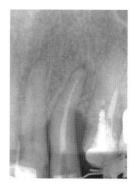

6-58B

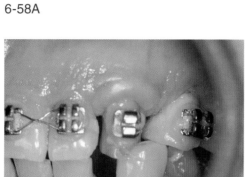

6-58C

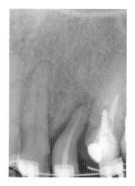

6-58D

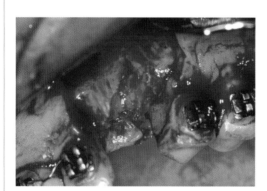

6-58E

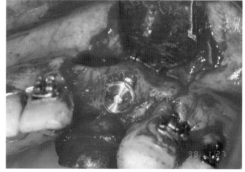

6-58F

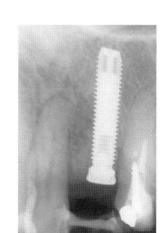

6-58G

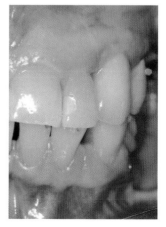

6-58H

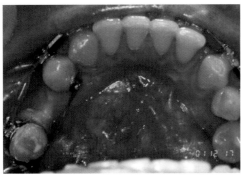

6-59A

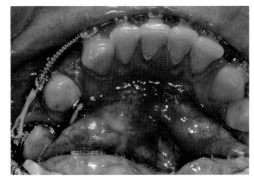

6-59B

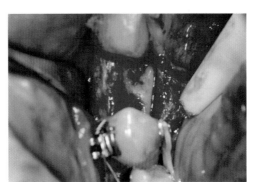

6-59C

6-59D

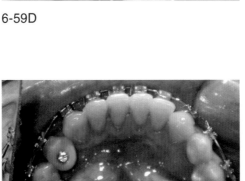

6-59E

6-59F

Fig. 6-59

6-59A. This case illustrates orthodontic movement through atrophic bone areas. Observe the compromised ridge on the distal of lower first premolar.

6-59B. At the same time that tooth is pushed to distal, mesial aspect shows adequate bone thickness.

6-59C. Final situation showing adequate space for implant placement.

6-59D. Observe bone thickness on the proposed site.

6-59E and F. Occlusal view of implant platform and (F) four months after osseointegration, serving as orthodontic anchorage.

bone height. According to the principles of tooth movement, two distinct phenomena can be created: tension and compression areas with osseous deposition and resorption, respectively. However, Thylander[62] and Geraci and cols.[16] demonstrated that, when there is a slow movement and the oral hygiene is adequate, no attachment loss is seen and bone levels remain intact. Based on the cited above, it is possible to obtain adequate height and bone thickness through orthodontic movements. The rationale is to move a tooth with good bone levels to the atrophic site. New adequate bone in height and thickness will be formed on the tension site; on the front side, bone crest narrowing is apparent, without attachment loss. Finally, the atrophied space will be occupied by the tooth, and the new bone site will receive a dental implant (Figs. 6-60A to H).

Conclusions

Osseointegration can provide comfort, esthetics and function. However, therapy in the esthetic zone requires greater attention. Clinical crown height, soft tissue topography, papillary formation, and emergence profile are related to hard/soft tissue levels. An accurate diagnosis along with surgical or orthodontic treatment provides good natural esthetics. Once osseointegrated, implants cannot be moved. This is extremely important considering patient expectations and the need for extensive occlusal correction. Good communication between different specialties is fundamental to achieve success in multidisciplinary treatment.

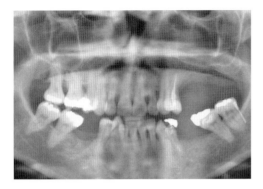

6-60A

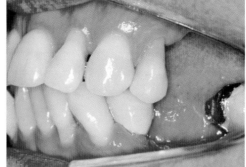

6-60B

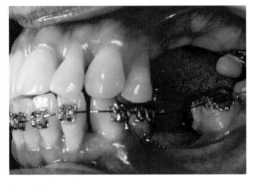

6-60C

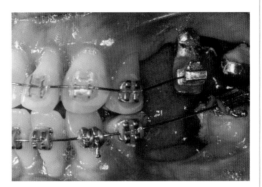

6-60D

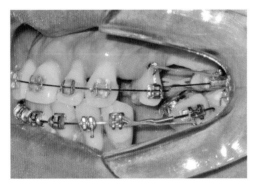

6-60E

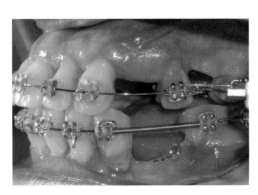

6-60F

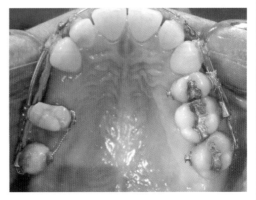

6-60G

Fig. 6-60. This 37-year old patient had a history of periodontal disease and loss of teeth 25 to 27. Implant placement on the upper posterior arch was impossible (A and B). A iliac crest bone graft surgery was suggested but the patient refused to. The orthodontic movement of tooth 24 was proposed to create bone on mesial and distal aspects. Besides, orthodontic treatment had already been conducted on the lower arch. The likelihood of premolar resorption was great.

6-60C. The maxillary tuberosity was chosen to anchorage two transitional implants and molar crown.

6-60D. A transpalatal metallic bar was connected between the right first molar and a provisional restoration made upon the 2 temporary implants. The bar had an extension in "Y" shape to put a fake tooth with a tube near the tooth that was going to be moved.

6-60E. When the premolar moved distally about 4mm, the transpalatal bar was removed, and the provisional crown served directly as an anchorage.

6-60F and G. The lateral and oclusal photos show the increase of bone and soft tissue in vertical and horizontal dimensions, provided by the tooth movement. Note also that the premolar was leveled with the posterior anchorage, providing good oclusal plane for restoration.

6-60H. Panoramic radiograph near the end of orthodontic movement. Note the improvement in vertical bone level. By this time it is feasible to put two implants plus a molar cantilever and completely restore the posterior upper occlusion on left side. The tooth that already had some bone loss, undergone great resorption, caused by the extensive movement and high compression at the root apex.

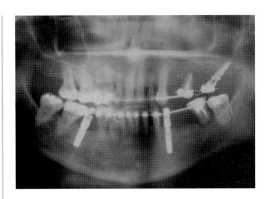

6-60H

References

1. AGAR, J.R.; CAMERON, M.A. Cement removal from restorations luted to titanium abutments with simulated subgingival margins. *J. Prosthet Dent,* 1997; 78:43-7.

2. ATWOOD, D.A. Bone loss of edentulous alveolar ridges. *J Periodontol* 1979; 50:11-21.

3. ATWOOD, D.A. Postextraction changes in the adult mandible as illustrated by microreadiographs of midsagittal sections and serial cephalometric roentgenograms. *J Prosthet Dent* 1963; 13:810-824.

4. ATWOOD, D.A. Reduction of residual ridges: A major oral disease entity. *J Prosthet Dent* 1971; 26:266-279.

5. BALSHI, T.J.; WOLFINGER, G.J. Two-implant-supported single molar replacement: interdental space requirements and comparison to alternative options. *Interior J Periodont Rest Dent* 1997; 17:427-435.

6. BELSER, U.; BUSER, D.; HESS, D.; SCHMIDT, B.; BERNARD, J.P.; LANG, N. Aesthetic implant restorations in partially edentulous patients – a critical appraisal. *J Periodontol 2000* 1998; 17:132-150.

7. BELSER, U.C.; BERNARD, J.P.; BUSER, D. Implant–Supported Restorations in the Anterior Region. *Pract. Periodont. Aesthet Dent.* 1996; 8:875-883.

8. BENNANI; BAUDOIN. *Estética e perfil de emergência na implantodontia.* Monique Revillion Dinato. Porto Alegre: Artmed, 2002.

9. BHASKAR, S.N. *Histologia e Embriologia Oral de Orban.* São Paulo: Artes Médicas, 10ª ed., 1989.

10. BINON, P.P. Implant and Components: Entering the New Millenium. *The Int. J. of Oral and Max. Implants,* v.15, n.1, 2000.

11. BRÅNEMARK, P-I; ZARB, G.A.; ALBREKTSON, T. Tissue Integrated Prostheses. *Osseointegration in Clinical Dentistry.* Quintessence Publ. Co., Chicago, 1985.

12. CARLSSON, G.E.; BERGMAN, B.; HEADGARD, B. Changes in the contour of the maxillary alveolar process under immediate dentures. A longitudinal clinical and x-ray

cephalometric study covering 5 years. *Acta Odontol Scand* 1967; 5:45-75.

13. CAWOOD, J.I.; HOWELL, R.A. A classification of the edentulous jaws. *Int J Oral Maxillofac Surg* 1988; 17:232-236.

14. DAVIES, J.E.; HOSSEINI, M.M. Histodynamics of Endosseous Wound Healing. In: DAVIES, J.E.; ed. *Bone Engineering* In squared incorporated, Toronto, Canadá, 2000.

15. DOUGLASS, J.B.; MEADER, L.; KA-PLAN, A.; ELLINGER, C.W. Cephalometric evaluation of the changes in patients wearing complete dentures. A 20-year study. *J Prosthet Dent* 1993; 69:270-275.

16. DUBRUL, E.L. *Sicher and Dubrul´s Oral Anatomy.* C.V. Mosby, 7th ed, 1980.

17. EL ASKARY, A.S. *Reconstructive Aesthetic Implant Surgery.* Blackwell Munksgaard, 2003.

18. EL ASKARY, A.S. *Cirurgia Estética Reconstrutiva na Implantodontia.* São Paulo: Ed. Santos, 2004.

19. ENOMOTO, H.; NOZAWA, K.; FURUKAWA, T.; TSURUMAKI, S.; TAKANO, M. *Achieving Tissue Esthetics and Cleansability of Implant-Supported Crowns in the Posterior Segments.* Quintessence Dental Technology 2002; 25:181-197.

20. ERICSSON, I.; LINDHE, J. Probing depth at implants and teeth. An experimental study in the dog. *J. Clin Periodontol* 1993; 20: 623-7.

21. FERNANDEZ, R.E.; BALSHI, T.J. One implant versus two implants, replacing a single molar: a three year comparative study. *Presented at the Annual Meeting of the Academy of Osseointegration.* Chicago, March 2-5, 1995.

22. FONTENELLE, A. Limitations in Adult Orthodontics. *In:* MELSEN, B. ed. *Current controversies in Orthodontics.* Chicago: Quintessence, 1991, p.147-179.

23. FRANCISCHONE, A.C., MONDEL-LI, J. The Science of beautiful smile.

Rev. Estética Dental Press Int., 2007; 4(2):97-106.

24. FRANCISCHONE, C.E.; VASCON-CELOS, L.N.; BRÅNEMARK, P-I. *Osseointegration and esthetics in sigle tooth reabilitation.* São Paulo: Quintessence, 2000.

25. FRANSCISCHONE, C.E.; VASCON-CELOS, L.W. *Free-metal restorations – Procera concept.* São Paulo: Quintessence, 2002.

26. GAILLUCCI, G.O.; BELSER, U.C.; BERNAND, J.; MAGNE, P. Modeling and characterization of the CEJ for optimization of esthetic implant design. *Int J Periodontics Restorative Dent* 2004; 24:19-29.

27. GARBER, D.A. The esthetic implant: letting restoration be the guide. *J Am Dent Assoc* 1995; 126:319-325.

28. GARBER, D.A.; BELSER, U.C. Restoration-driven implant placement with restoration-generated site development. *Comp Cont Dent Educ* 1995; 16:796-804.

29. GARG, A.K. *Prática da Implantodologia.* Editorial Premier Livros, 2001.

30. GERACI, T.F.; NEVINS, M.; CROS-SETTI, H.W.; DRIZEN, K.; RUBEN, M.P. Reattachment of the periodontium after tooth movement into an osseous defect in a monkey. *Int. J. of Periodontics Restorative Dent.* 1990; 10:185-197.

31. HERMAN, J.S.; COCHRAN, D.L.; NUMMIKOSKI, P.V.; BUSER, D. Crestal bone changes around titanium implants. A radiographic evaluation of unloaded non-submerged and submerged implants in the canine mandible. *J. Periodontol* 1997; 68:1117-1130.

32. HOBO, S.; ICHIDA, E.; GARCIA, L.T. *Osseointegração e Reabilitação Oclusal.* São Paulo: Quintessence, 1997.

33. HOM, B.; TURLEY, P. The effects of space closure of the mandibular first molar areas in adults. *Am. J. Orthod. Dentofac. Orthop.* 1984; 85:457-469.

34. JANSON, M.; PASSANEZZI, E.; JANSON, R.R.P.; PINZAN, A. Trata-

mento Interdisciplinar II – Alterações Verticais no Periodonto Induzidas Ortodonticamente. *Revista Dental Press de Ortod. Ortop. Facial* 2002; 7:85-105.

35. JOHNSON, K. A study of the dimensional changes occurring in the maxilla after tooth extraction: Part I: Normal healing. *Aust Dent J* 1963; 8:428-433.

36. KAN, J.Y.K.; RUNGCHARASSAENG, K. Interimplant papilla preservation in the esthetic zone: a report of six consecutive cases. *Int J Periodont Restorat Dent* 2003; 23:249-259.

37. KINSEL, R.P.; LAMB, R.E. Development of gingival aesthetics in the terminal dentition patient prior to dental implant placement using a full-arch transitional fixed prosthesis: a case report. *Int J Oral Maxillofac Implants* 2001; 16:583-89.

38. KOIS, J.C. Predictable single tooth peri-implant esthetics: Five diagnostic keys. *Compend Contin Educ Dent.* 2001; 22:199-206.

39. KOKICH, V. Anterior dental esthetics: An orthodontic perspective III. Mediolateral relationships. *J. Esthet. Dent.* 1993; 5:200-207.

40. LAZZARA, R.J. Managing the soft tissue margin: the key to implant aesthetics. *Pract Periodontics Aesthet Dent* 1993; 5:81-7.

41. LEKHOLM, U.; JEMT, T. Principles for single tooth replacement. In: ALBREKTSSON, T.; ZARB, G.A. *The Brånemark Osseointegrated Implant.* Chicago: Quintessence Publishing Co., 1989.

42. LOMBARDI, R. The principles of visual perception and their application to dental esthetics. *J. Prosth. Dent.* 1973; 23:358-382

43. LONDON, R.M. The esthetic effects of implant plataform selection. *Comp Cont Dental Educ* 2001; 22:675-682.

44. MANKOO, T. EVOLVING. *Implant Concepts in Complex Restorative Challenges.* Quintessence Dental Technology, v.25, p.198-212.

45. MCNEILL, C. *Science and Practice of Occlusion.* Chicago: Quintessence, 1997.

46. MELSEN, B.; Current. *Controversies in Orthodontics.* Chicago: Quintessence, 1991.

47. MJÖR, I.A.; FEJERSKOV, O. *Embriologia e Histologia Oral Humana.* Editorial Médica Panamericana, 1990.

48. PALLACI, P.; ERICSSON, I. *Esthetic Implant Dentistry. Soft and Hard Tissue Management.* Chicago:Quintessence Publishing Co., 2001.

49. PAREL, S.M.; SULIVAN, D.Y. *Esthetics and Osseointegration.* Dallas: Taylor Publishing, 1989.

50. PASSANEZZI, E.; JANSON, W.A.; NAHÁS, D.;CAMPOS JR., A. Newly Forming Bone Autografts to Treat Periodontal Infrabony Pockets: Cinical and Histological Events. *Int. J. of Period. Rest. Dent.,* 1989; 9:141-153.

51. POTASHNICK, S.R. Soft tissue modelling for the esthetic single-tooth implant restoration. *J Esthet Dent* 1998; 10:121-131.

52. RANGERT, B.R.; SULLIVAN, R.; JEMT, T.M. Load factor control for implants in the posterior partially edentulous segment. *Int J Oral Maxillofac Implants* 1997; 12:360-370.

53. RENOUARD, F.; RANGERT, B. Fatores de risco no tratamento com implantes. *Evolução Clínica e Conduta.* São Paulo: Quintessence, 2001.

54. SALAMA, H.; SALAMA, M.; KELLY, J. The Orthodontic-Periodontal connection in implants site development. *The Implant Report* 1996; vol. 8:923-932.

55. SPIEKERMAN, H.; DONATH, K.; HASSELL, T.; JOVANOVIC, S.; RICHTER. *Implantology.* Thieme Medical, 1995, p.220-224.

56. STEPOVICH, M.A. Clinical study of closing edentulous spaces in the mandible. *Angle Orthod.* 1979; 49:227-223.

57. STRUB, J.R.; GABERTHUEL, T.W.; GRUNDER, U. The role of attached

gingival in the health of periimplant tissue in dogs. 1 Clinical finding. *Int J Periodontics Restorative Dent.* 1991; 11:317-333.

58. TALLGREN, A. The continuing reduction of the residual alveolar ridges in complete denture wearers: a mixed-longitudinal study covering 25 years. *J Prosthet Dent* 1972; 27:120-132.

59. TARNOW, D.; NICOLAS, E.; FLETCHER, P.; FROUM, S.; MAGNER, A.; CHO, S.; SALAMA, M.; SALAMA, H.; GARBER, D.A. Vertical distance from the crest of bone to the height of interproximal papilla between adjacent implants. *J Periodontol* 2003; 74:1785-1788.

60. TARNOW, D.P.; CHO SC WALLACE, S.S. The effect of inter-implant distance on the height of inter-implant bone crest. *J Periodontol* 2000; 71:546-549.

61. TARNOW, D.P.; MAGNER, A.W.; FLETCHER, P. The effect of the distance from the contact point to the crest of bone on the presence or absence of the interproximal papilla. *J. Periodontol* 1992; 63:995-996.

62. THILANDER, B. Infrabony Pockets and Reduced Alveolar Bone Height in Relation to Orthodontic Therapy. *Seminars in Orthodontics* 1996; 2:55-61.

63. WEISGOLD, A.S.; ARNOUX, J.P.; LU, J. Single-tooth anterior implant: a world of caution. Part I, *J Esthet Dent* 1997; 9:225-233.

64. WEISGOLD, A.S.; ARNOUX, J.P.; LU, J. Single-tooth anterior implant: a world of caution. Part I, *J Esthet Dent* 1997; 9:225-234.

65. WHEELER, S.L.; VOGEL, R.E.; CASELLINI, R. Tissue preservation and maintenance of optimum esthetics: a clinical report. *Int J Oral Maxillofac Implants* 2000; 15:265-271.

66. WISE, M.D. Failure in the restored dentition. *Management and Treatment.* Chicago: Quintessence Publishing Co., 1995.

67. WORTHINGTON, P.; LANG, B.R.; RUBENSTEIN, J.E. Osseointegration in dentistry. *An overview.* Chicago: Quintessence Publishing, 2003.

68. ZARB, G.A.; BOLENDER, C.L.; CARLSSON, G.E. BOUCHER'S. *Prosthodontic Treatment for Edentulous Patients.* Mosby, 11th ed., 1997.

69. ZARB, G.A.; LEKHOLM, U.; ALBREKTSSON, T.; TENENBAUM, H. *Aging, Osteoporosis and Dental Implants.* Chicago: Quintessence Publishing, 2002.

70. ZINNER, I.D.; PANNO, F.V.; SMAIL, S.A.; LANDA, L.S. *Implant Dentistry: from Failure to Success.* Chicago: Quintessence Publishing, 2003.

71. ZITZMANN, N.U.; MARINELLO, C.P. Anterior single-tooth replacement: clinical examination and treatment planning. *Pract Periodont Aesthet Dent* 1999; 11:847-858.

72. ZUHR, O.; SCHENCK, G.; SCHOBERER, U.; WACHTEL, H.; BOLZ, W.; HÜRZELER, M.B. Maintenance of the Original Emergence Profile for Natural Esthetics with Implant-Supported Restorations. Quintessence Dental Technology 2002; 25:144-154.

7

THE USE OF INTRA-ORAL DONOR SITES ON ALVEOLAR OSSEOUS RECONSTRUCTION

Helcio Ganda Lira

Hugo Nary Filho

Mariza Akemi Matsumoto

Introduction

In recent years, implantology has received much attention due to its success on treatment of compromised patients. The increasing demand for implant therapy has lead clinicians to face issues never highlightened. In most cases, a multidisciplinary team has become paramount for esthetic and functional oral rehabilitation.

At the same time, several studies show excellent implant survival on tissues with sufficient bone quantity and quality.[1,4] Since this is a surgical prerequisite, biomechanical optimization of atrophic areas requires some type of osseous reconstruction.

The deficient alveolar ridge causes incorrect implant placement, poor soft tissue levels and finally, unsatisfactory esthetic results (Tarnow, 1992).

The literature has shown favorable outcomes for osseous reconstructions compared to non-grafted sites. Several possibilities are available, such as autologous, heterologous, and xenogenous bone grafts, as well as alloplastic implants, bone guided regeneration, and osseous distraction techniques. Amongst them, the autologous bone grafts have been widespread used in buccomaxillofacial and implant surgery. This modality is highly-recomended in the literature due to its predictable outcome (Tollman, 1995; Lekholm, 1999; Shliephake, 1997 and Fugazzoto, 1998).

The autologous bone, as a graft material, possesses three fundamental properties to new bone formation: conduction, induction and osteogenesis; in this way, it becomes a vital and functional tissue. However, these phenomena do not occur with the same intensity. Even with these drawbacks, bone substitutes do not present the same favorable results in larger areas,[3] being more adequate to fill osseous cavities or small defects.[14,20,46,49] In this sense, the generation of autologous bone segments is the success key for reconstructive procedures, and the literature has reported two techniques: onlay[47] and inlay/interpositional[28] bone grafts.

The main factor for materials choice and surgical approach is the defect morphology. The number of remaining walls for graft nourishment is a basic tenet in transplantation.

Concomitantly, intra-oral donor sites became a classic indication due to its less complexity, cost and morbidity. Major areas include mandibular symphysis, body and ramus. Also, bone can be harvested from maxillary tuberosities, zygomatic areas, maxillary/mandibular torus, and alveolar healing sockets as well. The developmental origin of autologous bone is another characteristic that favors biological success. Classical studies done in the 80's by Zins & Whitaker, de Kusiak, Zins & Whitaker observed that differences on graft volume, healing and vascularization were related to its embryonic development (endochondral or intramembranous type). Also, intramembranous type was favored in all aspects. Thus, several studies were conducted to elucidate this behavior[5,15,18,38] contributing to the concept that, instead of embryonic origin, bone architecture and corticomedular content govern adequate healing graft pattern. In this way, intra-oral donor sites have more favorable results than extra-oral areas. However, the surgeon has limited bone quantity that cannot be overestimated. Besides, larger alveolar segments than four teeth cannot be adequately rehabilitated.[36,48]

Another aspect important to surgical success is the interface between receptor site and bone block graft. The literature has shown several methods to prepare the receptor site with the aim to promote local revascularization and bone integration,[4,11,16,17] enhancing graft volume. However, attempts do reduce gap at this interface are equally important. The graft must be reshaped and molded to the recipient site. Additional procedures include the use of particulate bone or blood clot to fill the existing gaps.

In the last decade, a rich-platelet plasma gel (PPR) was developed to enhance bone repair and quality. Its action was due to the releasing of growth factors such as platelet-derived growth factor (PDGF), transforming growth factor beta (β-TGF) and insulin-like growth factor 1 (IGF-1).[29,43,50] Since then, PPR has been used alone or in combination with other materials to fill bone cavities or defects.[24,30,40,44,51] Miranda[31] (2005) showed the use of PPR in addition to block bone grafts in the rabbit calvaria. In the control group, graft and PPR were directly positioned over the receptor bed; in the first experimental group, graft was directly positioned over the receptor bed. In the second experimental group, particulate bone was used to fill the gaps. Regardless of previous treatment at the interface, bone repair and graft incorporation were seen after 60 days (Figs. 7-25A to C). However, a more exuberant granulation tissue was observed in the group treated with PPR (Figs. 7-26 A to C), suggesting the action of growth factors during the initial healing periods.

Preoperative evaluation

Case selection is performed through clinical, imaging and laboratorial analysis. Patient's medical history provides intra and postoperative risks. Clinical evaluation includes local examining of hard and soft tissue alterations. The morphology of donor and recipient site, as well as the topography of mandibular canal can be assessed in CT scans. Casts related in the semi-adjustable articulator are necessary to evaluate the amount of bone graft for implant placement and tooth positioning.

Mandibular symphysis

The mandibular symphysis region has the most adequate characteristics for reconstructive implantology. Easier access, absence of cutaneous incisions, less surgery time, and the possibility to perform it in an outpatient setting are offered advantages.[8,34,35] However, the only drawback associated is the bone quantity found in this region.

Besides, most patients are concerned with facial esthetics. Studies related to the morbidity of this area show that the removal of a block graft does not result in esthetic alterations to the soft tissue profile, even though complete recovery of bone contour is not achieved.[22,23] Complications such as pulp inflammation of lower anterior teeth can be avoided by preoperative radiographic and clinical evaluation. Accurate diagnosis of this area can be obtained with periapical, panoramic, and lateral cephalometric views. They will provide antero-posterior shymphiseal dimensions, as well as the available bone. Labial ptosis and numbness can also be prevented taking care during surgical procedures.

Anatomic characteristics

The triangular, curve-shaped anatomy of mandibular symphysis favors anterior alveolar ridge.[36,37] The mental foramina delimitate the extent of bone removal, comprising an area of 2 to 3cm.[9] Edentulous patients in this area can be treated unless alveolar bone resorption be accentuated.

Surgical Technique (Figs. 7-1 to 7-13)

Bilateral mental nerve blocks are preferred to manipulate hard and soft tissues in this region. Also, the flour or the mouth should be infiltrated to block lingual nerve. The labial mucosa in the canine region is incised through the periosteum. During tissue divulsion, is important to visualize mental foramina in order to protect them during bone removal. Osteotomies are performed with fissure burs at low-speed rotation or oscillating saws with abundant saline solution, which provide a fine and regular cut. Graft size is determined by the extent of osseous defect to be corrected. It is recommended to keep the superior osteotomy 5mm away from the root apices to avoid damage to the teeth.

Usually, osteotomy should be made up to the initial cancellous portion of the outer cortical plate. After, chisels are used to remove bone block. Sometimes the surgical hammer can be employed. However, care must be taken not to damage TMJ or dental structures. Thus, the block bone graft must be kept in a sodium lactate Ringer or saline solution until its placement in the recipient site.

The remaining bony lodge must be copiously irrigated to eliminate small fragments and osseous debris from surgical procedure. Also, bone spikes are reshaped.

The wound closure requires great attention to avoid labial ptosis and suture dehiscence. According to this, layered suture seems to be the ideal technique being the periosteum sutured first, followed by muscular and mucosal layers. Resorbable synthetic materials are recommended. Finally, to improve patient comfort and reduce postoperative swelling, compression dressing pad and adhesive tapes are used in the next days.

Fig. 7-1A and B. Frontal view of anterior teeth (A). The patient presents insufficient alveolar bone thickness in the edentulous site for implant placement (B).

Fig. 7-2. A full-thickness flap is performed. No releasing incisions are placed.

Fig. 7-3. Initial incision on labial mucosa exposing the donor site.

Fig. 7-4A and B. Divulsion is conducted through the periosteal layer.

Fig. 7-5. Incision placed at the periosteal base; muscle layer is dettached.

Fig. 7-6A. The mandibular symphysis is fully exposed.

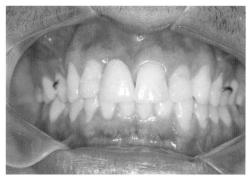

7-1A

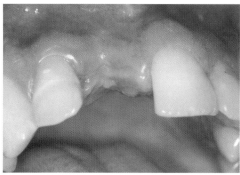

7-1B

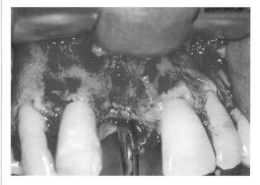

7-2

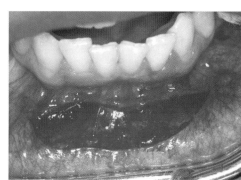

7-3

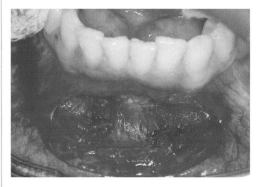

7-4A

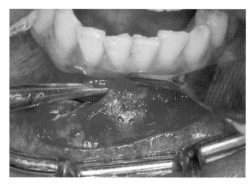

7-4B

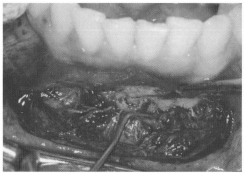

7-5

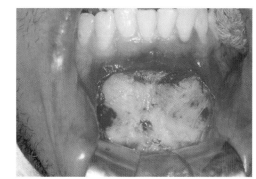

7-6A

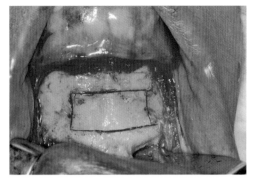

7-6B

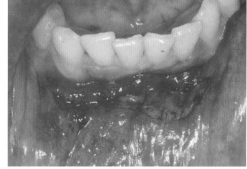

7-6C

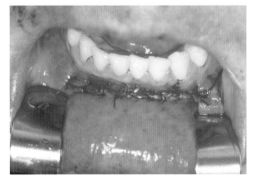

7-7

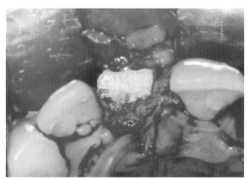

7-8A

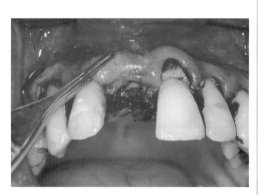

7-8B

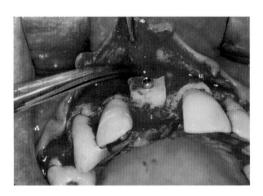

7-9A

7-9B

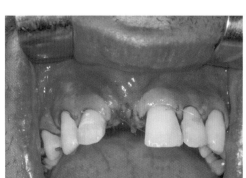

7-10

Fig. 7-6B and C. Vertical and horizontal osteotomies are performed with an oscillatory saw delimitating bone graft to be removed. Suturing of muscle layers (C).

Fig. 7-7. The mucosal layer is finally sutured.

Fig. 7-8A and B. Block graft adapted and fixated in the recipient site with a titanium micro-screw.

Fig. 7-9A and B. A free tension flap is not possible due to the bone graft volume. Submucosal dissection is mandatory (B).

Fig. 7-10. Flap is sutured over the graft.

Fig. 7-11. Clinical aspect of atrophic bone in the edentulous site (A). Observe alveolar ridge deficient in height and thickness (B), as confirmed after flap elevation (C).

Fig. 7-12. Mental nerve area exposed. Observe surgical osteotomies performed with an oscillatory saw (A); bone graft removed (B); The graft is contoured, adapted and fixed with the aid of a titanium micro-screw (C).

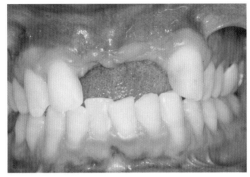

7-11A

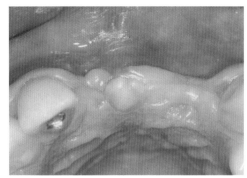

7-11B

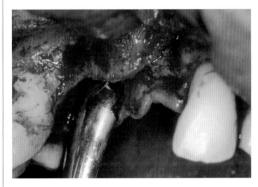

7-11C

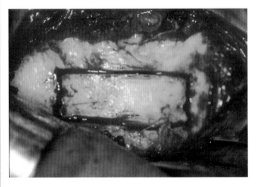

7-12A

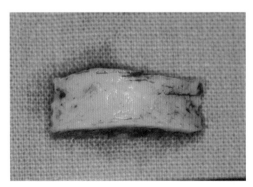

7-12B

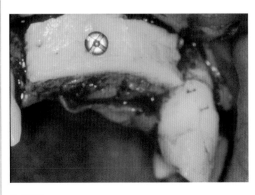

7-12C

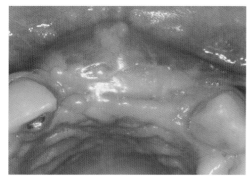

7-13A

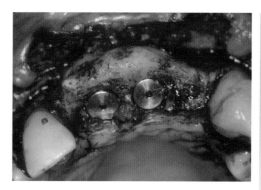

7-13B

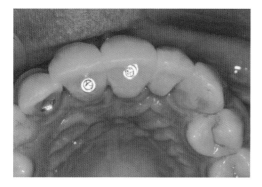

7-13C

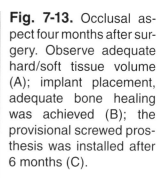

Fig. 7-13. Occlusal aspect four months after surgery. Observe adequate hard/soft tissue volume (A); implant placement, adequate bone healing was achieved (B); the provisional screwed prosthesis was installed after 6 months (C).

Mandibular body and ramus

The posterior mandibular region also offers adequate donor sites. Similar to the symphiseal area, bone grafts from mandibular body and ramus can maximize esthetic and functional results in localized osseous atrophy (Siebert Classification). They have been considered excellent options for treatment of jaws atrophy.[6,23,36,42] This graft is composed of cortical and cancellous bone with good integration to the recipient site. Misch (2000)[36] states that, in cases of posterior mandibular atrophy, it is possible to work in the same surgical area reducing the amount of anesthesics, time, and morbidity. Material removed from this site can be used either as onlay veneer grafts, bone fillings (maxillary sinus), or secured by titanium mesh and membrane barriers in cases of guided tissue regeneration. Crawford (2001)[13] cites the use of bone cores removed with a trephine bur. They can be triturated, compacted with membranes or fixed with screws.

According to Misch (2000)[36] the main indications for mandibular posterior grafts are:

❑ moderate to severe localized bone defects;
❑ edentulous areas corresponding up to four lost dental units;
❑ bone width augmentation in the posterior mandibular region; single edentulous site;
❑ indication for third molar removal along with graft necessity;
❑ combination with other donor sites for extensive reconstructions;
❑ craniofacial reconstructions

On the other hand, contra-indications include the following:

❑ total width of inferior ramus up to 10mm; superior path of mandibular canal; pathology related to the lower third molar; limited mouth opening;
❑ previous sagital ramus osteotomy;
❑ large alveolar defects.

Anatomic considerations

This area deserves special attention regarding the mandibular canal. In the retromolar region, bone height and thickness above the inferior alveolar nerve are 11.00±2.2mm and 14.2±1.9mm, respectively, in dentate individuals without the lower third molar[37] (Fig. 7-14). At least, 3mm of bone must remain above the inferior alveolar nerve in the retromolar harvested area. Also, invasion of lingual cortical plate in the ramus region can damage lingual nerve and associated blood vessels.

The clinical consequences of retromolar foramina were investigated by Sawyer and Kiely (1991)[41] and Pyle et al. (1999)[39]. Prevalence rates were similar and equal to 7.8%. Also, differences on gender, race, and inspected sites were not statistically significant. However, researchers believe that accessory nerves can be conduced through these foramina, which explain failures on inferior alveolar block anesthesia and suggests potential implications during retromolar surgery.

Retromolar region can be associated to pathological alterations as described by Izutsu et al.[21] and Courrier et al.[12] These authors observed sebaceous gland neoplasms in the minor salivary glands.

The surgical limits of the donor site are the coronoid process superiorly, the lower molars distally, the mandibular canal inferiorly, and the thickness of the mandibular ramus. Although the coronoid process can be regarded as a donor area by some authors (Wood, 1988) to fill sinusal cavities, small available bone and morbidity are frequent complications.

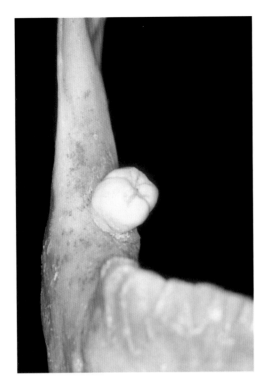

7-14A

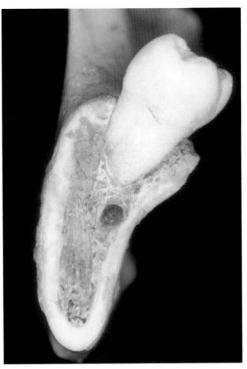

7-14B

Fig. 7-14. Dry skull frontal view of retromolar site (A); Cross-sectional view at the molar level showing root apex close to the mandibular canal (B).

Surgical technique (Figs. 7-15 to 7-24)

Sedation, exposure and recipient site preparation must be made before graft removal to evaluate bone quantity and morphology of the donor area. After mandibular regional block, anesthetic solution is infused below buccal periosteum to facilitate mucoperiosteal undermining. According to Capelli[10] (2003), incisions can be made in the following manner:

1. *Intrasulcular approach*: an incision is initiated mesially to the external oblique line at the height of the occlusal

plane avoiding lingual artery and the fat pad. After, the incision is extended anteriorly through the retromolar area, running laterally through the buccal molar fold distally to premolars. This approach can be used for non-compromised lower molars.

2. *Submarginal approach*: an incision is initiated as described above, but at the molar level, it runs submarginally on the buccal side below the attached gingiva to the height of the second premolar. This type is used with prosthetic crowns or cervical restorations on the molar vestibular area.

3. *Supracrestal approach*: for edentulous areas, the incision runs anteriorly along the alveolar ridge crest to the best area for surgical access.

Osteotomy is initiated at the base of coronoid apophysis, parallel to the external oblique line, at a distance of 4 to 6mm toward medial, extending anteriorly to the first molar area. Vertical osteotomies are placed perpendicularly anterior and posterior to height of 1cm. The inferior osteotomy is performed with part of the round bur just delineating the fracture line. Block displacement is done with a hammer and chisel or Smith forceps. The surgeon must be extremely careful because the neurovascular bundle can be adhered to the osseous block. After removal, bone block is kept in a saline so-

lution. Bleeding at the donor site is minimized with an appropriate hemostatic material. Sutures are placed according to the incision type. For the intrasulcular approach, an interrupted, single suture is done; submarginal and supracrestal techniques received a continuous and scalloped suture.

The bone graft must be contoured and adapted to the recipient bed. Lag titanium screws are used to secure the graft in position. Gaps between the outer cortical bed and the endosteal graft surface are filled with particulate bone. It is very important to round bone margins to avoid damaging the overlying soft tissue. A tension-free flap must be obtained through an incision at the base of the mucosa.

Postoperative healing period is considered satisfactory and oftentimes without complications. A prospective studied by Nkenke et al.[37] evaluated morbidity at retromolar donor site. Mouth opening values in the pre and postoperative periods were 40.8±5mm and 38.9±3.7mm, respectively, being not clinically significant. No damage occurred to the lingual and alveolar inferior nerves. After 1 postoperative week, no changes in neural sensitivity were detected. Discomfort rated by a VAS (Visual Analogue Scale) was significantly lower than that associated with implant placement. The authors concluded that the retromolar

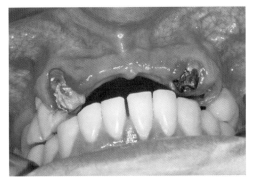

7-15A

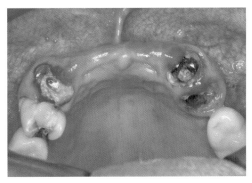

7-15B

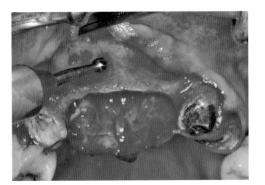

7-16A

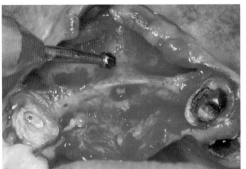

7-16B

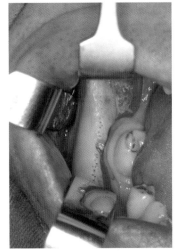

7-17

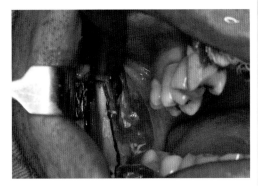

7-18A

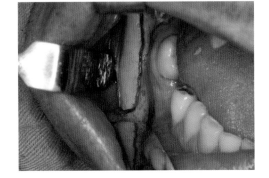

7-18B

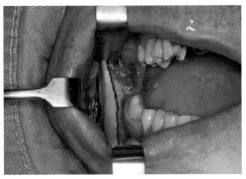

7-18C

Fig. 7-15A and B. Occlusal view of upper anterior region denoting the lack of adequate bone thickness.

Fig. 7-16A and B. Surgical exposure and debridement (A). Observe anterior maxillary atrophy. The incisive canal content (nasopalatine nerve and vessels) was removed.

Fig. 7-17. Surgical exposure of the donor site.

Fig. 7-18A, B and C. Ramus osteotomy. Anterior and posterior surgical limits have been defined.

Fig. 7-19. Donor site after graft removal (A). Observe the extent of the fragment removed (B and C).

Fig. 7-20. Closure of the donor site.

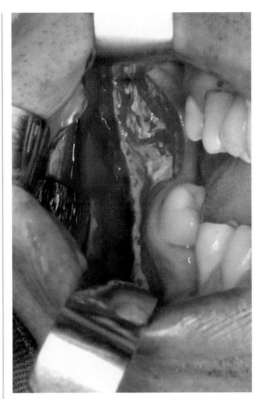

7-19A

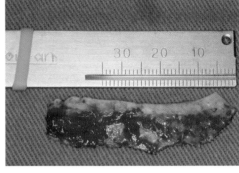

7-19B

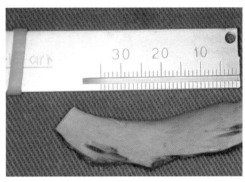

7-19C

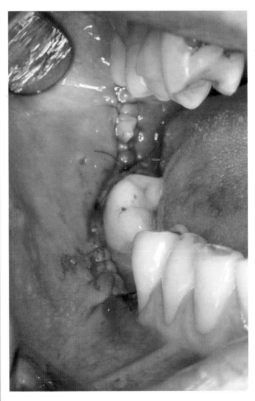

7-20

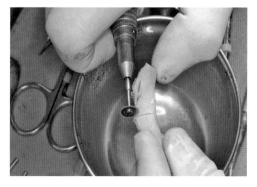

7-21A

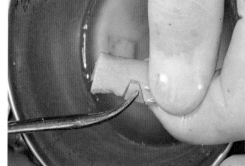

7-21B

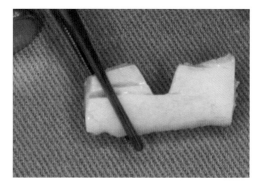

7-21C

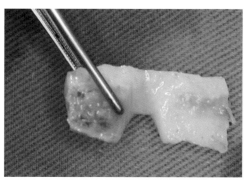

7-21D

Fig. 7-21A to D. A diamond saw at low-speed rotation is used to cut the graft (A). It must be contoured and well adapted to the recipient bed. The surgeon must handle the graft very carefully to avoid accidents (B). A V-shape configuration is made for the anterior nasal spine region (C and D).

Fig. 7-22A and B. A portion of the graft is triturated and packed between graft and alveolar ridge crest (A and B).

Fig. 7-23A and B. The block bone graft is adapted to the recipient site (A). Soft tissue flap must advanced to obtain tension-free suture (B).

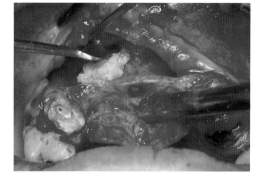

7-22A

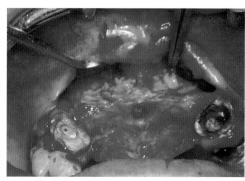

7-22B

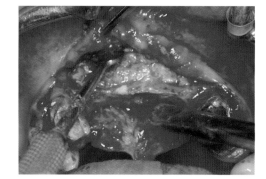

7-23A

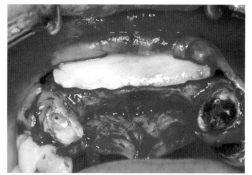

7-23B

Fig. 7-24. A titanium screw is used to secure the graft in position.

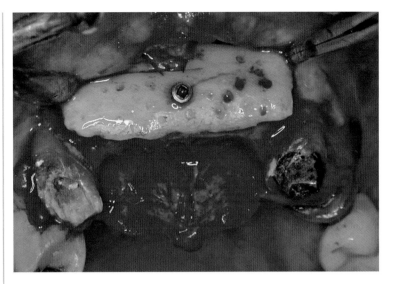

7-24

site offers a good option for bone graft with minimal discomfort and low risk of postoperative complications.

Perspectives in intra-oral grafts

The success of intra-oral bone grafts is confirmed by several clinical and research articles. The great issue is which donor area will attend the biologic, morphologic and dimensional requirements for the recipient site. Although intra-oral bone grafts have numerous advantages regarding its architecture, harvesting, morbidity, and cost-benefit ratio, each case has to be thoroughly evaluated to avoid serious complications.

Reshaping of the edentulous area poses a great challenge beyond esthetic and functional demands. However, it has to meet patient expectations. Failures such as graft rejection or poor dentogingival prosthesis may be due to surgical technique or incorrect indication. This problem has to be carefully discussed with our patients. Addressing therapeutic possibilities and the use of reverse planning certainly will improve their final prognosis. It is an strategy that involves all psychological, financial, esthetic and surgical aspects. Thus, good results in buccomaxillofacial procedures before implant placement can be managed exploring surgical limitations of each case. In this way, predictability of graft tech-

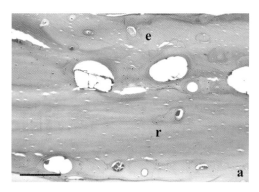

7-25A

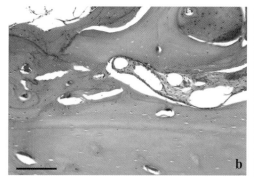

7-25B

Fig. 7-25. Histological section of the inferface between graft (e) and recipient bed (r) after 60 days, showing adequate bone healing in the control (A) and experimental groups particulate and PPR (B and C, respectively). (Hematoxilin-eosin stain. Bar=400µm.)

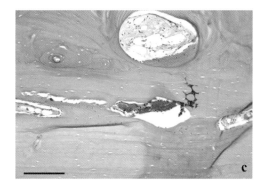

7-25C

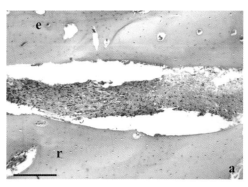

7-26A

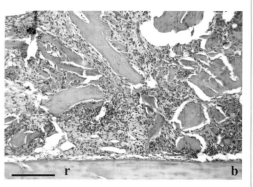

7-26B

Fig. 7-26. Histological section of the interface between graft (e) and recipient bed (r) 7 days postoperative. Observe a exuberant granulation tissue and osteogenesis (*) in the PPR group (C) compared to control (A) and particulate group (B). (Alcian Ponceau stain. Bar = 400µm.)

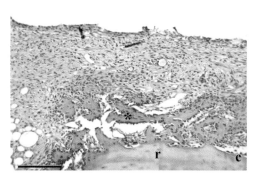

7-26C

References

1. ADELL, R.; ERIKSSON, B.; LEK-HOLM, U.; BRÅNEMARK, P-I; JEMT, T. A long-term follow-up study of osseointegrated implants in the treatment of totally edentulous jaws. *Int J Oral Maxillofac. Implants.* 1990; 5:347-359.

2. ADELL, R. et al. A 15- year study of osseintegrated implants in the treatment of the edentulous jaw. *International Journal of Oral Surgery 1981;* v. 10, p.387-416.

3. AL-RUHAIMI, K.A. Bone grafts substitutes: a comparative qualitative histologic review of current osteoconductive grafting materials. *International Journal of Oral and Maxillofacial Implants.* 2001; 16: 105-114.

4. ALBERIUS, P.; GORDH, M.; LINDBERG, L.; JOHNELL, O. Effect of cortical perforation of both graft and host bed on onlay incorporation to the rat skull. *European Journal of Oral Science,* 104:5-6, 1996.

5. ALONSO, N. et al. Cranial versus iliac onlay bones grafts in the facial skeleton: a macroscopic and histomorphometric study. *J. Craniofac. Surg.,* v.6, n.2, p.113-8, Mar. 1995.

6. BEDROSSIAN, E.; TAWFILIS, A.; ALIJANIAN, A. Veneer Grafting: a technique for augmentation of the resorbed alveolus prior to implant placement. A clinical report. *International J Oral Maxillofac. Implants* 2000; 15:853-858.

7. BEHNIA, H.; KHERADVAR, A.; SHAHROKHI, M. An anatomic study of the lingual nerve in the third molar region. *J.Oral Maxillofac. Surg.,* v.58, n.6, p.649-651, Jun. 2000.

8. BORSTLAP, W.A.; HEIDBUCHEL, K.L.W.M.; FREIHOFER, H.P.M.; KUIJPERS-JAGTMAN, A.M. Early secondary bone grafting of alveolar cleft defects. *J Craniomaxillofac Surg,* 18: 201-205, 1990.

9. BUHR, W.; COULON, J.P. Limits of the mandibular symphisis as a donor site for bone grafts in early secondary cleft palate osteoplasty. *Int J Oral Maxillofac Surg,* 25:389-393, 1996.

10. CAPELLI, M. Autogenous bone graft from the mandibular ramus: a technique for bone augmentation. *Int. J. Periodontics. Restorative. Dent.,* v.23, n.3, p.277-285, Jun. 2003a.

11. CARVALHO, P.S.P.; VASCONCELLOS, L.W.; PI, J. Influence of bed preparation on the incorporation of autogenous bone grafts: a study in dogs. *International Journal of Oral and Maxillofacial Implants,* 15: 565-570, 2000.

12. COURRIER, B.; PLANTIER, F.; KUFFER, R. Ulcerated mass of the retromolar area. *Oral Surg. Oral Med. Oral Pathol. Oral Radiol.Endod.,* v.93, n.6, p.635-639, Jun 2002a.

13. CRAWFORD, E.A. The use of ramus bone cores for maxillary sinus bone grafting: A surgical technique. *J Oral Implantology,* 27(2):82-88, 2001.

14. FUGAZZOTTO, P.A.; VLASSIS, J. Long-term success of sinus augmentation using various surgical approaches and grafting materials. *Int J Oral Maxillofac Implants,* v.13, n.1, 52-58, jan./fev., 1998.

15. GLOWACKI, J. Craniofacial onlay bone grafting: a prospective evaluation of graft morphology, orientation and embryologic origin/Discussion/. *Plast. Reconstr. Surg.,* v.85, n.1, p.15, Jan. 1990.

16. GOLDSTEIN, J.; MASE, C.; NEWMAN, M.H. Fixed membranous bone graft survival after recipient bed alteration. *Plastic and Reconstructive Surgery* 91:589-596, 1993.

17. GORDH, M.; ALBERIUS, P.; LINDBERG, L.; JOHNELL, O. Bone graft incorporation after cortical perforations of the host bed. *Otolaryngology Head and Neck Surgery,* 117:664-670, 1997.

18. HARDESTY, R.A.; MARSH, J.L. Craniofacial onlay bone grafting: a pro-

spective evaluation of graft morphology, orientation and embryonic origin. *Plast. reconstr. Surg.*, v.85, n.1, p.5-14, Jan. 1990.

19. HOLZLE, F.W.; WOLFF, K. D. Anatomic position of the lingual nerve in the mandibular third molar region with special consideration of an atrophied mandibular crest: an anatomical study. *Int. J. Oral Maxillofac. Surg.*, v.30, n.4, p.333-338, Aug. 2001.

20. HÜRZELER, M.B. et al. Reconstruction of the severely resorbed maxillar with dental implants in the augmented maxillary sinus: a 5-year clinical investigation. *Int J Oral Maxillofac Implants*, v.11, n.4, 467-475, jul./ ago., 1996.

21. IZUTSU, T.; KUMAMOTO, H.; KIMIZUKA, S.; OOYA, K. Sebaceous adenoma in the retromolar region: report of a case with a review of the English literature. *Int.J. Oral Maxillofac. Surg.*, v.32, n.4, p.423-426, Aug. 2003b.

22. JENSEN, J.; SINDET-PEDERSEN S. Autogenous mandibular bone grafts and osseointegrated implants for reconstruction of the severely atrophied maxilla: a preliminary report. *J Oral Maxillofacial Surg*, 49:1277-1287, 1991.

23. JOVANOVIC, S.A. Bone rehabilitation to achieve optimal aesthetics. *Pract Periodontics Aesthet Dent.* 1997; 1:41-51.

24. KASSOLLIS, J.D.; ROSEN, P.S.; REYNOLDS, M.A. Alveolar ridge and sinus augmentation utilizing platelet rich plasma in combination with freeze-dried bone allograft: Case series. *Journal of Periodontology*, 71:1654-1661, 2000.

25. KIESER, J.; KIESER, D.; HAUMAN, T. The course and distribution of the inferior alveolar nerve in the edentulous mandible. *J. Craniofac. Surg.*, v.16, n.1, p.7-9, Jan. 2005.

26. KIESSELBACH, J.E.; CHAMBERLAIN, J.G. Clinical and anatomic observations on the relationship of the lingual nerve to the mandibular third molar region. *J.Oral Maxillofac. Surg.*, v.42, n.9, p.565-567, Sept. 1984.

27. KUSIAK, J.F.; ZINS, J.E.; WHITAKER, L.A. The early revascularization of membranous bone. *Plast. Reconstr. Surg.*, v.76, n.4, p.510-16, Oct. 1985.

28. LUSTMANN, J.; LEWINSTEIN, I. Interpositional bone grafting technique to widen narrow maxillary ridge. *Int J Oral Maxillofacial Implants*, 10:568-XXX, 1995.

29. MARX, R.E.; CARLSON, E.R.; EICHSTAEDT, R.M.; SCHIMMELE, S.R.; STRAUSS, J.E.; GEORGEFF K.R. Platelet-rich plasma. Growth factor enhancement for bone grafts. *Oral Surgery Oral Medicine Oral Pathology Oral Radiology and Endodontics* 85:638-646. 1998..

30. MAZOR, Z.; PELEG, M.; GARG, A.K.; LUBOSHITZ, J. Platelet–rich plasma for bone graft enhancement in sinus floor augmentation with simultaneous implant placement: *Patient series study. Implant Dentistry* 13:65-72, 2004.

31. MIRANDA, S.R. Comparação histológica da região de interface de enxertos ósseos autógenos com ou sem PRP e osso triturado. Dissertação de mestrado em Odontologia – Área de concentração em Cirurgia e Traumatologia Bucomaxilofacial, Universidade do Sagrado Coração, 2005.

32. MISCH, C.M. Ridge augmentation using mandibular ramus bone grafts for the placement of dental implants: presentation of a technique. *Pract Period Aesthet Dent.* 1996; 8:127-135.

33. MISCH, C.M. Comparison of intraoral donor sites for onlay grafting prior to implant placement. *Int J Oral Maxillofacial Implants*, 12:767-776, 1997.

34. MISCH, C.M.; MISCH, C.E.; RESNIK, R.R.; ISMAIL, Y.H. Reconstruction of maxillary alveolar defects with mandibular symphisis grafts for dental implants: a preliminary procedural report. *Int J Oral Maxillofacial Implants*, 7:360-366, 1992.

35. MISCH, C.M.; MISCH, C.E. The repair of localized severe ridge defects for implant placement using mandibular bone grafts. *Implant Dentistry*, 4(4):261-267, 1995.

36. MISCH, C.M.; MISCH, C.E. Enxertos ósseos autógenos de áreas doadoras intra-orais em Implantologia. *In:* MISCH C.E. *Implantes Dentários Contemporâneos.* 1a ed., São Paulo: Ed. Santos, Cap. 31, p.497-508, 2000.

37. NKENKE, E.; RADESPIEL-TROGER, M.; WILTFANG, J.; SCHULTZE-MOSGAU, S.; WINKLER, G.; NEUKAM, F.W. Morbidity of harvesting of retromolar bone grafts: a prospective study. *Clin Oral Implants Res*, v.13, n.5, p.514-521, Oct. 2002b.

38. PINHOLT, E.M. et al. Revascularization of calvarial, mandibular, tibial and iliac bone grafts in rats. *Ann. Plast. Surg.*, v.33, n.2, p.193-7, Aug. 1994.

39. PYLE, M.A.; JASINEVICIUS, T.R.; LALUMANDIER, J.A.; KOHRS, K.J.; SAWYER, D.R. Prevalence and implications of accessory retromolar foramina in clinical dentistry. *Gen. Dent.*, v.47, n.5, p.500-503, Sept.1999.

40. ROSENBERG, E.S.; DENT, H.D.; TOROSIAN, J. Sinus grafting using platelet-rich plasma: Initial case presentation. *Practical Periodontics & Aesthetic Dentistry*, 12:843-850, 2000.

41. SAWYER, D.R.; KIELY, M.L. Retromolar foramen: a mandibular variant important to dentistry. *Ann. Dent.*, v.50, n.1, p.17-18, 1991.

42. SETHI, A.; KAUS, T. Ridge augmentation using mandibular block boné grafts: preliminary results of an ongoing prospective study. *International J Oral Maxillofacial Implants*, 2001; 16: 378-388.

43. TAYAPONGSAK, P.; O'BRIEN, D.A.; MONTEIRO, C.B.; ARCEO-DIAZ, L.Y. Autologous fibrin adhesive in mandibular reconstruction with particulate cancellous bone and marrow. *Journal of Oral and Maxillofacial Surgery*, 52:161-165, 1994.

44. THOR, A. Reconstruction of the anterior maxilla with platelet gel, autogenous bone, and titanium mesh: a case report. *Clinical Implant Dentistry Related Research*, 4:150-155, 2002.

45. TOLMAN, D.E. Reconstructive procedures with endosseous implants in grafted bone: a review of the literature. *Intern Journal of Oral and Maxillofacial Implants* 1995, 10(3): 275-294.

46. TONG, D.C. et al. A review of survival rates for implants placed in grafted maxillary sinuses using meta-analysis. *Int J Oral Maxillofac Implants*, v.13, n.2, mar./abr., 1998.

47. TRIPLETT, R.G.; SCHOW, S.R. Autologous bone grafts and endosseous implants: complementary techniques. *Journal of Oral Maxillofacial Surgery*, 54:487-494, 1996.

48. TRIPLETT, R.G.; SCHOW, S.R. Regeneração óssea com osso coletado da região mandibular anterior. *In:* NEVINS M.; MELLONIG J.T. *Implantoterapia: Abordagens clínicas e evidências de sucesso.* São Paulo: Quintessence, Cap. 15, p.209-218, 2003.

49. WHEELER, S.L. Sinus augmentation for dental implants: the use of alloplastic materials. *J Oral Maxillofac Surg*, v.55, n.11, p.1287-1293, nov., 1997.

50. WHITMAN, D.H.; BERRY, R.L.; GREEN, D.M. Platelet gel: an autologous alternative to fibrin glue with applications in oral and maxillofacial surgery. *Journal of Oral and Maxillofacial Surgery*, 55:1294-1299, 1997.

51. WILTFANG, J.; KLOSS, F.R.; KESSLER, P.; NKENKE, E.; SCHULTZE-MOSGAU, S.; ZIMMERMANN, R.; SCHLEGEL, K.A. Effects of platelet-rich plasma on bone healing in combination with autogenous bone and bone substitutes in critical- size defects. An animal experiment. *Clinical Oral Implants Research*, 15:187-193, 2004.

52. ZINS, J.E.; WHITAKER, L.A. Membranous versus endochondral bone: implications for craniofacial reconstruction. *Plast. Reconstr. Surg.*, v.72, n.6, p.778-85, Dec. 1983.

8

LOADING OR IMMEDIATE FUNCTION ON OSSEOINTEGRATED IMPLANTS

Carlos Eduardo Francischone Jr.

Ricardo Falcão Tuler

José Antonio de Siqueira Laurenti

Introduction

Osseointegration has changed several esthetic, phonetic, and functional concepts in dentistry. The first Bråmenark et al.[11] protocol stated that a non-loading functional period (first-stage surgery) was necessary to obtain adequate bone healing. After a six-month period, implants could be exposed and prosthetic rehabilitation initiated. Long-term clinical experience and research studies improved our knowledge on bone-implant interface. Since then, some authors have been shown their results on immediate loading.

For the immediate loading technique, micromovements greater than 20µm (primary stability) cannot be tolerated (Skalak, 2001). Good surgical technique, bone quality and rigid splinting of implants are mandatory.[7,8,11,19,31,33]

First, the immediate loading protocol was used to rehabilitate edentulous mandibular arches. Now, this concept may be used to rehabilitate the edentulous maxilla. Although it involves a more complicated anatomy, less dense bone, as well as esthetic and phonetic considerations, its clinical success has been demonstrated.[38] Besides, promising results on immediate loading of partial and single edentulous sites have generated a great excitement and opened new frontiers in research. However, theses cases are more complex because adequate soft tissue contours and functional integration have to be matched.

Nevertheless, available literature only presents short-term studies on immediate loading for single tooth restorations.[13-15,17,25] More research is need to develop predictable surgical and prosthetic treatment applicable to all cases.

Loading or immediate function on implants

Based on the bioengineering studies by Prof. Richard Skalak, P-I Brånemark began extensive research on immediate loading in 1980. It was verified that micromovements greater than 20μm would compromise the bone-implant interface. Also, due to the mandibular mechanical capacity to withstand loading, implants should be rigidly splinted soon after accurate installation. It is important to remember that before the osseointegration principles have been spread to the scientific community, Professor Brånemark had already conducted experiments on immediate loading. Only after a couple of years this matter was finally brought up.

The immediate loading concept has been better understood and can be considered a safe option to rehabilitate total or partially edentulous patients, as related by Henry, Rosenberg,[19] Salama et al.,[29] Balshi and Wolfinger,[7] Schnitman et al.,[32] Piatelli et al.,[26,27] Wood and Hajjar,[42] Chiapasco et al.,[12] Tarnow, Emtiaz and Claasi,[34] Randow et al.,[28] Horiuchi et al.,[20] Lima,[24] Tuler,[35] Andre,[3] Krekmanov,[23] Francischone Junior,[17] Cunha,[13] and Vasconcelos.[38]

Fracischone[16] highlights the importance of primary and secondary stability, as well the fundamental role of primary stability on immediate function. The primary stability is a key mechanical factor related to implant design, surgical technique, and bone density. On the other hand, secondary stability refers to biological aspects as surgical and implant tissue responses, as well as the wound healing process. According to the medical dictionary, load is static, while what is found in the mouth is dynamic. Thus, immediate function is a more adequate term than load.

Rehabilitation techniques in immediate function

Edentulous mandibles

An implant-supported fixed total prosthesis is advisable for completely edentulous arches.

Patients treated in this way report masticatory satisfaction, comfort, and esthetics. In other situations, an overdenture can be indicated. This will depends on anatomic limitations, maxilomandibular relationships, health conditions, socioeconomic factors, lack of motor skills, etc.

FIXED PROSTHESIS

The standard protocol for edentulous mandibles includes a fixed prosthesis supported by four to five implants. During treatment planning, it is important to verify the esthetic aspect of inferior dentures. Try-in of artificial teeth comprises the labial support, centric relation, vertical dimension, freeway space, facial proportions, and comfort. When all these are accepted, denture must be duplicated to create a multifunctional guide (Fig. 8-1). The stent provides adequate implant positioning in the patient's mouth. It registers vertical occlusal dimension transferring it to a semi-adjustable articulator, at the same time that the relationship between soft tissue contour and implant analog is captured.

The lingual portion of multifunctional guide must be removed (Fig. 8-2) for surgical access. Four to five implants can be placed in the anterior region. Actually, four implants provide the same success level of five to six implants in this treatment modality (Fig. 8-3).

First, an incision is made along the crest from the first molar region to the opposite site. After mucoperiosteal flap elevation (Fig.8-4) mental foramina are localized and the symphyseal region exposed. The distance between the most distal implant and the foramen must be 5mm. (Fig. 8-5). In some cases, flattening of alveolar crest is necessary before implant placement. However, one must not remove the dense portion of bone ridge, because it provides adequate thickness (5mm) to this region (Fig. 8-6).

Initial cortical perforation with a round bur no. 2 is followed by osseous site preparation (Adell et al.[1]). Sequential drilling under copious saline irrigation is used to enlarge the proposed implant bed. Buccal and lingual fenestrations must be avoided, as well as trauma to anatomical structures.

Now, fixtures are installed (Fig. 8-7). Decision regarding the use of a thread tapper is delegated to the surgeon according to bone quality and implant design.

Considering all immediate loading procedures made within 24 to 48 hours and laboratorial steps to fabricate definitive prosthesis, abutments must be tightened to 20Ncm torque providing adequate seating. The abutment height is selected according to the thickness of the surrounding mucosa (Fig. 8-8). Finally, flaps

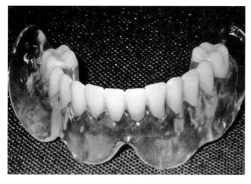

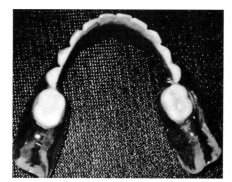

8-1

8-2

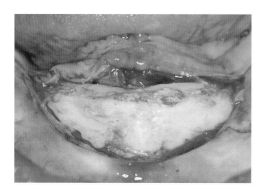

8-3

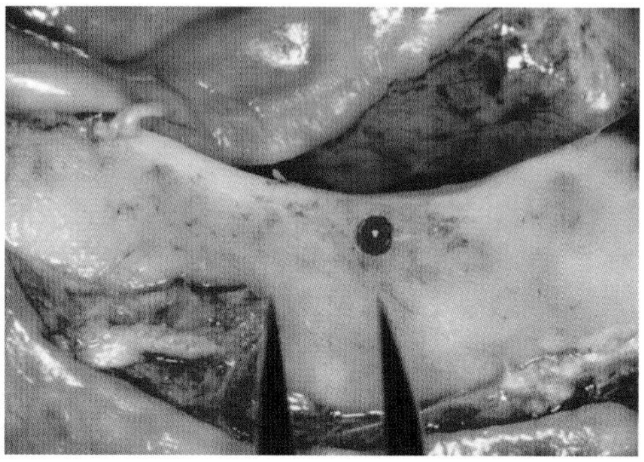

8-4

Fig. 8-1. The removable denture with artificial teeth is duplicated to fabricate a multifunctional guide.

Fig. 8-2. The lingual portion of the multifunctional guide is removed. Posterior portions serve as tissue stops for seating and stabilization.

Fig. 8-3. Mucoperiosteal flap elevation exposing bone tissue and mental foramina.

Fig. 8-4. Adequate distance from the mental foramen for implant placement.

Fig. 8-5. Installation of four implants between the mental foramina.

Fig. 8-6. Adequate bone thickness must be ≤5mm.

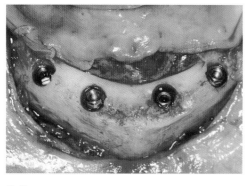

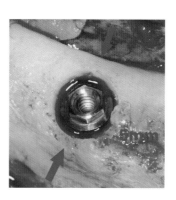

8-5

8-6

are closed with Vicryl 4-0 interrupted sutures (Poliglactin 910) (Fig. 8-9).

In the prosthetic phase, square impression copings receive autopolymerizing acrylic resin prefabricated bars and are connected to the abutments. Thus, impression copings are splinted together and to the multifunctional guide (Fig. 8-10). The stent serves as an impression tray, interocclusal record and still provides interplay between soft tissue and implants (Fig. 8-11).

Afterwards, all laboratorial steps (infra-structure wax-up, investment, casting, soldering, tooth arrangement, finishing and polishing) are executed and must follow strict criteria to obtain passive-fit structures (Fig. 8-12). Accurate seating of implant-supported prostheses is fundamental, being defined as maximum contact at the im-

Fig. 8-7. Implant installation with the transfer screws (A). Observe adequate implant positioning slightly below crestal level (B).

Fig. 8-8. Prosthetic abutments are tightened to 20Ncm torque (A). Final view of installed abutments.

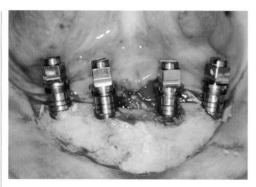

8-7A

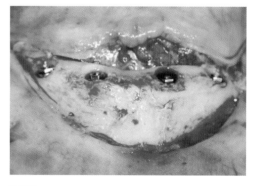

8-7B

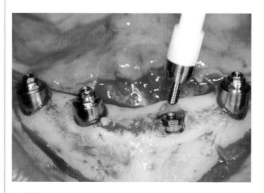

8-8A

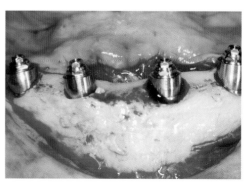

8-8B

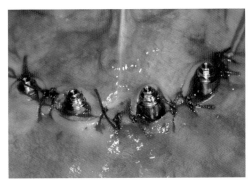

8-9

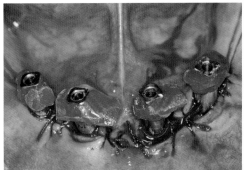

8-10A

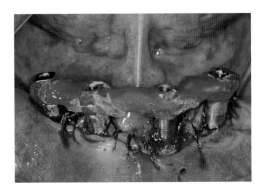

8-10B

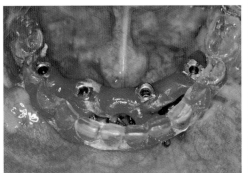

8-10C

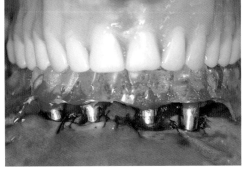

8-10D

Fig. 8-9. After flap closure, impression procedures are initiated.

Fig. 8-10. Square impression copings with prefabricated acrylic bars positioned over the abutments (A); the components are splinted together (B); and to the multifunctional guide (C). The maxillomandibular relationship is obtained (D).

plant-abutment interface, without abutment stress and screw overload. Many authors (Jemt,[21] Goll[18], Weinberg,[40] Sellers,[30,] Jimenez; Aparicio,[5]) in the literature have provided critical appraisal on passive fit and developed alternative techniques to overcome this problem.

Fig. 8-11. An impression is made with light-body silicone material injected around prosthetic abutments.

Fig. 8-12. Final screwed prosthesis in place.

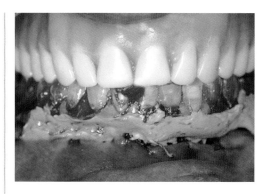

8-11

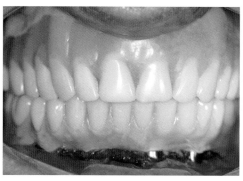

8-12

THE BRÅNEMARK NOVUM CONCEPT

This treatment philosophy was published in 1999 by Brånemark et al. The aim is to reduce time period between implant placement and prosthesis connection (same day teeth) through the use of rigid implant splinting during surgery. Prefabricated metallic components eliminate impression, casting and soldering steps. Surgical predrilled bars provide accurate implant positioning (Fig. 8-13A to C). After implant installation, flap is sutured, the silicon stent positioned and the mesobar screwed to the abutments. The silicon stent serves to mould soft tissue beneath the bar and around implants (Fig. 8-13D).

Surgical candidates must present interforaminal distance greater than surgical bar and bone width ≥ 6mm (Fig. 8-14) for complete seating. Thus, osseous flattening is performed at the alveolar crest using abundant irrigation. Otherwise, implants are placed according to anatomic limits. A prefabricated prosthetic bar is inserted over its surgical counterpart (Fig. 8-15). A centric registration record is obtained with a putty silicon impression material. After, prosthetic bar is mounted in a semi-adjustable articulator for tooth arrangement (Fig. 8-16). Teeth are tried in the mouth. Aspects such as vertical dimension, occlusal contacts, as well as tooth form, shade and position are checked. Laboratorial steps (processing, finishing, and polishing) are made and the final prosthesis delivered to the patient in the same day (Fig. 8-18).

It is important to point out that the Brånemark Novum presents success levels similar to conventional protocols. However, indications must be done on individual basis.

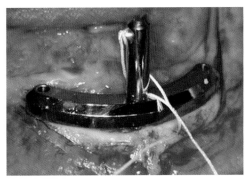

8-13A

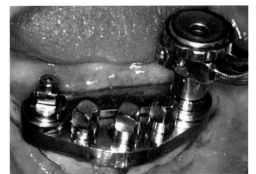

8-13B

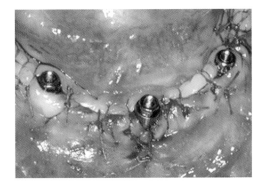

8-13C

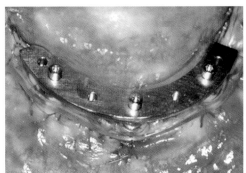

8-13D

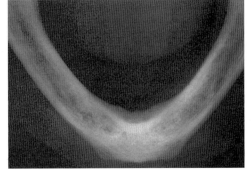

8-14

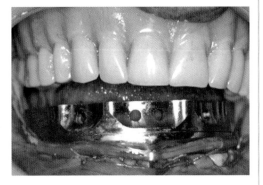

8-15

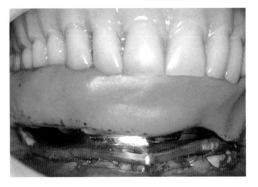

8-16

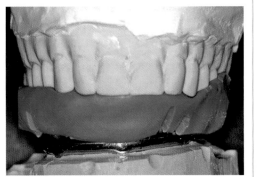

8-17

Fig. 8-13

8-13A. Surgical predrilled guide for bone site preparation.

8-13B. Torque wrench for implant positioning.

8-13C. Installed implants.

8-13D. Surgical bar and silicone pad installed.

Fig. 8-14. Occlusal radiograph showing interforaminal distance and the bone thickness.

Fig. 8-15. Prefabricated prosthetic bar installed over the surgical bar.

Fig. 8-16. Centric relation registered with a dense silicone material.

Fig. 8-17. Master casts mounted in the semi-adjustable articulator.

PROVISIONAL FIXED PROSTHESIS

Another alternative to the rehabilitation of edentulous patients is the IOL (Immediate Occlusion Loading) system. In this technique, the own patient prosthesis is duplicated to fabricate a surgical guide (Fig. 8-19). The IOL system comprises a prosthetic abutment, retentive titanium cylinder, and distal extension bars. The advantages are: low cost, easy fabrication, and reduced surgical time. However, its provisional characteristic demands a new prosthesis after the osseointegration period with rigid implant splinting through a metallic infra-structure. Surgical steps are shown in figure 8-20.

After, prosthetic cylinders are connected to the abutments. First, the intaglio surface of the prosthesis is relieved and the cylinders adjusted to the interocclusal distance. The surgical field is isolated with a sterilized rubber dam. Distal extension bars are inserted in the terminal abutments (Fig. 8-21). The abutments and bars are secured to the prosthesis with pink autopolymerizing acrylic resin (Fig. 8-22). Prosthesis is removed and abutment replicas connected. Finishing and polishing are conducted in the usual manner, while the patient receives protection caps. Once completed, prosthesis is delivered (Fig. 8-23).

OVERDENTURES

The lower denture can be converted in a two-implant supported bar overdenture (Fig. 8-24). Two implants can be placed in the lateral incisor position. In this way, additional implants will be placed to the posterior if the patient wishes a fixed implant-supported prosthesis. Also, a fifth implant can be inserted in the midline.

Soon after implant installation, prosthetic abutments are tightened with a 20Ncm torque. Now, the prosthesis is relieved and serves as an individual tray (Fig. 8-26). Then, laboratory phases are developed as usual and the overdenture is delivered to the patient (Fig. 8-27). Finally, there are several attachments that can be used with this modality.

Edentulous Maxilla

The maxillary arch presents anatomic variations and bone quality quite different from mandibular arch. Areas with bone height up to 7mm are very common. Moreover, factors as lip line, muscular support, esthetics and phonetics have to be addressed before considering immediate function treatment. During surgery, it is important to overtreat the surgical site to guarantee primary implant stability.[38]

Krekmanov,[23] and Vasconcelos[38] pointed out that adequate

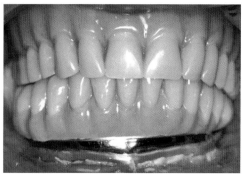

8-18A

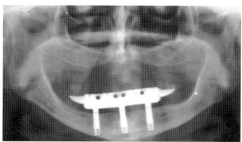

8-18B

Fig. 8-18. Clinical (A) and radiographic (B) aspects of fixed prosthesis installed on the same day.

Fig. 8-19

8-19A. Lower complete denture.

8-19B. Surgical guide tried in the mouth.

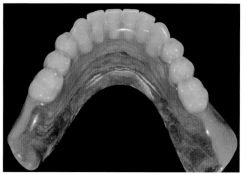

8-19A

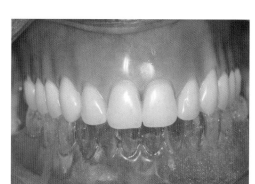

8-19B

Fig. 8-20

8-20A. Incision and mucoperisoteal elevation.

8-20B. IOL implant installation.

8-20C. Prosthetic abutments connected to the IOL implants.

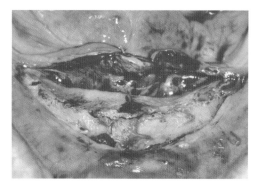

8-20A

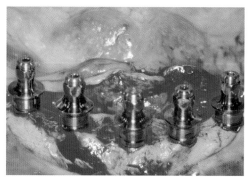

8-20B

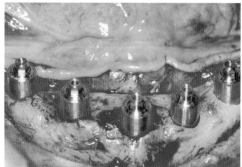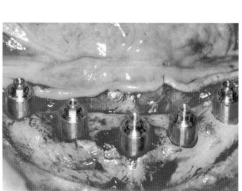

8-20C

Fig. 8-21

8-21A. Provisional cylinders connected to the abutments.

8-21B. Rubber dam and distal extension bars in position.

Fig. 8-22. Provisional cylinders secured in the prosthesis with pink acrylic resin.

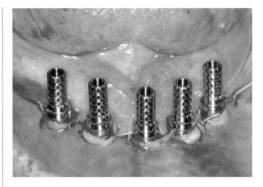

8-21A

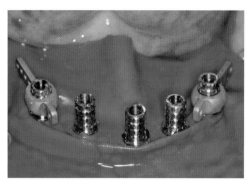

8-21B

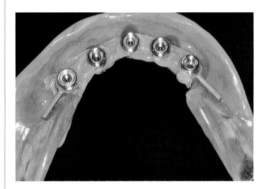

8-22

Fig. 8-23

8-23A. Frontal view of inferior prosthesis.

8-23B. Occlusal contact points are checked.

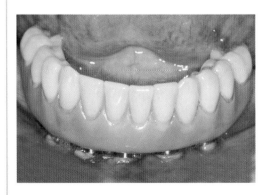

8-23A

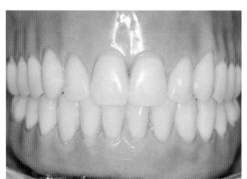

8-23B

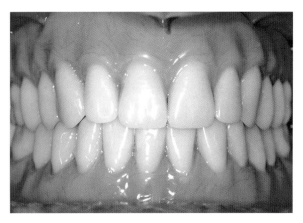

8-24

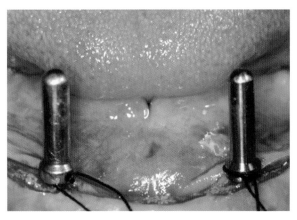

8-25

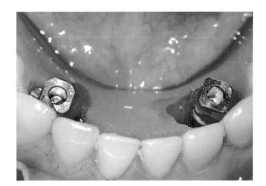

8-26A

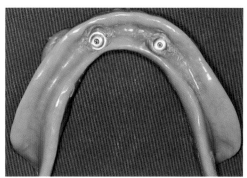

8-26B

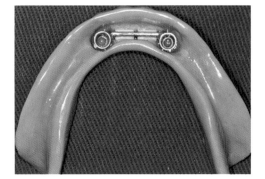

8-27A

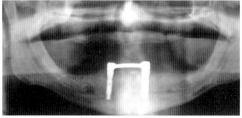

8-27B

Fig. 8-24. Final view. Esthetics, phonetics and function are integrated.

Fig. 8-25. Guide pins for implant placement.

Fig. 8-26

8-26A. The lower denture acts like an individual tray. Square impression copings are connected to the implants.

8-26B. Intaglio view of the splinted cylinders.

Fig. 8-27

8-27A. Two overdenture bar-clips are installed.

8-27B. Panoramic view of implants connected to the bar.

bone height and thickness for implant installation can be found in the intercanine region. This precludes the need for complex surgeries, bone grafts or zygomatic fixations. In this technique, the most distal implants are angulated to the mesial portion reducing the cantilever effect. Then, two to four fixtures are installed in the anterior region (Fig. 8-28). Also, longer implants can be placed increasing primary stability. It is important to remember that although maxillary bone represents the bulk of facial appearance, its rehabilitation is difficult to perform. Severely resorbed posterior maxillae with compromised bridgework can beneficiate from this treatment (Fig. 8-29).

Single-tooth restorations

Certainly, single-tooth restorations represent the patient's expectations to replace unitary loss in a short period of time. This is possible where there is adequate bone/soft tissue quantity and quality to support prosthesis and maintain gingival architecture. According to Touati,[36] papilla formation is guided by emergency profile, directly related to form, size and contour of restoration (Fig. 8-30). Clinicians must be extremely careful when the implant placement involves esthetic regions.[17]

The sequence on figure 8-31 illustrates the lack of bilateral upper incisors indicated for immediate function. Two implant designs were installed: standard (Fig. 8-32A) and TiUnite MKIII (Fig. 8-32B). The latter represents a new thread design and surface treatment concepts claimed to improve secondary stability and clinical outcome.

After, impression making procedures are performed. An square coping is connected to the top of the implant and master casts obtained with artificial gingiva and type IV stone. Provisional crowns were fabricated and installed either in the same day or in the morning after (Figs. 8-33A and B). Both restorations remained undisturbed during osseointegration period. No significant alterations were observed for gingival architecture (Fig. 8-34). Thus, final abutment and prosthetic crowns were installed.

Francischone,[17] Cunha[13] verified slightly higher ISQ values for standard than TiUnite MK III, being no significant differences observed during postoperative, 6 months and one-year periods. They concluded that implant type does not necessary influence the implant success rate on immediate function, being 95.8% in this situation.

Another example is a patient with poor dental esthetics on tooth 11. The tooth was extracted avoiding tissue trauma and the implant immediately placed (Fig. 8-35). The implant was three-di-

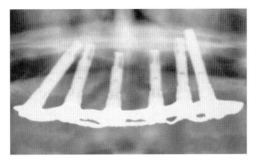

8-28

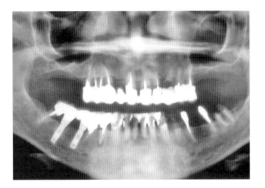

8-29A

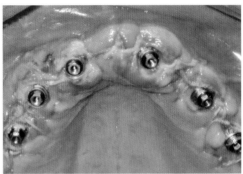

8-29B

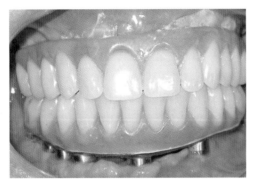

8-29C

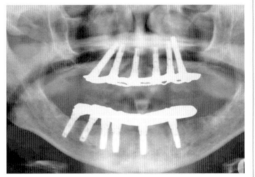

8-29D

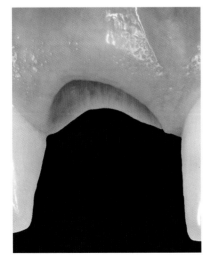

8-30A

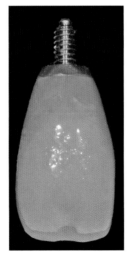

8-30B

Fig. 8-28. Panoramic radiograph showing the inclination of distal implants to the anterior region.

Fig. 8-29. Panoramic view of initial case planned for immediate function (surgical procedure by Dr. Laercio W. Vasconcelos).

8-29A. Compromised bridgework with great bone loss on both arches.

8-29B. occlusal view after abutment connection.

8-29C. Clincal aspect of final prosthesis.

8-29D. Final radiograph showing implant positioning.

Fig. 8-30A and B. Papilla formation is dictated by emergence profile.

Fig. 8-31A and B.
Clinical and radiographic aspects for implant installation on regions 22 and 12.

Fig. 8-32

8-32A. Standard implant type installed on region 12.

8-32B. MK III TiUnite implant type installed on region 22.

Fig. 8-33A and B.
Provisional crowns cemented.

Fig. 8-34. Periapical radiographs (A and C) and frontal view (B) after osseointegration.

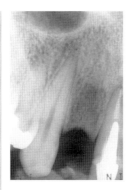
8-31A

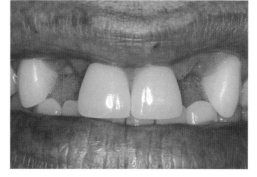
8-31B

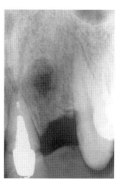
8-31C

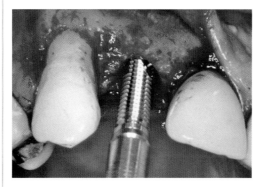
8-32A

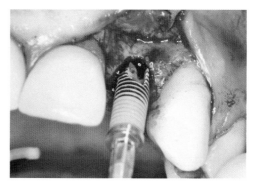
8-32B

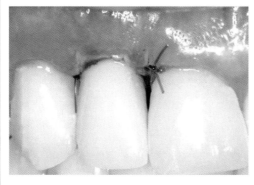
8-33A

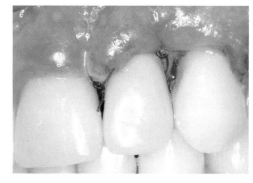
8-33B

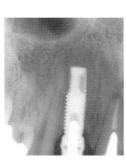
8-34A

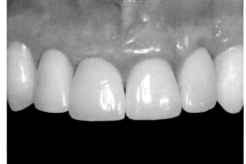
8-34B

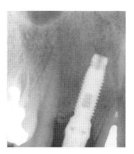
8-34C

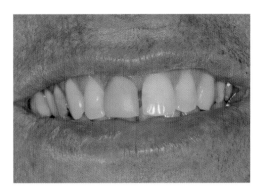

8-35A

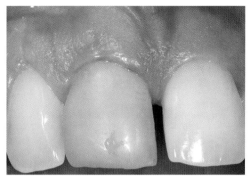

8-35B

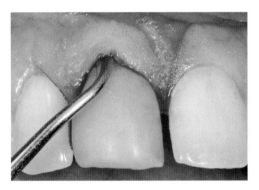

8-35C

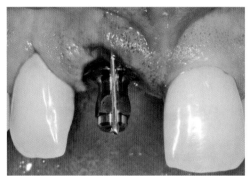

8-35D

Fig. 8-35. Extraction of tooth 11 and immediate implant placement.

mensionally positioned. After four months, a connective tissue graft surgery was performed to maintain adequate gingival architecture and fabricate provisional crown (Fig. 8-36). Four months were added until the provisional restoration be inserted. An impression coping is connected and impression made. However, it is very difficult to obtain the contour of the adjacent soft tissues. A clinical hint is to screw provisional crown to the implant analog embedded in putty silicon material. The provisional crown is removed and an impression coping connected. Autopolimerizing acrylic resin is added around the impression coping (Fig. 8-38).

The pick-up procedure uses customized impression coping and favors all laboratorial steps

Fig. 8-36. Prosthetic abutment over the top the implant (A). Abutment contouring is necessary (B). Suture of connective tissue graft (C). Provisional crown after four months (D).

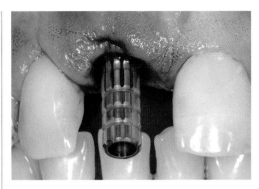

8-36A

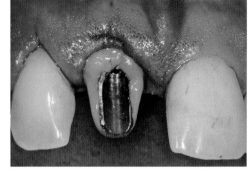

8-36B

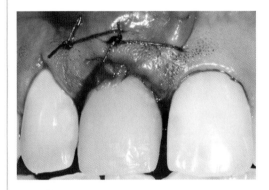

8-36C

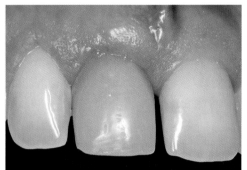

8-36D

(Fig. 8-39). In this case, zirconia abutments and alumina copings were used to achieve esthetic excellence. The esthetic abutment is tightened to 32Ncm torque. Thus, alumina coping is transferred from the mouth and veneer porcelain applied (Fig. 8-40). Color selection, interocclusal relationship and a new pick-up impression are made. After, definitive prosthesis is cemented (Fig. 8-41).

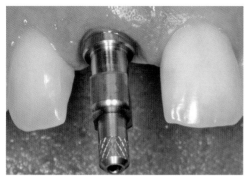

8-37

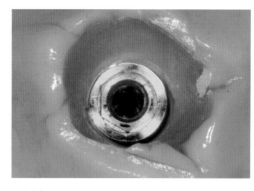

8-38A

Fig. 8-37. An impression coping is added to the implant.

Fig. 8-38

8-38A. Negative impression of emergence profile.

8-38B. Now, the same impression coping is connected to the implant analog.

8-38C. Acrylic resin is added around the impression coping.

8-38D. Customized impression coping to capturing emergence profile.

8-38E and F. customized coping in the mouth.

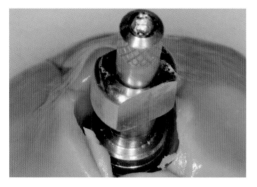

8-38B

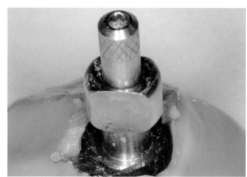

8-38C

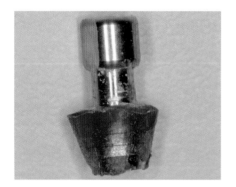

8-38D

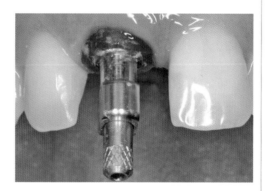

8-38E

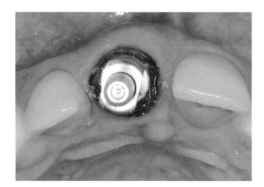

8-38F

Fig. 8-39

8-39A. A transfer impression is made.

8-39B. Master model with artificial gingival.

8-39C. Zirconia abutment prepared.

8-39D. Alumina coping in the master model.

Fig. 8-40

8-40A. Zirconia abutment connected to the implant.

8-40B. Alumina coping try-in in the mouth.

8-40C. Pick-up impression.

Fig. 8-41. Final prosthesis installed. Observe harmonious aspect between gingival adjacent tissue and crown emergence profile (clinical case done by Dr. Luis Guillermo Peredo Paz).

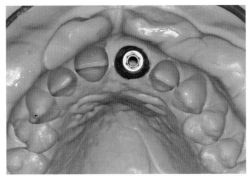
8-39A

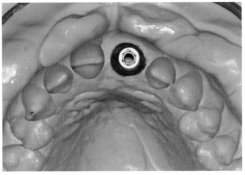
8-39B

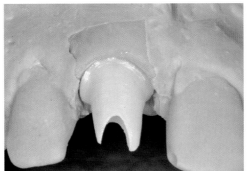
8-39C

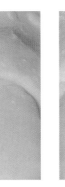
8-39D

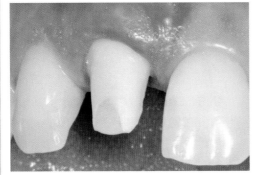
8-40A

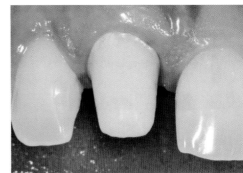
8-40B

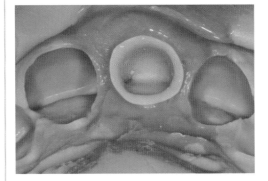
8-40C

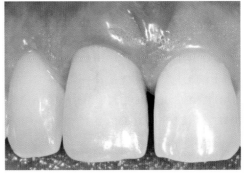
8-41

Final Considerations

Implants have been used for immediate function in both jaws with considerable long-term success regarding biological limits. The reverse planning favors correct surgical and prosthetic rehabilitation. For this, bone quantity and quality are extremely important because they provide high primary stability. Otherwise, unfavorable prognosis is likely to occur.

The rehabilitation of partial and single tooth loss with osseointegrated implants under immediate loading is a valid alternative. Bahat and Daftary[6] stated that lip line, periodontal biotype, osseous crest topography, the contours of crown restoration, and soft tissue augmenting procedures have to be considered in this modality. However, further studies are necessary to confirm short-term clinical data.

It is important to bear in mind that the same osseointegration principles must be followed during immediate loading procedure: patient rigorous selection criteria, avoidance of traumatic surgery, implant type and design, and finally, multidisciplinary collaboration.

Finally, judicious treatment planning is helpful to adequate surgical technique and prosthetic components. Although immediate loading has demonstrated high success level, one must consider that a two-stage protocol still is an excellent option for osseointegration treatment.

Referências

1. ADELL, R.; LEKHOLM, U.; ROCKLER, B.; BRÅNEMARK, P-I. et al. A 15-year study of osseointegrated implants in the treatment of edentolous jaw. *Int. J. Oral Maxillofac. Surg.,* v.10, p.387-416, 1981.
2. ALBREKTSSON, T. et al. Osseointegrated titanium implants. Requirements for ensuring a long-lasting direct bone-to-implant anchorage in man. *Act Orthop. Scand.,* v.2, n.52, p.155-70, 1981.
3. ANDRÉ, R.A. Análise comparativa da estabilidade inicial e tardia de dois implantes retentores de sobredentadura mandibular submetidos à carga imediata, por meio de freqüência de ressonância, 139p. *Dissertação de Mestrado em Implantologia – Universidade do Sagrado Coração.* Bauru – SP 2003.
4. ANDREAZA, H.C. Comparação entre torque de inserção e freqüência de ressonância, em implantes unitários Standard e TiUnite, submetidos à carga imediata. *Dissertação de Mestrado – Universidade do Sagrado Coração.* Bauru – SP, 2002.
5. APARICIO, C. A new method for achieving passive fit of an inte-rim restoration supported by Brånemark implants: A technical note. *Int. J. Oral Maxillofac. Implants,* v.10, p.614-8, 1995.
6. BAHAT, O.; DAFTARY, F. Surgical reconstruction – a prerequisite for long-term implant success: A philosophic approach. *Pract Periodont Aesthet Dent,* 7(9):21-32, 1995.
7. BALSHI, T.J.; WOLFINGER, G.J.

Imediate loading of Brånemark implants in edentulous mandible: a preliminary report. *Implant Dent.*, v.6, n.2, p.83-8, Summer 1997.

8. BERNARD, JP. et al. Osseointegration of Brånemark fixtures using a single-step operating technique. A preliminary prospective one-year in edentulous mandible. *Clin. Oral implants Res.*, v.6, p.122-9, 1995.

9. BRÅNEMARK, P-I.; BREINE, U.; ADELL, R.; HANSSON, B. O.; LINDSTROM, J.; OHLSSON, A. Intra-Osseus Anchorage of Dental Protheses. I – Experimental Studies. Scand. *J. Plast. Reconstr. Surg.*, Stockholm, v.3, p.81-100, 1969.

10. BRÅNEMARK, P-I.; HANSSON, B.O.; ADELL, R.; BREINE, U.; LINDSTROM, J.; HALLEN, O.; OHMAN, A. Osseointegrated implants in the treatment of edentolous jaw. Experience from a 10-year period. Scand. *J. Plast. Reconstr. Surg.*, suppl. 16, p.1-132, 1977.

11. BRÅNEMARK, P.I. et al. Brånemark Novum – a new treatment concept for rehabilitation of the edentulous mandible. Preliminary results from a prospective clinical follow-up study. *Clin. Implant Dent. Relat. Res.*, v.1, p.2-16, 1999.

12. CHIAPASCO, M. et al. It retained mandibular overdentures with immediate loading. A retrospective multicenter study on 266 consecutive cases. *Clin. Oral Implant Res.* v.8, p.48-57, 1997.

13. CUNHA, H.A.; FRANCISCHONE, C.E.; NARY FILHO, H.; OLIVEIRA, R.C. A comparison between cutting torque and ressonance frequency in the assessment of primary stability and final torque capacity of standard ant ti unite single-tooth implants under immediate loading. *Int J Oral Maxillofac Implants.* 2004 Jul-Aug, 19(4): 578-85.

14. ERICSSON, I. et al. Immediate functional loading of Brånemark single-tooth implants. An 18-month clini-cal pilot follow-up study. *Clinical Oral Implants Research,* v.11, p.26-33, 2000.

15. ERICSSON, I.; NILSON, H.; NILNER, K. Immediate functional loading of Brånemark single tooth implants. A 5-year clinical follow-up study. *Appl. Osseointegration Res.,* v.2, p.12-16, 2001.

16. FRANCISCHONE, C.E. Função ou Carga Imediata? *Implant News,* v.1, n.1, p.16-17, 2004.

17. FRANCISCHONE JR, C.E. Análise da freqüência de ressonância de implantes unitário Brånemark Standard e MK TiUnite, submetidos à carga imediata. *Dissertação de Mestrado – Universidade do Sagrado Coração.* Bauru – SP, 2002.

18. GOLL, G.E. Production of accurately fitting full-arch implant frameworks: part I – clinical procedures. *J. Prosthet. Dent.,* v.66, n.3, p.377-84, 1991.

19. HENRY, P.; ROSENBERG, I. Single stage surgery for rehabilitation of the edentulous mandible: preliminary results. *Pract Periodontics Aesthet. Dent.* v.6, n.9, p.15-22, 1994.

20. HORIUCHI, K. et al. Immediate loading of Brånemark system implants following placement in edentulous patients: A clinical report. *Int. J. Oral Maxillofac. Implants,* v.15, n.6, 2000.

21. JEMT, T. Failures and complications in 391 consecutively insertsd fixed prostheses supported by Brånemark implants in edentulous jaws: a study of treatment from the time of prosthesis placement to the first annual checkup. *Int. J. Oral Maxillofac. Implants,* v.6, n.3, p.270-6, 1991.

22. JIMENEZ, V.; TORROBA, P. Diseño de prótesis sobre implants para conseguir un ajuste pasivo: técnica del cilindro cementado sobre prótesis atornilladas. *Actualidad Implantol.,* v.1, n.5, p.27-32, 1992.

23. KREKMANOV, L.; KAHN, M.; RANGERT, B.; LINDSTROM, H. Tilting of posterior mandibular and

maxillary implants for improved protesis support. *The International Journal of Oral & Maxillofacial Implants*, v.15, n.3, 2000.

24. LIMA, E.G. Avaliação da estabilidade de implantes submetidos à carga imediata através da freqüência de ressonância. *Dissertação de Mestrado – Universidade do Sagrado Coração.* Bauru – SP, 2002.

25. MALÓ, P.; RANGERT, B.; DVARSATER, L. Immediate funcition of Brånemark implants in the esthetic zone: a retrospective clinical study with 6 months to 4 year of follow up. Disponível em: http://clinicamalo@mailtelepac.pt, 2000.

26. PIATTELI, A. et al. Bone reaction to early occlusal loading of two stage titanium plasma-sprayed implants: a pilot study in monkeys. *Int. J. Periodont. Res. Dent.,* v.17, n.2, p.163-69, 1997a.

27. PIATTELLI, A. et al Immediate loading of titanium plasma-sprayed screw-shaped implants in man: A clinical and histological report of 2 cases. *Journal of Periodontology,* v.68, p.591-597, 1997b.

28. RANDOW, K. et al. Immediate functional loading of Brånemark dental implants. A 18-month clinical follow-up study. *Clin. Oral Implants Res.,* v.10, p.8-15, 1999.

29. SALAMA, H. et al. Immediate loading of bilaterally splinted titanium root-from implants in fixed prosthodontics. A technique reexamined two cases report. *Int. J. Periodontics Restorative Dent.,* v.15, p.345-61, 1995.

30. SELLERS, G.C. Direct assembly framework for osseointegrated implant prosthesis. *Maxillofac. Prosthet. Dent. Implants,* v.62, n.6, p.662-8, 1989.

31. SCHNITMAN, P.A. et al. Immediate fixed interium prostheses supported by two-stage threaded implants : methodology and results. *J. Oral Implants,* v.16, p.96-105, 1990.

32. SCHNITMAN, P.A. et al. Ten-year results of a Brånemark implants im-

mediately loaded with fixed prostheses at implant placement. *Int. J. Oral Maxillofac. Implants,* v.12, n.4, p.495-503, Jul., 1997.

33. SKALAK, R. Biomechanical considerations in osseointegrated prostheses. *J. Prost. Dent.;* n.49, p.843-848, 1983.

34. TARNOW, D.P.; EMTIAZ, S.; CLASSI, A. Immediate loading of threaded implants at stage 1 – surgery in edentulous arch: ten consecutive cases reports with 1-to 5-year data. *Int. J. Oral Maxillofac. Implants,* v.12, n.3, p.319-24, 1997.

35. TULER, R.F. Avaliação da aplicabilidade de prótese modificada sobre reabilitações totais inferiores, tipo protocolo, implantossuportadas, em sistema de carga imediata. Estudo clínico e radiográfico. *Dissertação de Mestrado - Universidade do Sagrado Coração.* Bauru – SP, 2002.

36. TOUATI, B.; GUEZ, G.; SAADOUN, A.P. Aesthetic soft tissues integration and optimized emergence profile: Provisionalization and customized impression coping. *Pract Periodont Aesthet Dent,* v.11, n.3, p.305-314, 1999.

37. VASCONCELOS, L.W. et al. Implantes inclinados no sentido póstero-anterior da maxila: apresentação de um caso clínico. *Revista APCD,* v.57, n.6, p.434-8, 2003.

38. VASCONCELOS, L.W. Avaliação clínica, pelo método da freqüência de ressonância de implantes instalados por meio de técnica cirúrgica modificada na maxila e submetidos à função oclusal imediata. Faculdade de Odontologia de Araçatuba FOA-UNESP. Tese-Doutorado, 2005.

39. VASCONCELOS, L.W. Aprendizado Constante. *Implant News,* v.1, n.1, p.20-21, 2004.

40. WEINBERG, L.A. The biomecanics of force distribution in implant-supported prostheses . *Int. J. Oral Maxillofac. Implants,* v.8, n.1, p.19-31, 1993.

41. WOLF, S.M.R. O significado psi-

cológico da perda dos dentes em su-jeitos adultos. *Revista da APCD,* v.52, n.4, p.307-316, Jul/Ago 1998.

42. WOOD, G.D.; HAJJAR, A. A retro-spective surgery of patients trea-ted with one-stage (ITI) enous implants. *Dent. Update,* v.24, n.1, p.19-23, Jan/Feb. 1997.

9

Autogenous Bone Grafts on Implantology

Laércio W. Vasconcelos
Gustavo Petrilli
Laura P.G. Paleckis

Introduction

Oral implantology has had a tremendous impact in therapeutic options. Totally or partial edentulous areas can be rehabilitated regarding anatomy, function and esthetics. However, more refined prosthetic techniques emerged to achieve excellent results.

The resorption phenomena after toot loss compromises bone volume. Thus, osseous reconstruction is necessary to further implant placement in adequate prosthetic positions.

In this sense, autogenous bone is still considered the "gold standard" material. Part of its cellular viability is lost during healing but revascularization occurs and the graft is incorpo-rated to the recipient bed. Then, adequate setting for implant placement is made. One draw-back is that a second surgical site must be confectioned for bone harvest, increasing the likeli-hood of morbidity.

Intra and extra-oral donor sites are available. Besides, the graft can be used in several mac-roscopic ways: block (cortical, cancellous, and corticocancel-lous) or particulate (triturated or bone chip) forms.

Bone graft success involves diverse aspects, such as adequate postoperative healing and long-term osseous stability. It means that the implants will remain os-seointegrated to a bone grafted area withstanding occlusal forc-es via dental prosthesis.

To achieve this, knowledge of the healing process and adequate surgical technique are imperative to correctly handle bone grafts.

Biological aspects of autogenous bone graft repair and revascularization

Repair and revascularization of bone grafts depends on its density and architecture. Thus, cancellous bone is first characterized by blood clot and granulation tissue formation at bone-implant interface. After, proliferating capillary vessels invade bone trabeculae and sometimes anastomosis can be formed with graft nourishment. Viable osteoblasts from graft and that of recipient bed begin to secrete osseous matrix at interfacial and subjacent areas, surrounding non-viable bone cores. Through osteoinduction, growth factors exert its effects on stem and osteogenic cells, favoring osseous neoformation. The remodeling phase is characterized by bone resorption and new bone deposition during few months (Fig. 9-1).

On the other hand, osseous repair in cortical bone follows a different path. The initial phase is characterized by inflammation and granulation tissue at the interface, but its dense archi-tecture precludes rapid vessel proliferation, retarding revascularization. Thus, osteoclastic activity can be seen on preexisting Volkmann and Havers canals to facilitate angiogenesis (Fig. 9-2). In this way, osteoblasts invade graft and bone neoformation begins. This is a slow process and non-vital and vital new bone areas can be found at the same time. The osseous repair is centripetal and localized in the osteons rather than interstitial lamellae. The corticocancellous block has both repair mechanisms with fast healing of cancellous layer and bulk strength of cortical area.

Particulate bone graft can be obtained either triturated or in the shaved form (bone chips). Bone particles offer lesser obstacles to fluid penetration from recipient bed and facilitate vessel proliferation similar to the cancellous type. Also, bone resorption velocity depends on particle size.

Several authors investigated differences between grafts from endochondral (iliac crest) and intramembranous (mandible, calvaria) origin. Faster revascularization was observed in the former due to its architecture and wide marrow spaces, contrary to the intramembranous type which pursues more dense cortical and cancellous spaces.

Patients undergone bone graft must be followed during all postoperative period. Time

Fig. 9-1. Cancellous bone (OE) involved by granulation tissue (TG) densely vascularized with immediate osseous neoformation (Masson 100x).

Fig. 9-1. For grafts other than bone block types, healing is initiated through resorption lacunae (arrow) at the interface to vascularize it (Masson 100x).

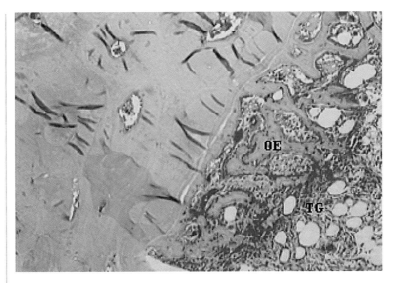

9-1

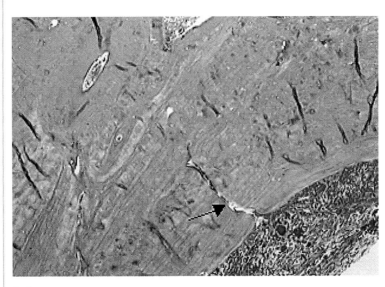

9-2

necessary for osseointegration can vary from 5 to 6 months depending on size and form of the bone grafted. Areas with particulate grafts can be reentered faster than block grafts, and corticocancellous block faster than cortical ones. Also, time to reentry still depends on individual bone characteristics. For example, a less dense, richer cancellous iliac crest bone with a thin cortical plate must be exposed early than a more cortical bone with restricted marrow spaces. Otherwise, bone loss will be greater in the former. Besides, drilling for implant placement must be thoroughly performed. New burs will avoid stressing the graft-recipient bed interface. The use of a screwtap is also recommended. In this case, primary stability will be achieved at the expenses of basal bone.

Wearing of removable appliances is important for social and professional activities. However, pressure over the grafted area can cause resorption, mobility and bone sequestration. Remaining teeth can act as terminal abutments for provisional restorations. Complex situations involve edentulous patients who will not wear their complete dentures for four months. After, the prosthesis can be relieved but just for esthetic purposes.

Bone graft success is a multifactorial issue. Several factors can be enlisted: anamnesis, treatment planning, donor site selection, recipient bed preparation, graft fixation and its coverage. Close patient follow-up and implant placement after bone healing have influence in the outcomes.

Anamnesis

Before surgery, patients must be screened regarding medical past and actual conditions, age, deleterious habits (for example, smoking) as well as their psychological predicament to the treatment planned. Intra-oral examination includes bone defects, adjacent teeth and periodontal status. Imaging and laboratorial exams are also necessary. Panoramic, periapical, Waters projection, lateral cephalometric views and CT scans are helpful. Stereolithographic techniques can also be employed to provide accurate three-dimensional bone reconstruction of the affected area. Laboratorial exams and medical evaluation (e.g., cardiac or other systemic conditions) add important information. Medically compromised patients must undergone treatment with a physician before bone graft surgery.

Surgical planning

By definition, bone graft surgeries are pre-prosthetic procedures. Thus, reverse planning will provide the need for surgery. After, intra and extra-oral photographic documentation is made, as well as maxillary and mandibular casts are related in the semi-adjustable articulator. The diagnostic wax-up is efficient, because it provides ideal prosthetic position and the amount of bone volume. A surgical guide is very helpful in the intraoperative period. This treatment sequence improves final treatment prognosis and yields satisfactory results.

Donor site selection

Bone requirements will dictate donor site selection. Width augmentation and small unilateral maxillary sinus graft procedures can be performed with intra-oral sites. Height and width augmentation and bilateral maxillary sinus grafts will require extra-oral donor sites. Insufficient bone quantity can be viewed as a clinical complication. Donor site election is close related to bone size and shape defect. Extra-oral donor sites include iliac bone crest, cranial vault; intra-oral sites comprehend retromolar and interforaminal areas.

The bone iliac crest is the most used area for osseous reconstructions due to its abundant cortical and cancellous bone. In addition, donor and recipient areas can be prepared at the same surgical time.

Cranial vault is constituted by a three-layered bone tissue, being outer and inner cortical plates interposed by diploe. It is indicated for large reconstruction areas. Generally, parietal or occipital bones are the recommended choice.

The retromolar area offers cortical bone, with little or no cancellous component. It can be used for onlay and inlay techniques as well as filling with particulate bone. The size and thickness of the graft depend on the anatomy of this area. Surgical access is limited. Patients must present with minimal bone height usually found in robust mandibles. An L-shape bone graft can be removed from this region.

Interforaminal area comprehends both cortical and cancellous bone reinforced at the mental protuberance region. Surgical access is facilitated. Its semi-curved shape can be used for onlay, inlay, bone filling, sinus lifting procedures, and to close gaps between graft and recipient bed. A radiological examining is important to verify incisive and canine root lengths, localization of mental foramen emergence, and bone available in this area.

Surgical technique – general aspects

Graft removal

ILIAC BONE CREST

Surgical intervention must be done in an hospital setting under general anesthesia or deep sedation. A muldisciplinary team must be composed of: plastic surgeon, orthopedist or general surgeon. Buccomaxillofacial surgeon or implantodontist as well as medical nurses complete the surgical staff. The graft is removed from antero-posterior iliac crest

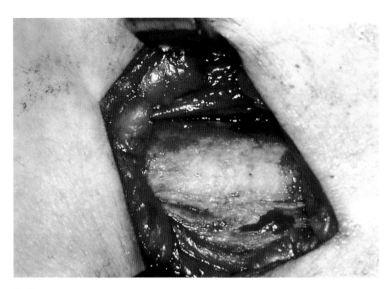

9-3

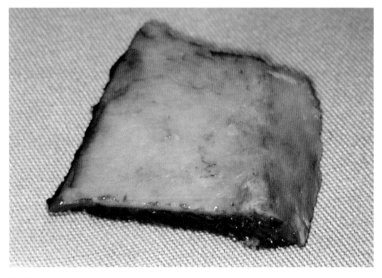

9-4

Fig. 9-3. Bone iliac crest surgical access.

Fig. 9-4. Corticocancellous bone block removed.

area (Figs. 9-3 and 9-4). A multilayered incision is performed to reach osseous crest. Striker saws or cylindrical burs at low-speed rotation under copious saline irrigation with chisels are used to remove the graft. Prefabricated occlusive molds corresponding to the form of the residual ridge, U-shaped, bicortical, cortical and cancellous blocks can be used to map the graft. Graft is removed and reshaped to better adapt to the recipient site. Donor site is rinsed and aspirated. A surgical drain is installed and remains in position for 24 hours. Resorbable sutures are placed in deep planes. Non-resorbable material is used to approximate superficial plane. Although a frequent procedure, related complications are minimal and due to surgical techniques or to the extent of graft removal. Patients stay for 1 or 2 days at the hospital to stimulate lower limb movements. When bone graft size is not considerable, surgery can be made under intravenous sedation and infiltration anesthesia.

CRANIAL VAULT

The procedure is conducted at hospital setting under general anesthesia. A multidisciplinary team (plastic surgeon, neurosurgeon and buccomaxillofacial professional) is necessary. Skin shaving is not mandatory unless good anti-septic techniques been available. Coronal incision runs to the periosteum, with subsequent divulsion and bone tissue exposure.

Osteotomy is made with 700 fissure burs or saws under copious saline irrigation. Chisels are added. Surgery depth is determined by bleeding and tactile perception of a less resistant area (cancellous bone). Graft can be U or stripe-shaped. When necessary, cancellous bone can be harvested too. Graft is remodeled, adapted, and secured to the compromised site.

Accidents and complications are rare. The most common finding is significant bleeding due to section of parietal branch of superficial temporal artery which can be controlled or avoided. The integrity of inner cortical plate is paramount. Compared to the iliac graft procedure, surgeons need more time to harvest the cranial vault. Only after graft removal the recipient site is prepared.

Vertical augmentation is difficult due to the density of cranial vault, because the graft cannot be contoured to an L-shape. Its indications comprehend width augmentation or during maxillary sinus lifting with adjunctive particulate bone filling.

RETROMOLAR REGION

Intra-oral graft procedures can be done in an outpatient setting under local anesthesia or conscious sedation. Lingual and alveolar inferior nerves are blocked along with buccal nerve. Incision is placed at the buccinator's fold, medial to the oblique line. In this way, buccinator muscle is detached without fiber sectioning and further suture dehiscence. Divulsion must involves a great area. The inferoposterior surgical limit is masseter muscle fiber attachment. Osteotomies are made with 700 fissure burs at low-speed rotation under copious saline irrigation. Superior, mesial and distal areas are delimited. Just part of the oblique line is included because likelihood to compromise this area is great (half of the buccal mandibular thickness is enough). Vertical osteotomy runs obliquely to the vestibular avoiding mandibular canal structures and nerve bundles. Its inferior limit is located above the masseter muscle fibers, where surgical access is made possible. Chisels are used to elevate bone graft because its difficult access prevents the use of burs. Mandibular body must be well supported to give confidence during surgical procedure (Figs. 9-5 and 9-6).

Possible accidents and complications include damage to the alveolar inferior nerve, with temporary or permanent numbness, hemorrhage and swelling. Lingual nerve can be damage during flap elevation. Mandibular fracture occurs after inadequate management of surgical elevators or due to the lack of postoperative care.

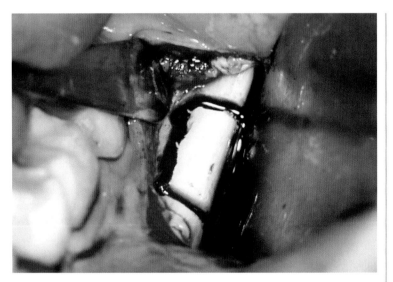

9-5

Fig. 9-5. Surgical access and graft removal at the retromolar area.

Fig. 9-6. Size of block graft.

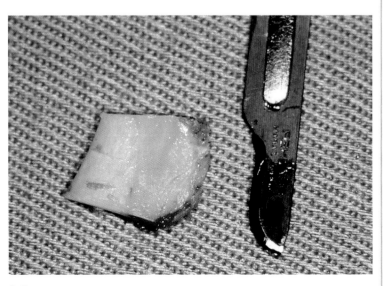

9-6

Interforamen region

Bilateral block of inferior alveolar nerves are preferred along with infiltrative anesthesia at the incisive region. Also, mandibular nerves are bilaterally anesthetized; sometimes, sublingual nerves are blocked too. Incision must be placed at labial site. First, mucosal and muscular planes are included (orbicular oriis). The scalpel blade is runs parallel to the bone ridge along the premolar area. Second, the blade is perpendicular positioned to bone ridge and flap is dissected to the mandibular base. There is an increased risk for soft tissue prolapse as well as swelling and hematoma at the submentonian region. Alternatively, incision can be executed at the bone crest involving dental papilla with broad flap elevation. Besides, there is a risk for suture dehiscence, gingival recession and root exposure of involved teeth when this incision is made.

Osteotomies are made with 700 fissure burs under copious saline irrigation, located 0.5mm above the root apex and medial to the canine roots. The lingual cortical plate defines depth of osteotomy. Chisels are inserted to elevate block bone graft. Cancellous remaining bone can be harvested with curettes or special collectors. After surgical lodge management, dissected planes are sutured. Non absorbable sutures are placed for intermediary layers. The patient stays with mouth closed during all procedure, which facilitates technique and provides comfort.

The most common accidents and complications include hemorrhage, hematoma, swelling, temporary or permanent labial paresthesia, apicectomies and dental necrosis.

Recipient site preparation

The recipient site must be examined regarding to the bone defect limits and its surgical exposition. Incision must be carried out at the alveolar crest avoiding dental papilla. A mucoperiosteal flap must be created to provide adequate nourishment to the wound area. Next, donor site area is accessed and adequate amount of bone graft is harvested. Once the graft is properly contoured to the defect, the recipient site is activated through decorticalization and perforation. In this way, the influx of nutrients and osteogenic cells is facilitated to the graft (Fig. 9-7). Once the recipient site is prepared, the graft can be contoured and adapted.

The graft must be carefully adapted to the recipient site. The corticocancellous block with wide internal spaces must be firmly positioned to avoid structural collapse leading to final volume loss. Also, this favors osteoconduction because it eliminates dead spaces and permits passage of osteogenic cells to the interior of the graft.

Revascularization occurs from the recipient site to the bone graft. The cancellous portion in contact with the recipient site accelerates this process. The outer layer must be perforated to facilitate revascularization with additional effect provided by periosteum.

Graft margins must be rounded to avoid flap irritation during closure. Dead spaces must be avoided and, in this case, can be filled with particulate or cancellous bone.

Block Graft Fixation

Rigid fixation of bone graft is related to incorporation, consolidation and volume maintenance. Drilling and lag screws facilitate graft revascularization (Fig. 9-8). Fixation offers resistance to shearing forces that prevent proliferation of new vessels at the bed-graft interface. Fibrous tissue due to bone block movement can be seen when the graft is not adequately secured.

The block must be secured with screws of adequate length. A round bur is used to create a small depression to adapt the screw head at the desire fixation site. This avoids trauma, osseous resorption, and screw exposure in the oral cavity. Progressive site drilling is made and the screw

stabilized. Great care must be taken to avoid graft movement. Large blocks can be fixed in two points. Dead spaces are filled with triturated bone particles to prevent fibrous tissue apposition between graft and recipient site.

Particulate bone graft is indicated either to alveolar or bone defect filling, as well as to maxillary sinus lifting. It can be retrieved from bone chips or triturated particles. Bone chips from shaved areas have a smaller particle size. Manual or mechanical fragmentation generates larger bone particles.

During healing process, particles are completely resorbed (Fig. 9-9) or encapsulated into a new formed bone matrix. The resorption process is inversely proportional to the particle size. Thus, bone grafts with smaller particle size will have considerable volume loss. This must be taken into account for exclusively use of shaved bone.

When bone particles are used, they must be carefully packed into the defect. During sinus lifting procedures, creation of a cortical plate "roof" is useful to the upper limit of the defect, facilitating uniform filling of the defect.

Graft Covering

A tension-free flap completely covering the bone graft is fundamental to an undisturbed

Fig. 9-7. Recipient bed perforation facilitates graft incorporation and creates an early site for new formed bone (NO) (hematoxilin-eosin staining, 50X).

Fig. 9-8. Seven-day postoperative aspect. Observe early bone formation (arrow) onto the screw fixation head (Masson, 100X).

Fig. 9-9. Shaved bone particle (P) at the beginning of resorption process. Seven-day postoperative aspect (Masson, 160X).

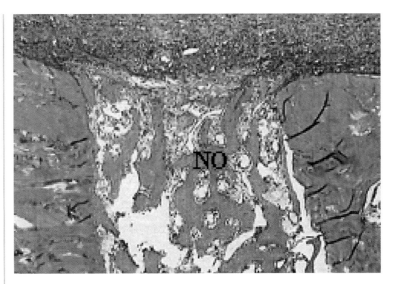

9-7

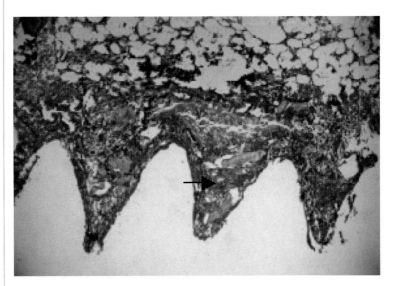

9-8

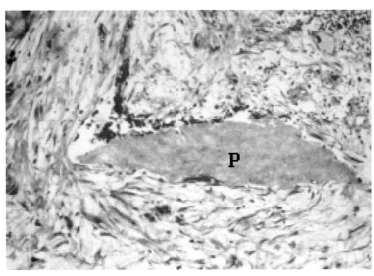

9-9

healing process. Now, there is an increased volume and the overlying soft tissue must be gently manipulated at this area. The underlying periosteum and the base of the flap must be released to achieve good protection. Meticulous suture is critical to avoid dehiscence and graft exposure.

Maxillary Sinus Lifting

Bone deficiency in height and width is commonly seen after posterior tooth loss in the maxillary arch. This prevents implant placement. After teeth removal and decreasing on masticatory force transmission, anatomic alterations occur in the maxillary sinuses. Sinus wall becomes thinner and pneumatization is evident due to osteoclastic process at the sinus membrane. In addition, there is concomitant alveolar bone resorption.

The use of short implants on the posterior maxilla diminishes long-term success rate. That is why graft procedures are necessary before sinus lifting.

For small reconstructions, intra-oral donor sites (frequently the retromolar area). Large reconstructions can be benefit from iliac crest areas, especially in bilateral cases.

Graft can either be used in particulate or block configuration. The triturate bone is packed into the sinus wall cavity for si-

nus lifting. On the other hand, the block form is fixed to the buccal area to increase thickness and sometimes bone height in cases of irregular occlusal plane.

Sinus elevation may or not be simultaneous to implant placement. Two approaches can be used: in the first technique, bone graft is performed previous to implant placement. In the second technique, bone graft and implants are placed in the same surgical stage. Implant installation is only possible when a minimum of 5mm-bone height is found.

The first technique provides more predictable results because implants are installed 5 to 6 months after graft healing. In this way, masticatory forces only exert its effects on the grafted area after 12 months when advanced osseous remodeling can be found.

The immediate technique diminishes treatment period. However, it has a lower success than mediate technique. A study conducted at the Sao Paulo Brånemark Osseointegration Center showed that implant success rate with immediate technique was of 90% compared to the 95% in the mediate technique.

After graft removal, an incision is placed along the alveolar crest in the posterior maxillary area. Vertical releasing incisions are made and a mucoperiosteal flap is elevated to expose the anterior maxillary sinus wall. Os-

Fig. 9-10. Access is provided to the left maxillary sinus wall. A small membrane perforation is visualized.

Fig. 9-11. The cancellous portion of an osseous lamina is adapted to form the roof of the cavity.

Fig. 9-12. Triturated bone is packed into the prepared site. Also, block graft is secured to increase bone width and thickness.

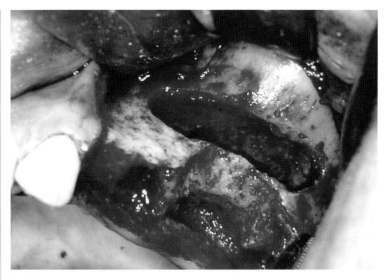

9-10

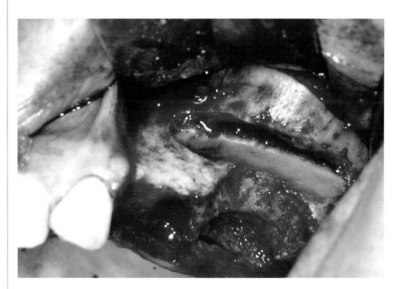

9-11

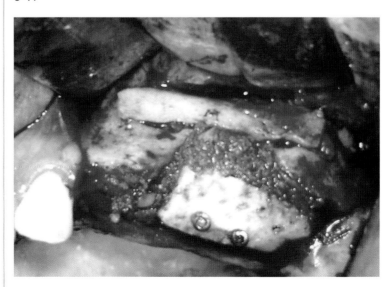

9-12

teotomy is initiated with a low-speed diamond round bur under copious saline irrigation. Once sinus mucous membrane is visualized, its elevation is done with specific curettes to the desired level.

Now, an osseous lamina is inserted parallel to the alveolar crest creating the roof of the bony lodge. (Figs. 9-10 to 9-12). Triturated bone is packed under the lamina. If membrane perforation is detected, the defect can be closed with a bone lamina or block.

When simultaneous implant placement is desired, triturated bone can be packed the posterior cavity wall. Implants are placed and the cavity is completely filled with bone. Finally, flap is repositioned and sutured without tension.

Total maxillary reconstruction

This constitutes one of the great challenges in Oral Implantology and Buccomaxillofacial Surgery. Several surgical issues have to be addressed. Surgeon's experience along with patient cooperation represents the main factors that influence final outcome of this complex procedure. Risks need to be carefully considered.

The first description of total maxillary reconstruction had a horse-shoe bone block graft secured to the maxilla with the aid of titanium screws. Thus, reported success rates for implants varied from 25 to 75%.

After, researchers recommended bone graft reconstruction followed by 5 to 6 month time intervals to provide complete bone healing. Advantages of implant placement on mature bone include adequate surgical positioning and prosthetic treatment, as well as better lip support and esthetics. However, postoperative complications and problems on soft and hard tissue stability after treatment have been described even in non-compromised cases.

Based on the stated above, patients need to advised about invasive nature and failure risk of this complex procedure. It is very important to explain that patients cannot wear their total prosthesis in the next 30 days until a new prosthesis being made and relined with soft lining material. Also, is important that the definitive prosthesis design meets the patient's expectations. Even with bone augmentation, some pink material has to be added for lip support and adequate tooth length.

Anamnesis, physical examination and laboratorial tests are highly recommended before surgical procedure. Also, stereolithographic models improve treatment planning because it enables three-dimensional view of anatomic landmarks and overlying defects. Thus, accurate diagnosis is provided for maxillary reconstruction. Bone height and width augmentation is made possible through osseous block grafts associated to sinus lifting procedures. Depending on the anatomy of the recipient site, grafts can be divided or used as single blocks.

Iliac crest is the best donor area for large defects because it provides adequate amount of corticocancellous bone. The recipient site is prepared at the same time of graft removal. An incision is made along the alveolar bone crest with two vertical releasing incisions on the posterior maxillary area. A mucoperiosteal flap is elevated exposing the recipient bed. The piriform aperture is contoured; zygomatic and canine buttress areas are shown. This maneuver facilitates flap repositioning after graft surgery.

Maxillary sinus lifting (if indicated) is performed as usual. A block graft is adapted to the recipient site. This will provide bone height and width augmentation. The graft can be either divided or U-shaped. Titanium screws are used to secure the graft in position. Cancellous bone is packed into dead spaces between graft and recipient bed (Figs. 9-13 to 9-18).

Last, flap is repositioned without tension. Horizontal releasing incisions enhance soft tissue resilience and favor perfect graft coverage. Carefully tissue apposition is necessary to finalize the procedure (Fig. 9-19).

During osseous healing, close patient follow-up is important to identify complications as suture dehiscence or thread exposure. Periodical prosthesis relining with soft material avoids trauma to the reconstructed region. Another option is to use a fixed prosthesis incorporating abutment teeth and tuberosity sites (Figs. 9-20 to 9-23).

Implants are placed after 5-6 months (Figs. 9-24 and 9-25). However, additional 5 to 6 months are necessary prior to abutment connection. Then, final prosthesis is initiated (Figs. 9-26 to 9-37).

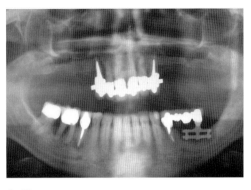

9-13

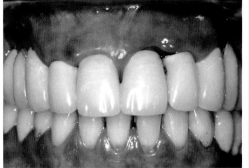

9-14

Fig. 9-13. Initial panoramic view.

Fig. 9-14. Frontal view showing posterior deficient areas.

Fig. 9-15. Alveolar maxillary ridge after surgical exposure.

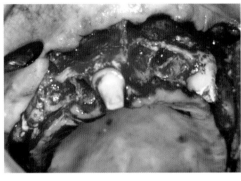

9-15

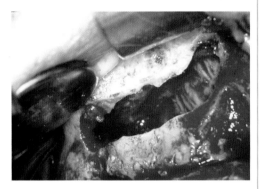

9-16

Fig. 9-16. Access to the right maxillary sinus is completed. Note sinus membrane elevation.

Fig. 9-17. Triturated bone is packed into the cavity.

Fig. 9-18. Block graft stabilization. Dead spaces are filled with cancellous bone. Observe increase in height and thickness.

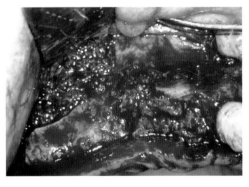

9-17

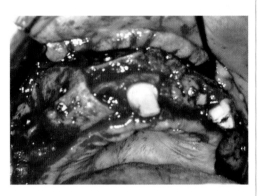

9-18

Fig. 9-19. Sutures are placed without tension.

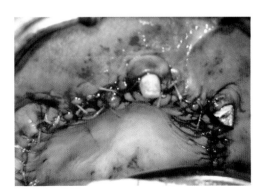

9-19

Mandibular Reconstruction

Initially, implant protocols aimed to restore completely edentulous mandible. Even with increased bone resorption between mental foramina, implants can achieve high success rates. On the other hand, posterior areas pose some problems to osseous reconstruc-tion. Sometimes, mandibular canal is close to the alveolar crest or insufficient bone height prevents implant installation. Also, the centrifugal resorption pattern leads to inadequate bone thickness. For this, bone graft can be performed. However, the choice of donor site area depends on defect size, being the iliac bone crest the more reasonable option oftentimes. The main incision is

Fig. 9-20. Tuberosity and tooth-borne provisional fixed prosthesis.

Fig. 9-21. Frontal view of provisional prosthesis.

Fig. 9-22. Occlusal view of provisional prosthesis.

Fig. 9-23. Panoramic radiograph after bone block graft.

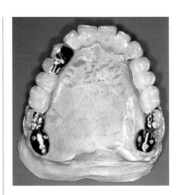

9-20

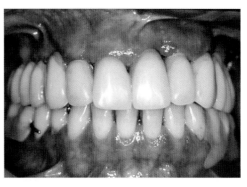

9-21

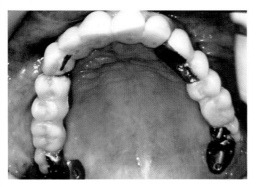

9-22

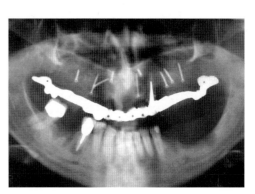

9-23

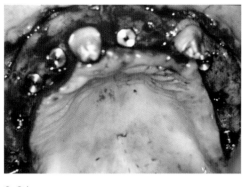

9-24

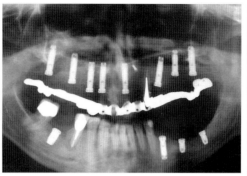

9-25

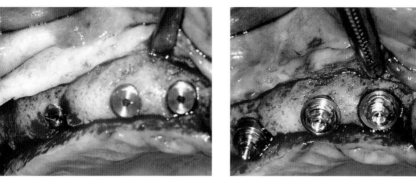

9-26   9-27

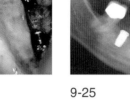

9-28   9-29

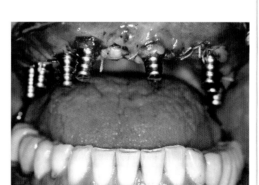

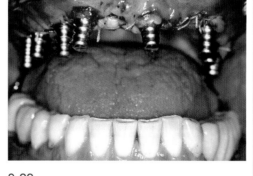

9-30   9-31

Fig. 9-24. Implants are installed after 6 months.

Fig. 9-25. Panoramic radiograph after implant placement.

Fig. 9-26. Implants are exposed after 6 months. Observe adequate bone surrounding titanium fixtures.

Fig. 9-27. Abutment installation.

Fig. 9-28. Square impression copings are splinted with autopolymerizing acrylic resin to capture three-dimensional implant position.

Fig. 9-29. Transfers are screwed for impression procedure.

Fig. 9-30. Impression made with multifunctional guide to record maxillomandibular relation.

Fig. 9-31. Prosthesis is delivered three days after implant exposure.

Fig. 9-32. Soft tissue aspect after healing.

Fig. 9-33. Metallic infrastructure try-in.

Fig. 9-34. Metalloceramic prosthesis installed.

Fig. 9-35. Definitive prosthesis.

Fig. 9-36. Patient's smile.

Fig. 9-37. Final radiographic view.

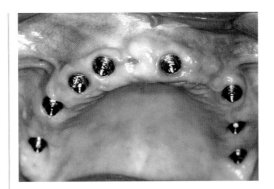

9-32

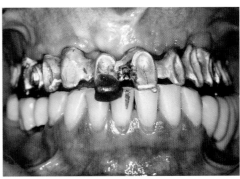

9-33

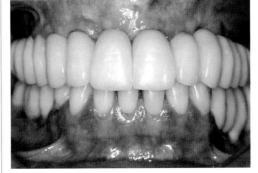

9-34

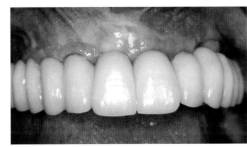

9-35

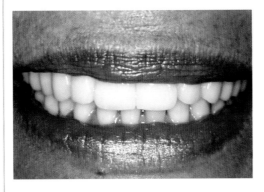

9-36

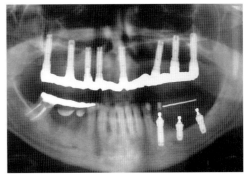

9-37

placed laterally to the mandibular ridge, along with two releasing mesial and distal incisions. Mucoperiosteal flap elevation exposes recipient bed. Care must be taken to avoid mental nerve emergence. Graft is adapted and carefully secured to the recipient site (Figs.9-38 to 9-41).

Clinicians have to bear in

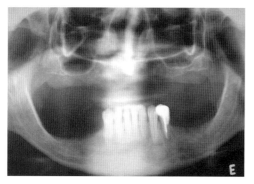

9-38

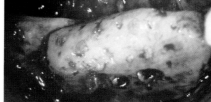

9-39

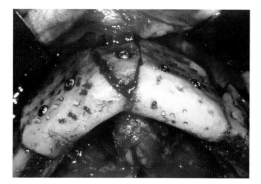

9-40

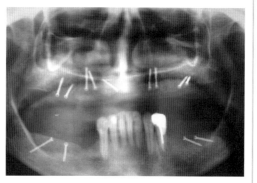

9-41

Fig. 9-38. Initial panoramic view.

Fig. 9-39. Autogenous block graft secured to the right mandibular ridge.

Fig. 9-40. U-shaped graft is divided and secured to the maxillary arch.

Fig. 9-41. Panoramic radiograph soon after graft surgery.

mind that recipient site activation (cortical perforation) is very important because vascularization is less intense in the mandibular arch. Flap closure and suture are performed as already described. Removable prosthesis must not be used during osseous healing. After 5 to 6 months, implants can be installed (Figs. 9-42 to 9-48). Additional period (4-6 months) is required for osseointegration (Figs. 949 to 9-54).

Bone grafts aiming esthetic needs

An excellent esthetic outcome is fundamental to the implant success. In addition to bone quantity and quality, as well as gingival architecture, the presence of osseous crest and relation with adjacent teeth must be considered during treatment planning.

Bone availability is the main factor for ideal implant position-

Fig. 9-42. After six months, the right grafted area is exposed.

Fig. 9-43. Implants are installed in the same area.

Fig. 9-44. After six months, the left grafted area is exposed.

Fig. 9-45. Implants are installed in the same area.

Fig. 9-46. Maxillary grafted area is exposed.

Fig. 9-47. Implant placement.

Fig. 9-48. Panoramic radiograph after implant installation.

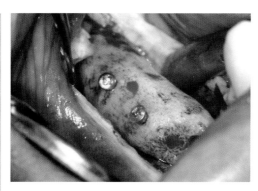

9-42

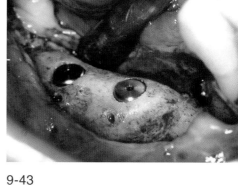

9-43

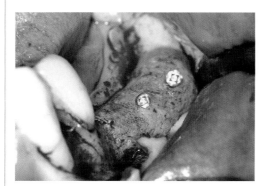

9-44

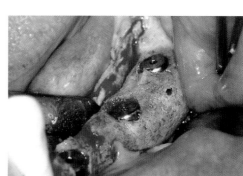

9-45

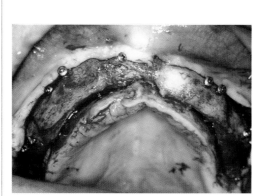

9-46

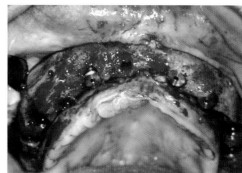

9-47

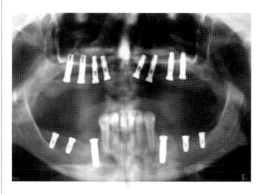

9-48

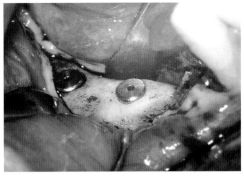

9-49

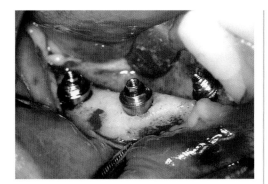

9-50

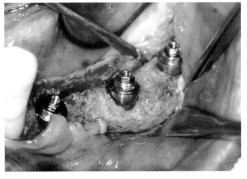

9-51

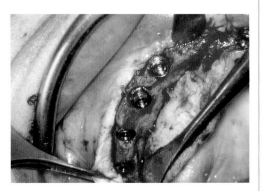

9-52

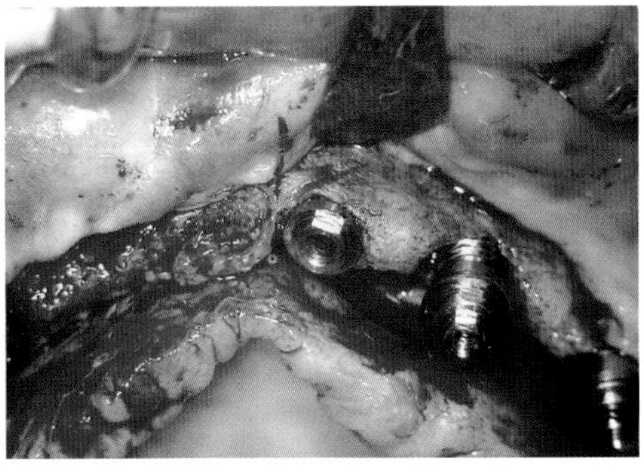

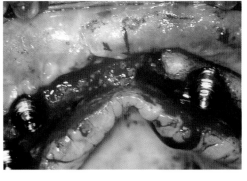

9-53

9-54

Fig. 9-49. On the right side, implants are exposed. Note the lack of bone resorption around implants.

Fig. 9-50. Abutment immediately connected to the implants

Fig. 9-51. Abutments connected on the left side.

Fig. 9-52. Implants exposed on maxilla. Less bone resorption is seen in the posterior areas due to the gingival thickness and reduced occlusal load.

Fig. 9-53. Bone resorption around implants due to total prosthesis.

Fig. 9-54. An implant in the anterior region was lost.

ing which leads to an acceptable esthetic result in prosthetic rehabilitations.

Bone resorption on esthetic areas can be classified as follows:

❑ mild alveolar bone resorption and gingival tissue alterations: implants can be installed without bone grafts. In some cases, vertical soft tissue augmentation is necessary to improve esthetics;

❑ moderate alveolar bone resorption and gingival tissue alterations: a buccal bone graft is necessary to accurately positioning the implants. After 5-6 months, implants can be placed in ideal positions;

❑ large alveolar bone resorption and gingival tissue alterations: bone graft previous to implant placement is mandatory.

Bone grafts aiming esthetics are necessary in mild to moderate defects and be harvested from intra-oral sites. The retromolar area is the preferred site (Figs. 9-55 to 9.66)

Prosthetic protocol for grafted areas

When the implants are exposed in previous grafted areas, unnecessary trauma must be avoided. It is recommended to connect the definitive abutments immediately. The use of provisional prosthesis is not indicated because this will generate traumatic forces on implants. Also, rigid splinting of implants must be achieved as soon as possible.

Final considerations

Surgical planning for edentulous maxilla has considerably included autogenous bone grafts. Predictable and safe results can be achieved when basic principles are strictly followed. However, the risk of treatment morbidity is significant at the donor sites. Nevertheless, advances in bone engineering shows promises. In the near future, patients will benefit from less invasive reconstruction techniques. Otherwise, bone graft continues to be the best option to improve osseointegration outcomes.

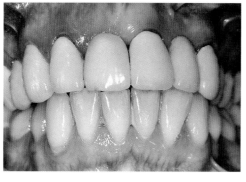

9-55

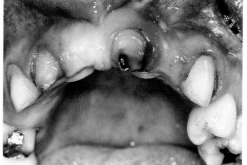

9-56

Fig. 9-55. Initial case, frontal view.

Fig. 9-56. The metalloceramic prosthesis was removed.

Fig. 9-57. An implant was installed in the region of 11. The need for bone graft in the region of 22 has been addressed.

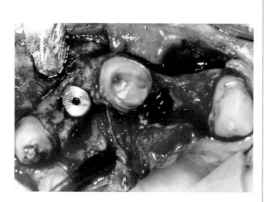

9-57

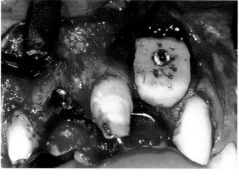

9-58

Fig. 9-58. Occlusal view of the bone defect.

Fig. 9-59. Bone grafted from retromolar area to cover the defect.

Fig. 9-60. The site was reopened after 5 months.

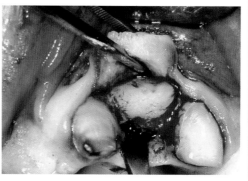

9-59

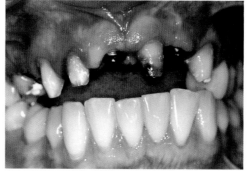

9-60

Fig. 9-61. Implant placement

Fig. 9-62. The implants are exposed after 5 months of osseointegration.

9-61

9-62

Fig. 9-63. Abutments connected to implants.

Fig. 9-64. Occlusal view of implant positioning and gingival architecture.

Fig. 9-65. Definitive prosthesis in place.

Fig. 9-66. Final frontal view.

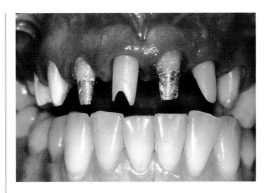

9-63

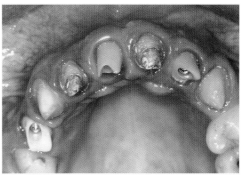

9-64

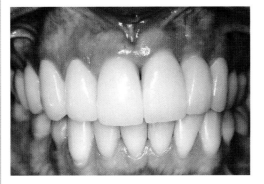

9-65

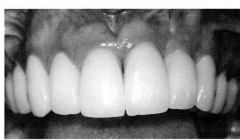

9-66

References

1. ALBREKTSSON, T. Repair of bone grafts. *Scand J Plast Surg* v.14, p.1-12, 1980.
2. BACH, D.R. et al. Cranial, iliac, and demineralized freeze-dried bone grafts of the mandible in dogs. *Arch Otolaryngol Head Neck Surg.* v.117, p.390-395, 1991.
3. BLOCK, M.S. et al. Bone maintenance 5 to 10 years after sinus grafting. *J Oral Maxillofac Surg,* v.56, n.6, p.706-714, 1998.
4. BURCHARDT, H.; ENNEKING, W.F. Transplantation of bone. *Surg Clin North America.* v.58, n.2, p.403-427, 1978.
5. CARVALHO, P.S.P. et al. Influence of bed preparation on the incorporation of autogenous bone grafts: a study in dogs. *Int J Oral Maxillofac Implants.* v.15, n.4, p.565-570, 2000.
6. CHEN, N.T. et al. The roles of revascularization and resorption on endurance of craniofacial onlay bone grafts in the rabbit. *Plast Reconstr Surg.* v.93, p.715-724, 1994.
7. CYPHER, T.J.; GROSSMAN, J.P. Biological principles of bone graft healing. *J Foot Ankle Surg,* v. 35, n.5, p.413-417, 1996
8. FISCHER, J.; WOOD, M.B. Experimental comparison of bone revascularization by musculocutaneous and cutaneous flaps. *Plast Reconstructive Surg,* v.79, p.81-88, 1987.

9. FONSECA, R.J. et al. Revascularization and healing of onlay particulate autologous bone grafts in primates. *J Oral Surg,* v.38, n.8, p.572-577, 1980.

10. HARDESTY, R.A.; MARSH, J.L. Craniofacial onlay bone grafting: A prospective evaluation of graft morphology, orientation and embryonic origin. *Plast Reconstr Surg,* v.85, n.1, p.5-15, 1990.

11. LEW, D. et al. Comparative study of osseointegration of titanium implants in corticocancellous block and corticocancellous chip grafts in canine iliium. *J Oral Maxillofac Surg,* v.52, p.952-958, 1994.

12. LORENZETTI, M. et al. Bone augmentation of th inferior floor of the maxillary sinus with autogenous bone or composite bone grafts: a histologic-histomorphometric preliminary report. *Int J Oral Maxillofac Imp* v.13, p.69-76, 1998.

13. LOZANO et al. The early vascularization of onlay bone grafts. *Plast Reconstructive Surg,* v.58, p.302-305, 1976.

14. MOWLEM, R. Bone grafting. *British Journal of Plastic Surg.* v.8, p.293-304, 1963.

15. NATHANSON, A. The early vascularization of an autogenous bone inlay into an artificial defect in the rabbit mandible. *Acta Otolaryngol* v.85, p.135-148, 1978.

16. PALECKIS, L.G.P. Reparação inicial de enxertos ósseos autógenos em bloco ou em partículas. Estudo microscópico em mandíbula de cães. Araçatuba, 2004. 121p. *Tese (Doutorado em Cirurgia e Traumatologia Bucomaxilofacial)* – UNESP – SP.

17. PALLENSEN, L. et al. Influence of particle size of autogenous bone grafts on the early stages of bone regeneration: a histologic and stereologic study in rabbit calvarium. *Int J Oral Maxillofac Surg,* v.17, n.4, p.499-506, 2002.

18. PINHOLT, E.M. et al. Revascularization of calvarial, mandibular, tibial, and iliac bone grafts in rats. *Ann Plast Surg,* v.33, n.2, p.193-197, 1994.

19. SULLIVAN, W.G.; SZWAJKUN, P.R. Revascularization of cranial versus iliac crest bone grafts in the rat. *Plast Reconstr Surg,* v.87, p.1105-1109, 1991.

20. THOMPSON, N.; CASSON, J. Experimental onlay bone grafts to the jaws. *Plast Reconstr Surg* v.46, p.341-349, 1970.

21. TOLMAN, D.E. Reconstructive procedures with endosseous implants in grafted bone: a review of literature. *Int J Oral Maxillofac Implants,* v.10, p.275-294, 1995.

22. TRUETA, J. The roles of the vessels in osteogenesis. *J Bone Joint Surg,* v.45B, p.402-416, 1963.

23. ZIDE, M.F. Autogenous bone harvest and bone compacting for dental implants. *Compend Contin Educ Dent.* v.21, p.585-590, 2000.

10

FUNDAMENTALS OF ZYGOMATIC IMPLANTS AS A SURGICAL ALTERNATIVE IN THE TREATMENT OF ATROPHIC MAXILLAE

Luis Rogério Duarte

Hugo Nary Filho

Introduction

Maxillary reconstruction approaches present some risk factors since they demand good surgical technique, soft tissue quality, patient cooperation, and excellent medical conditions. However, undisturbed healing cannot be found in all individuals. In some cases, contamination or exposure results in graft partial or total loss, aggravating the initial pre-treatment condition. Long-term stability of hard and soft tissues in the at-rophied maxilla is still an intricate question even for the most successful cases.[1,39,56] Besides, it has implications on implant positioning as well as esthetic and functional requirements.[16,36,40.51] Thus, attempts to achieve a predictable prognosis in patients with severely resorbed maxilla undergone bone graft surgery are elusive. Besides, related postoperative discomfort requires alternative techniques.[62,74]

The development of zygomatic fixture (ZF) represents an excellent alternative for these cases. Initially, it was used for maxillectomized patients due to large trauma or tumor resection. Most of these patients only had anchorage areas in the zygomatic body or frontal process.[37,76] Longer fixtures and modified angulations at the top of the implant were necessary to provide prosthetic treatment. Later, zygomatic fixtures were used to rehabilitate atrophied maxilla. This approach provides less expensive, time-consuming, and more simplified treatment with the same success levels of conventional fixations. Promising results have encouraged the use of ZFs.[47] Although fewer and short-term studies have been reported on immediate function with ZF implants[17,18], its use appears to be quite logical: rigid splinting of inclined implants distributes axial and oblique loads to stabilize complete prosthesis. Brånemark, Gröndahl & Worthington,[11] Sutton,[68] Misch,[48] Spiekerman[65] stated that rehabilitation of atrophied maxilla poses a great challenge. Moreover, large autogenous grafts from extra-oral sites are recommended.

Today, treatment options can be divided into two major groups; first, the use of anchorage/reconstruction techniques with prosthetic compensation. Second, the use of ZFs in severely compromised cases. In this way, patients continue to benefit from their implant-supported prostheses.

Anchorage and Osseointegration

In the initial stages of implant research, Brånemark stated that primary stability was the predominant factor to prevent axial or lateral micromovements, determining the biological phenomena called "osseointegration". The presence of osseous tissue around implants was fundamental to achieve maximum bone-to-implant contact. When anchorage techniques were developed to stabilize fixtures, it was believed that anchorage would be responsible for osseointegration after implant placement.

It seems reasonable to think that cases with obturator or significant added material to the prosthesis can show unfavorable biomechanical behavior, such as poor crown-to-implant ratio or large cantilever arms. Then, surgeons must strongly consider stable anchorage points to distribute applied loads. In this way, secondary stability is developed to maintain osseointegration levels. Resistant anatomic landmarks providing structural rigidity must be addressed. If delayed loading is planned, cross-arch metallic infrastructures represent a third factor in implant stability. On the other hand, they must be regarded as a secondary stability factor for immediate function.

Duarte et al.[19] stated that bicortical stabilization of ZFs with a total prosthesis soon after its placement (in immediate function) can facilitate osseointegration course and protects overall rehabilitation.

Indications

Zygomatic fixtures were first developed by Brånemark to rehabilitate maxillectomized patients or resection tumors. After, the ZF were regarded as a new surgical option. We now discuss its principal indications.

Large bone grafts in the completely edentulous maxilla

This would be a classical alternative to extensive osseous reconstructions. The anterior region is characterized by sufficient alveolar bone which permits at least two zygomatic fixtures. Ideally, four ZFs are necessary to biomechanically stabilize a polygonal figure (Figs. 10-1 to 10-4). In fact, the two anterior ZFs placed under the nasal fossa act like buttresses to the system and remain stable even when osseointegration fails.

Partial rehabilitation cases without sinus bone graft success

Poor inlay/onlay bone graft quality, site contamination or infection, implant failure due to immediate function and rupture of mucous membrane during sinus lifting without further repair possibilities are situations that compromise patient confidence. Besides, uncertainty regarding vascularization level of affected sites prevents a second attempt. An alternative is to install a ZF and more two conventional anterior and posterior implants. Also, the pterygoid bone is a viable option (Figs. 10-5 to 10-9). An implant-supported dentogingival prosthesis can be made to rehabilitate functional and esthetic needs.

Maxillectomized patients due to tumor resection

Patients suffering from large resection facial tumors have poor self-steem and social interactions. This represents a great effort during surgical and prosthetic management (Figs. 10-10 to 10-13). Attempts with autogenous bone grafts can be made, but the lack of soft tissue to achieve a free-tension flap closure and adequate vascularization is a concern because bone viability is fundamental. In some cases, when surgical management is impossible or patients do not accept it, the prosthesis design has to be modified and ZFs are a sound option. Two well-anchored zygoma fixtures can be

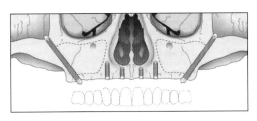

10-1

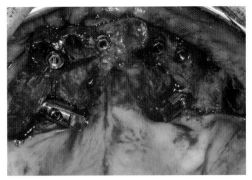

10-2

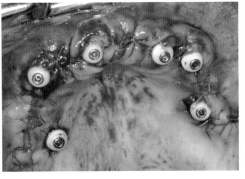

10-3

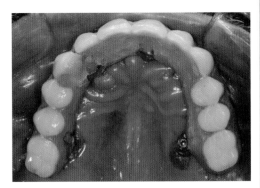

10-4

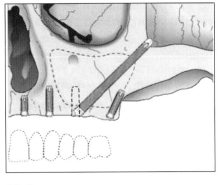

10-5

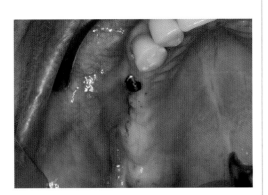

10-6

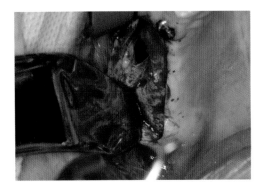

10-7

Fig. 10-1. Therapeutic option with two posterior ZF fixtures and four conventional implants in the anterior region.

Fig. 10-2. Fixtures installed.

Fig. 10-3. Implant exposure and Multi-Unit abutment connection.

Fig. 10-4. Installed prosthesis. (case conducted by Dr Luis Guillermo Peredo and Dr. Rogerio Luis Duarte).

Fig. 10-5. Alternative approach: zygoma fixure with three conventional implants to stabilize central fulcrum point.

Fig. 10-6. Posterior maxillary region where the ZF is indicated due to the failure of sinus bone graft surgery.

Fig. 10-7. Maxillary sinus wall fenestration found during attempt to fill the sinus.

Fig. 10-8. A ZF was installed in the maxillary tuberosity and pterygoid process.

Fig. 10-9. Close view of conventional implant on the tuberosity region and pterygoid process. (Case conducted by Dr. Luis Rogerio Duarte, Andre Carlos de Freitas and Maddy Crusoe at the Bahia Dental School, Bahia University, Brazil.)

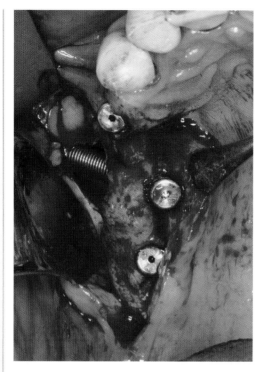

10-8

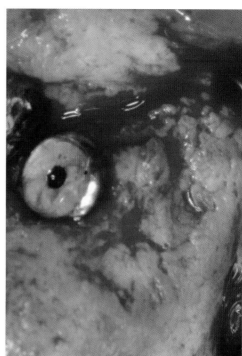

10-9

used for a maxillofacial device. This prosthesis behaves like a bar-retained overdenture. It can be removed to facilitate periimplant oral hygiene procedures.

Conversion of two to four-implant overdentures in fixed prostheses, using two additional ZF

Many overdenture cases can be turned into fixed prostheses. Overdentures are common due to insufficient bone in maxillary posterior region. Normally, inlay bone grafts can be planned but socio-economical issues prevent its use. Besides, a sinus graft procedure demands a donor area or bone substitutes. In this way, overdentures can be implant-retained and/or mucous-supported. In the maxillary arch, they are similar to fixed acrylic prosthesis except that palatal portion can be removed. This enhances oral hygiene measures and patients can better appreciate taste foods. After osseointegration period, abutments are immediately installed during exposure, a new prosthetic bar is made and the fixed-hybrid prosthesis delivered up to 48 hours. Cases of traumatic gingival inflammation can have a similar treatment. When prostheses are screwed, this is no longer a problem (Figs. 10-14 to 10-21).

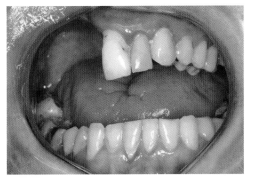

10-10

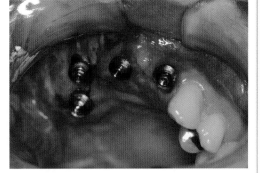

10-11

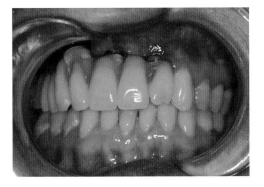

10-12

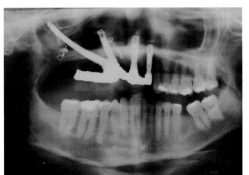

10-13

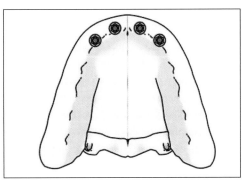

10-14

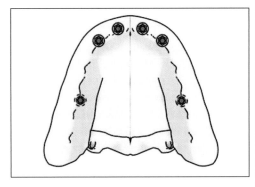

10-15

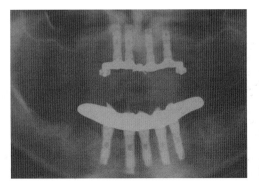

10-16

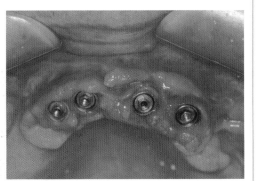

10-17

Fig. 10-10. This patient undergone maxillectomy due to tumor resection.

Fig. 10-11. Three conventional implants and one ZF are installed.

Fig. 10-12. Frontal view of the installed prosthesis.

Fig. 10-13. Panoramic radiograph. (Clinic case conducted by P-I Brånemark and Carlos Eduardo Francischone.)

Fig. 10-14. Implant positioning for maxillary overdenture.

Fig. 10-15. in this new approach, two zygoma fixtures are incorporated to final prosthesis design.

Fig. 10-16. Panoramic radiograph showing peri-implantitis and loss of the end abutment on the maxillary quadrant.

Fig. 10-17. Occlusal view of standard abutments.

Fig. 10-18. ZFs are installed on the second premolar areas.

Fig. 10-19. Panoramic radiograph after ZF placement and removal of compromised implant.

Fig. 10-20. Occlusal view of fixed prosthesis after ZF installation.

Fig. 10-21. Frontal aspect of rehabilitated patient.

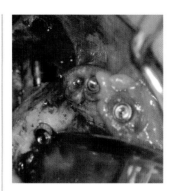

10-18

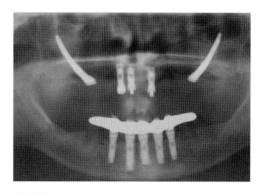

10-19

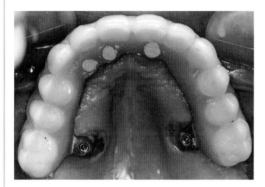

10-20

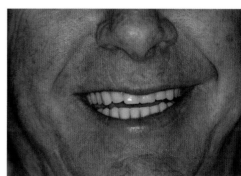

10-21

Failure of terminal implants in complete maxillary rehabilitations

Sometimes, oral rehabilitation of atrophied maxilla is limited by advanced lateral maxillary sinus wall position due to alveolar resorption and sinus expansion. According to Skalak and Rangert[10], increased occlusal forces are verified on terminal implants. When these fixtures are lost, the anterior region is overloaded. Zygomatic implants can help to achieve the original stability (Figs. 10-22 and 10-23). The new fixture can be incorporated to the existing metallic infra-structure by soldering procedures.

Failure of inclined distal implants and ZF installation due to anatomical impairment

Installation of inclined implants can be an alternative to the treatment of atrophied maxilla. Implants are positioned in the canine region and inclined to the second premolar or first molar. In fact, this configuration is very similar to a bracket and can provide immediate implant function. Surgeons must observe maxillary anatomical characteristics to indicate this technique (Fig. 10-22) and establish a polygonal configuration. It demands surgical experience because bone overlying the canine area can be damaged during sequential perforation. For this, ZFs can be positioned more posterior and superiorly having the same treatment philosophy in mind. Then, immediate loading can be achieved without further complications. The same technique can be used when distal implants are lost during osseointegration or function (Figs. 10-24 to 10-28).

Treatment philosophy for zygomatic fixtures on immediate function

Initially, zygomatic fixtures were left undisturbed during osseointegration period. From 2003, research at the Sagrado Coracao University (Bauru, Sao Paulo, Brazil) demonstrated the efficacy of ZFs under immediate loading. The first article published on immediate function with four zygomatic implants was made by Duarte et al.,[17] on January 2004. Two years later, Bedrossian et al.[4] published immediate function on two zygomatic implants. Similar surgical and prosthetic procedures are utilized in this technique. Standard or multiunit abutments can be employed. The treatment sequence is at follows: reverse planning, multifunctional guide, surgical procedure, abutment installation, impression making, master cast, wax-up, bar and artificial teeth try-in, as well as prosthesis adjustment and delivery (Figs. 10-29 to 10-37).

Severely anterior resorbed maxilla due to combination syndrome

In 2001, Prof. Brånemark suggested the use of four zygomatic fixtures to rehabilitate severely resorbed maxillae. This philosophy came from surgical background on maxillectomized cases where non-conventional anchorage points and innovative prosthesis design are necessary. In 2003, our team at the Sagrado Coracao University decided to study this therapy to the severely anterior resorbed maxilla. In these cases, the major issue is to

Fig. 10-22. Schematic drawing showing implant failure.

Fig. 10-23. FZ installation to substitute the compromised implant.

Fig. 10-24. Panoramic radiograph before prosthesis delivery.

Fig. 10-25. Panoramic radiograph after ZF placement on the right side.

Fig. 10-26. Implant rigid splinting for overdenture support.

Fig. 10-27. Overdenture fabricated with the Procera Implant Bridge system.

Fig. 10-28. Final panoramic view (Clinical case conducted by Drs. Mauricio Rigolizo, Hugo Nary Filho and Luis Guillermo Peredo-Paz).

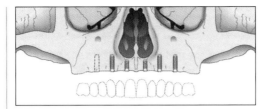

10-22

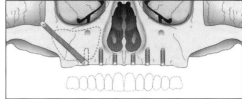

10-23

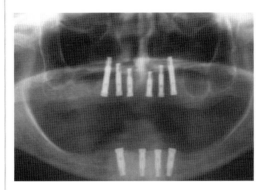

10-24

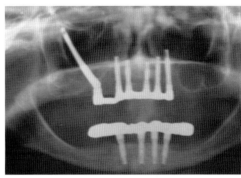

10-25

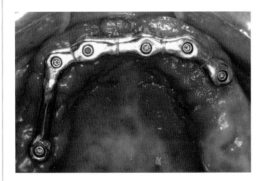

10-26

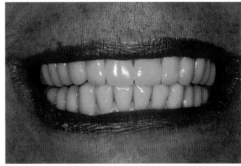

10-27

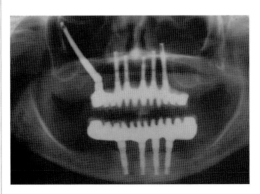

10-28

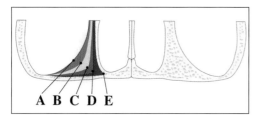

10-29

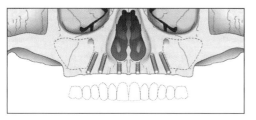

10-30

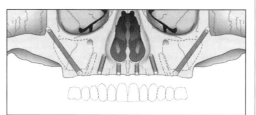

10-31

Fig. 10-29. Classification of canine buttress resorption (according to Bånemark et al., 1978).

Fig. 10-30. Schematic drawing showing theory of inclined implants.

Fig. 10-31. ZF installation maintaining anchorage and prosthetic compensation.

Fig. 10-32. ZF installed after no-successful placement of conventional inclined implant.

Fig. 10-33. Full dento-gingival fixed prosthesis over inclined implants and ZF. (Clinical case conducted by Luis Rogerio Duarte and Sergio Wendell.)

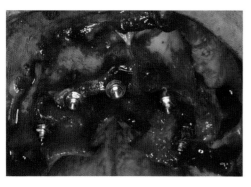

10-32

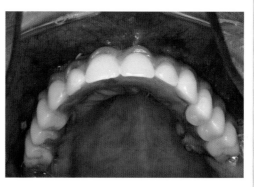

10-33

construct a polygon to stabilize and distribute occlusal forces. At least three directional planes must be splinted to neutralize deleterious forces on osseoin-tegrated implants. But how to achieve this if the anterior region does not provide such bone anchorage?

Based on the suggestions of

Fig. 10-34. Occlusal view, edendulous maxilla.

Fig. 10-35. Pre-operative panoramic radiograph.

Fig. 10-36. Two distal ZFs and four anterior conventional implants installed.

Fig. 10-37. Definitive prosthesis installed within 36 hours.

Fig. 10-38. Postoperative panoramic radiograph. (Clinical case conducted by Drs. Hugo Nary Filho, Luis Rogerio Duarte and Luis Guillermo Peredo Paz.)

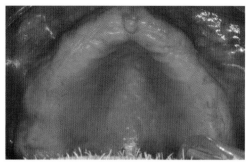

10-34

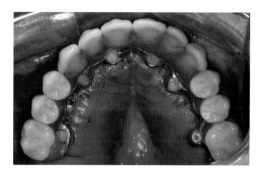

10-35

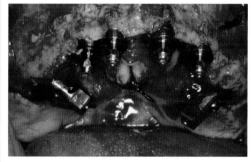

10-36

10-37

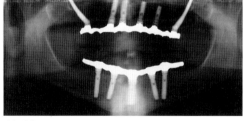

10-38

Prof. Brånemark, Duarte et al.[17,18] proposed a new prosthetic protocol with immediate implant function and prosthodontic rehabilitation supported by 4 ZF. Avoidance of provisionalization is necessary due to the extensive resorption in the anterior maxilla.

Basically, the first ZF is installed at the most superior portion of the zygoma adjacent to the lateral orbital wall; its alveolar portion remains at the incisive or canine area. The second ZF touches the outside of the zygomatic buttress and its head is positioned posterior and bucally to increase load-bearing area (Figs. 10-39 to 10-45).

The success rate of this technique was of 98% after twelve months in 20 patients. It demands adequate skills and a thorough knowledge of surgical face anatomy, such as orbital cavity, infratemporal fossa and associated important structures.

Accidents and complications with zygoma fixtures

Accidents and complications can be expected in some cases. Our clinical philosophy is based on research studies that show high success rates and solutions for every single case of edentulism. When studies reported that osseointegrated implants have a 97% success rate, it must be remembered that these numbers correspond to strictly rigid protocols to rehabilitate mandibular edentulous arch, according to Prof. Brånemark. From a scientific view, not all cases are prone to success and individual analysis is mandatory.

The ZF cases have shown success rates similar to conventional implants. However, complex techniques can bring some drawbacks. Attempts to solve complications involves specialties such as implantology, prosthodontics, surgery, ENT and radiologists.

Periimplant alterations. The zygoma fixture assumes a more palatal position than conventional implants due to the zygomatic bone inclination.[72] Thus, oral hygiene measures are difficult to perform in patients with fixed prosthesis. Plaque accumulation with chronic inflammatory changes can be seen. Long-term ZF success could be decreased due to bone loss in the infection sites. Indeed, the same facts can be observed in conventional implants. In 2004, Brånemark et al.[10] reported that 20% of installed fixtures had some type of soft tissue alteration without jeopardizing osseointegration. Our clinical experience confirms their findings (Figs. 10-46 and 10-47).

Another problem is the screw abutment orifice necessary due to fixture angulation. A gap can be formed, with passage of

Fig. 10-39. Schematic configuration for cases with combination syndrome (according to Brå-nemark, 2001).

Fig. 10-40. Panoramic view. Note severely anterior resorbed maxilla.

Fig. 10-41. A full-thickness flap is elevated to expose the atrophied maxilla.

Fig. 10-42. Surgical exploration after drilling. Observe thin maxillary region due to sinus pneumatization.

Fig. 10-43. Four ZFs are installed according to the proposed protocol.

Fig. 10-44. Definitive prosthesis installed within 48 hours.

Fig. 10-45. Postoperative radiograph after implant placement. (Cortesy by Drs. Luis Rogerio Duarte, Andre Carlos de Freitas e Roberto Brandao Lacerda.)

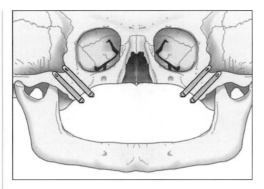

10-39

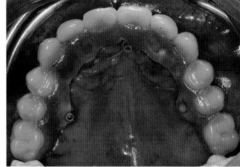

10-40

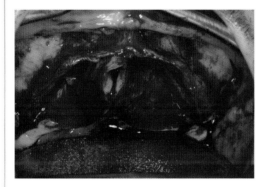

10-41

10-42

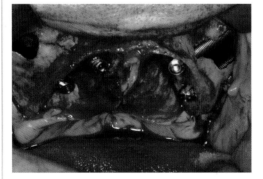

10-43

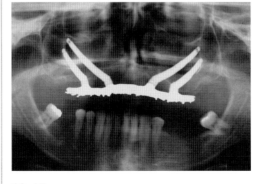

10-44

10-45

231

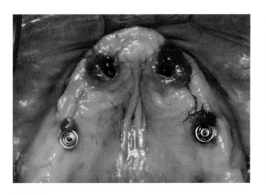

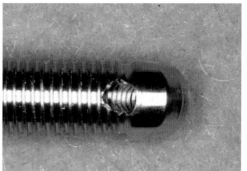

10-46

10-47

Fig. 10-46. Soft tissue inflammatory alterations after prosthesis removal.

Fig. 10-47. The screw abutment orifice.

fluid and bacteria. Nevertheless, there are no comparative studies to support this hypothesis. With new zygomatic fixtures introduction such problem was solved due to screw abutment elimination.

Periorbital lesions and postoperative hematoma

Soft tissue complications can occur at the upper face region due to the use of metallic aspiration cannulas, long burs, and surgical retractors. The drilling sequence is the most critical step. It demands high skilled surgeons, expertise and accurate anatomic knowledge to avoid trauma to the patient. Even thus, accidents may occur due to anatomical variations. Computerized tomography, extra-oral radiographs and stereolithographic models are auxiliary aids to prevent or solve accidents (Figs. 10-48 to 10-50).

With the increased use of ZF, other complications can be warranted in addition to that exposed in this chapter.

Fig. 10-48. Blood clot at the lateral canthal region soon after surgical placement of zygoma fixture.

Fig. 10-49. Postoperative blood collection after three days.

Fig. 10-50. Water´s projection showing the proximity of ZF to the orbital cavity.

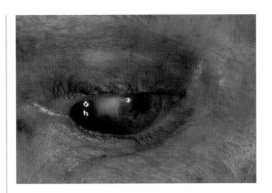

10-48

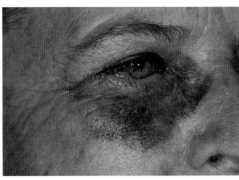

10-49

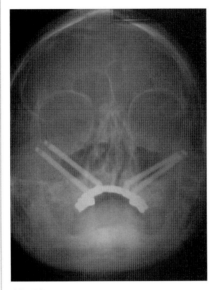

10-50

Final considerations and future directions for zygomatic fixations

The use of ZFs has become a common practice in the implantology field. However, surgical team experience is fundamental to achieve good prognosis. Its use must be strongly considered in cases of bone graft failure or tumor resections. Still, we cannot accept the indiscriminate use of ZFs in all cases. The zygoma fixtures constitute an irreversible procedure and must be properly indicated (Table 10-1).

Newer designs, cantilever beam optimization with inclined implants, and straight fixtures represent hardware modifications proposed by Prof. Brånemark to improve patient's safety as well as quality of life and longevity.

Table 10-1. Anchorage versus reconstructive techniques.

Factors	Zygoma fixtures	Bone grafts
Morbidity	Low	High
Cost	Low	High (three different steps)
Prosthetic needs	High	Low
Hygiene	Difficult	Fair
Esthetics	Good with dentogingival prosthesis	Good but unpredictable
Technical difficulties	High, demand skilled teams	High, demand skilled teams
Maintenance	Difficult	Fair
Predictability	High (95% according to the literature)	Controversial
Periimplant alterations	20% of the cases, according to the literature	Similar to ZFs, but without comparative studies
Treatment time	Reduced	Increased

References

1. ADELL, R.; LEKHOLM, U.; ROCKLER, B.; BRÅNEMARK, P.I. Fifteen year of the study of osseointegrated implants in the treatment of edentulous jaw. *Int. J. Oral Surg.*, 6:387-416, 1981.

2. AL-NAWAS, B. et al. Critical Soft Tissue Parameters of the Zygomatic Implants. *J. Clin. Periodontol.*, v.31, p.497-500, 2004.

3. BEDROSSIAN, E. et al. The Zygomatic Implants: Preliminary Data on Treatment of Severely Resorbed maxillae. A Clinical Report. *Int. J. Oral Maxillofac Implants*, v.17, p.861-865, 2002.

4. BEDROSSIAN, E. et al. Immediate function with zygomatic implant: a graftless solution for the patient with mild to advanced atrophy of the maxilla. *Int. J. Oral Maxillofac. Implants*, 21(6):937-42, 2006.

5. BEZERRA, F.J.B.; AZOUBEL, E. Alternativas cirúrgicas no tratamento da maxila atrófica. In: BEZERRA, F.J.B.; LENHARO, A. *Terapia clínica avançada em implantodontia.* São Paulo: Artes Médicas, 2002, p.159-192.

6. BIJLANI, M.; LOZADA, J.L. Immediately loaded dental implants-influence of early functional contacts on implant stability, bone level integrity, and soft tissue quality: a retrospective 3- and 6- year clinical analysis. *Int. J. Oral Maxillofac. Implants*, v.11, p.126-127, 1996.

7. BOTHUR, S.; JONSSON, G.; SANDAHL, L. Modified Technique Using Multiple Zygomatic Implants

in Reconstruction of the Atrophic Maxilla: a Technical Note. *Int. J. Oral Maxillofac Implants.*, v.18, p.902–904, 2003.

8. BOYES-VARLEY, J.G. et al. Surgical Modifications to the Brånemark Zygomaticus Protocol in the Treatment of the Severely Resorbed Maxilla: A Clinical Report. *Int. J. Oral Maxillofac Implants.*, v.18, n.2, p.232–237, 2003.

9. BRÅNEMARK, P.I. Fixture in Os Zigomaticum. *Gotemborg Brånemark Osseintegration Center.* 1999, 10p. Apostila.

10. BRÅNEMARK, P.I. et al. Zygoma Fixture in the Management of Advanced Atrophy of the Maxilla: Tecnique and Long-Term Results. *Scand J. Plast. Reconstr. Surg. Hand Surg.*, v.38, p.70-85, 2004.

11. BRÅNEMARK, P. I.; GRÖNDAHL, K.; WORTHINGTON, P. Osseointegration and Autogenous Onlay Bone Grafts: *Reconstruction of the Edentulous Atrophic Maxilla.* 1ª ed. Chicago: Quintessence Books, 2001, 160p.

12. COELHO, A.B.; TELLES, D.; FERREIRA, N.T. Guia Multifuncional: uma Abordagem Protética Racional da Carga Imediata sobre Implantes Osseointegrados. *In:* TELLES, D.; HOLLWEG, H.; CASTELLUCCI, L. *Prótese Total: Convencional e sobre Implantes.* 1ª ed. São Paulo: Ed. Santos, 2003, p.213-239.

13. COLOMINA, L. Immediate Loading of Implant-Fixed Mandibular Prostheses: a Prospective 18-Month Follow-up Clinical Study-Preliminary Report. *Implant. Dent,* v.10, n.1, p.23-29, 2001.

14. COOPER et al. A Multicenter 12-Month evaluation of single tooth implants restored 3 weeks after I stage surgery. *Int. J. Oral Maxillofac Implants.*, v.16, p.182-192, 2001.

15. CUNHA, H.A. et al. A Comparison Between Cutting Torque and Resonance Frequency in the Assessment of Primary Stability and Final Torque Capacity of Standard and TiUnit Single-Tooth Implants Under Immediate Loading. *Int. J. Oral Maxillofac Implants.*, v.19, p.578-585. 2004.

16. DESJARDINS, R.P. Prosthesis design for osseointegrated implants in the edentulous maxilla. *Int. J. Oral Maxillofac Implants.*, v.7, p.311-320, 1992.

17. DUARTE, L.R. et al. Reabilitação da maxila atrófica utilizando quatro fixações zigomáticas em sistema de carga imediata. *Implants News,* v.1, n.1, p.25-30, Jan/Fev. 2004.a

18. DUARTE, L.R.; NARY FILHO, H.; FRANCISCHONE, C.E.; PEREDO, L.G.; BRÅNEMARK, P-I. The establishment of a protocol for total rehabilitation of atrophic maxillae employing four zygomatic fixtures in a immediate loading system – a 30 month clinical trial and follow-up. *Clin. Impl. Dent Rel. Res.,* v.9, n.4, p.186-196, 2007.

19. DUARTE, L.R. Estabelecimento de protocolo para reabilitações totais da maxila atrófica utilizando fixações zigomáticas em sistema de carga imediata. 2005. (Ex. 176 fls.) Dissertação de Mestrado, USC, Bauru-SP.

20. EGER, D.E.; GUNSOLLEY, J.C.; FELDMAN, S. Comparison of Angled and Standard Abutment and their Effect on Clinical Outcomes: a Preliminary Report. *Int. J. Oral Maxillofac. Implants,* v.15, n.6, p.819-823, 2000.

21. ENGELMAN, M.J. Maxillay-Completely Edentulous. In: ENGELMAN, M.J. *Clinical Decision making and Treatment Planning in Osseointegration.* 1.ed. Ilenois: Quintessence, 1996, p.177-197.

22. ERIKSSON, A.R.; ALBREKTSSON, T. Temperature Threshold levels for Heat-Induced Bone Tissue Injury: a Vital Microscopic Study in the Rabbit. *Journal of Prosthetic Dentistry,* v.50, p.101-107, 1983.

23. FERRARA, E. D.; STELLA, J. P. Restorations of the Edentulous Maxilla: the Case for the Zygomatic Implants. *J. Oral Maxillofac. Surg.,* v.62, p.1418-1422. 2004.

24. FILHO, H.N.; ILG, J.P. Atrofia Severa da Maxila. *In:* DINATO, J.C.; POLIDO, W.D. *Implantes Osseointegrados: Cirurgia e Prótese.* 1ª ed. São Paulo: Artes Médicas, 2001, p.343-372.

25. FILHO, H.N.; FRANCISCHONE, C.E.; SARTORI, I.A.M. Considerações sobre o uso da fixação zigomática no tratamento de maxilas Atróficas. *In:* GOMES, L.A. *Implantes Osseointegrados: Técnica e Arte.* 1ª ed. São Paulo: Ed. Santos, 2002, p.143-155.

26. FILHO, H.N.; FRANCISCHONE, C.E.; SARTORI, I.A.M. Fixação zigomática. *In:* GOMES, L.A. *Implantes Osseointegrados: Cirurgia e Prótese.* 1ª ed. São Paulo: Artes Médicas, 2001, 529p.

27. FRANCISCHONE JÚNIOR, C.E.; TULER, R.F. Função ou carga imediata em osseointegração. *Bio Odonto,* v.1, n.2, mai./jun. 2004.

28. FREITAS, A.C. et al. Prototipagem Aplicada ao Planejamento Reverso das Fixações Zigomáticas. *Implants News,* v.2, n.2, p.25-30. mar./abr. 2005.

29. GAPSKI, R. et al. Critical Review of Immediate Implant Loading. *Clin. Oral Impl. Res.,* v.14, n.4, p.515–527, 2003.

30. HEITZ-MAYFIELD, L.J. et al. Does Excessive Occlusal Load Affect Osseointegration? An Experimental Study in the Dog. *Clin. Oral Impl. Res.,* v.15, p.259-268, 2004.

31. HENRY, P.J. A Review of Guidelines of Implants Rehabilitation of the Edentulous Maxilla. *J. Prosthetic Dent.,* v.87, p.281-288, 2002.

32. HENRY, P.; ROSEMBERG, I. Single stage-surgery for rehabilitation of edentulouos mandible: preliminary results. *Practical Periodontics and Aesthetic Dentistry.,* v.6, p.15-22, 1994.

33. HILDEBRAND, D. et al. Immediate Loading of Implants in Edentulous Jaws: a Serie of Case Reports. *Int. J. Oral Maxilofacial Surgery,* v.30, n. suppl A, p. S14, 2001.

34. HIRSCH, J.M. et al. A Clinical Evaluation of the Zygoma Fixture: One Year of Follow-Up at 16 Clinics. *J Oral Maxillofac Surg.,* v.62, p.22-29, 2004.

35. IVANOFF, C.J. et al. Influence of Bicortical or Monocortical Anchorage on Maxillary Implant Stability: a 15-Year Retrospective Study of Brånemark System Implants. *Int. J. Oral Maxillofac. Implants.,* v.15, n.1, p.103-110, 2000.

36. JEMT, T.; LEKHOLM, U. Implant Treatment en Edentulous Maxillae: a 5 Year Follow-up Report on Pacientes with Different Degrees of Jaw Resorption. *Int. J. Oral Maxilofac. Implants,* v.10, p.303-311, 1995.

37. JENSEN, O.T.; BROWND, C; BLACKER, J. Nasofacial Orostheses Supported by Osseointegrated Implants. *Int, J. Oral Maxilofac. Implants,* v.7, p.203-11, 1992.

38. JIMÉNEZ-LÓPES, V. *Carga ou Função Imediata em Implantodontia: Aspectos Cirúrgicos, Protéticos, Oclusais e de Laboratório.* São Paulo: Quintessence, 2005, 288p.

39. KAHNBERG, K-E.; NYSTRÖM, E.; BARTHOLDSSON, L. Combined Use of Bone Grafts and Brånemark Fixtures in the Treatment of Severely Resorbed Maxillae. *Int. J. Oral Maxillofac. Implants,* v.4, n.4, p.297-304, 1989.

40. KELLER, E.E.; TOLMAN, D.E.; ECKERT, S.E. Maxilary Antral-Nasal Autogenous Bone Graft Reconstruction of Compromised Maxilla: a 12-year Retrospective Study. *Int, J. Oral Maxilofac. Implants,* v.14, p.707-721, 1999.

41. KELLY, E. Changes Caused by a Mandibular Removable Partial Denture Opposing a Maxillary Complete Denture. *J Prosthet Dent.,* v.90, p.213-219. 2003.

42. KIM, Y. et al. Occlusal Considerations in Implant Therapy: Clinical Guidelines with Biomechanical Rationale. *Clin. Oral. Impl. Res.,* v.16, p.1-26, 2005.

43. KOSER, L.R.; DUARTE, L.R.; CAM-

POS, P.S.F. Emprego da Técnica de Fixação Zigomática como Alternativa para Maxila Atrésica. *Revista Brasileira de Implantodontia e Prótese sobre Implantes,* v.11, n.44, p.289-295, 2004.

44. LAMBERT, P.M.; MORRIS, H.F.; OCHI, S. Positive Effect of Surgical Experience with Implants in Second-Stage Implants Survival. *Journal of Oral and Maxillofacial Surgery,* v.55, p.21-18, 1997.

45. MALEVEZ, C. et al. Clinical Outcome of 103 Consecutive Zygomatic Implants: a 6-48-months Follow-up study. *Clin. Oral Impl. Res,* v.15, p.18-22, 2004.

46. MALEVEZ, C. et al. Use of Zygomatics Implants to Deal with Resorbed Posterior Maxillae. *Periodontology,* v.33, n.1, p.82-89, out. 2003.

47. MATSUMOTO, M.A. et al. Fixação Zigomática. *Pesquisa Odontológica Brasileira (Brazilian Oral Research)* v.14, p.21 supl. 2000 SBPqO – Universidade de São Paulo.

48. MISCH, C.E. Classificação e Planos de Tratamento para Arcos Parcial e Completamente edêntulos em Implantodontia. *In:* MISCH, C. E. *Implantes Dentários Contemporâneos.* São Paulo: Ed. Santos, 2000, p.163-174.

49. MISCH, C.E. Implants design considerations for the posterior regions of the mouth. *Contemporary Implants Dentistry,* v.8, p.376-378.

50. MORRIS, H.F.; MANZ, M.C.; TAROLLI, J.H. Success of Multiple Endosseous Dental Implant Designs to Second Stage Surgery Across Study Sites. *Journal of Oral and Maxillofacial Surgery,* v.55, p.76-82, 1997.

51. NARY FILHO, H.; ILG, J.P. Atrofia severa da maxila. In: DINATTO, J.C.; POLIDO, W.D. *Implantes Osseointegrados, Cirurgia e Prótese.* São Paulo: Artes Médicas, 2001, p.343-372.

52. NARY FILHO, H., FRANCISCHONE, C.E., SARTORI, I.A.M. Considerações sobre o Uso da Fixação Zigomática no Tratamento de Maxilas Atróficas. *Implantes Osseointegrados: Técnica e Arte.* São Paulo: Ed. Santos, 2002, p.143-156-155.

53. NKENKE, E. et al. Anatomic Site Evaluation of the Zygomatic Bone for Dental Implant Placement. *Clin. Oral Impl. Res.,* v.14, p.72-79, 2003.

54. NKENKE, E. et al. Morbidity of Harvesting of Bonegrafts from the Iliac Crest for Preprosthetic Augmentation Procedures: a Prospective Study. *Int. J. Oral Maxillofac. Surg,* v.33, p.157-163, 2004.

55. NOBEL BIOCARE. *Zygoma Fixtures Clinical Procedures.* Götemburg, Sweden, 2000.

56. NYSTRÖM, E.; KAHNBERG, K-E.; GUNNE, J. Bone Grafts and Brånemark Implants in the Treatment of the Severely Resorbed Maxilla: a 2-Year Longitudinal Study. *Int. J. Oral Maxillofac. Implants,* v.8, n.1, p.45-53, 1993.

57. PALMQVIST, S.; CARLSSON, G.E.; OWALL, B. The Combination Syndrome: a Literature Review. *J. Prosthet Dent.,* v.90, p.270-275, 2003.

58. PAREL, S.M. et al. Remote Implant Anchorage for the Rehabilitation of Maxillary Defects. *J. Prosthet Dent.,* v.86, p.377-381, 2001.

59. PETRUSON B. Sinuscopy in patients with titanium implants in the nose and sinuses. *Scand J Plast Reconstr Surg Hand Surg.,* v.38, p.86-93, 2004.

60. RANGERT, B.; JEMT, T. JORNEUS, L. Forces and Moments on Brånemark Implants. *Int. J. Oral Maxillofac. Implants,* v.4, p.241-247, 1989.

61. RANGERT, B.; RENOUARD, F. Fatores de risco no tratamento com implantes. *Evolução clínica e conduta.* São Paulo: Quintessence, 2001, 176p.

62. ROUMANAS, E. et al. Craniofacial defects and osseointegrated implants: Six-year Follow-up Report on the Success Rates of Craniofacial Implants at UCLA. *Int, J. Oral Maxilofac. Implants,* v.9, p.579-585, 1994.

63. RIGOLIZZO, M.B.; CAMILLI, A.; FRANCISCHONE, C.E.; PADO-VANI, C.R.; BRÅNEMARK, P. I.; ZIGOMATIC BONE: Anatomic Bases for Osseointegrated Implant Anchorage. Oral Maxillofac Implants 2005; 20:441-447.

64. SCHNITMAN, P.A. et al. Immediate Fixed Interium Prostheses Supported by Two-Stage Threaded Implants: Methodology and Results. *J. Oral Implants*, v.16, p.96-105, 1990.

65. SPIEKERMANN, H. et al. *Color Atlas of Dental Medicine – Implantology.* Tieme, 1995, 388p.

66. STEENBERGHE, D.V.; SVENSSON, M.Q.B.; BRÅNEMARK, P.I. Clinical Examples of What Can Be Achieved with Osseointegration in Anatomically Severely Compromised Patients. *Periodontology 2000*, v.33, n.1, p.90-99, out. 2003.

67. STELLA, J.P.; WANER, M.R. Sinus Slot Techinique for Simplification and Improved Orientation of Zygomaticus Dental Implants: a Technical Notes. *Int. J. Oral Maxillofac Implants*, v.15, p.889-893, 2000.

68. SUTTON, D.N. et al. Changes in Facial Form Relative to Progressive Atrophy of the Edentulous Jaws. *Int. J. Oral Maxillofac. Surg.*, v.33, p.676–682, 2004.

69. SZMUKLER-MONCLER, S. et al. Considerations Preliminary to the Application of Early and Immediate Loading Protocols in Dental Implatology. *Clin. Oral Impl. Res.*, v.11, p.12-25, 2000.

70. SZMUKLER-MONCLER, S. et al. Timing of Loading and Effect of Micromotion on Bone-Dental Implant Interface: Review of Experimental Literature. *J. Biomed. Mater. Res.*, v.43, p.192-203, 1998.

71. TAMURA, H.; SASAKI, K.; WATA-HIKI, R. Primary Insertion of Implants in the Zigomatic Bone Following Subtotal Maxillectomy Bull. *Tokyo dent Coll*, v.41, p.21-24, 2000.

72. UCHIDA, Y. et al. Measurement of the Maxilla and Zygoma as an Aid in Installing Zygomatic Implants. *Int. J. Oral Maxillofac Surg*, v.59, p.1193-1198, 2001.

73. VAN STEENBERGHE, D. et al. Accuracy of Drilling Guides for Transfer from Three-Dimensional CT- Based Planning to Placement of Zygoma Implants in Human Cadavers. *Clin. Oral Impl. Res.*, v.14, p.131-136, 2003.

74. VENTURELLI, A. A modified surgical protocol for placing implants in the maxillary tuberosity: clinical results at 36 months after loading with fixed partial dentures. *Int. J. Oral Maxillofac. Implants*, v.11, n.6, p.743-749, 1996.

75. VRIELINCK, L. et al. Imaged- Based Planning and Clinical Validation of Zygoma and Pterygoid Implant Placement in Patient with Severe Bone Atrophy Using Customized Drill Guides. Preliminary Results from a Prospective Clinical Follow-up Study. *Int. J. Oral Maxillofac Surg.*, v.32, p.7-14, 2003.

76. WEISCHER, T.; SCHETTLER, D.; MOHR, C. Titanium Implants in the Zygoma as Retaining Elements after Hemimaxillectomy. *Int. J. Oral Maxillofac. Implants*, v.12, n.2, p.211-214, 1997.

11

Soft Tissue Management on Implantology

José Bernardes das Neves

Introduction

The use of osseointegrated implants to substitute traumatized or root fractured teeth, cysts, odontogenic tumors, advanced periodontal disease, failures on root canal therapy, has becoming a good option for partially or complete edentulous patients.[1,2] However, anterior regions need accurate techniques[1] because dental prostheses with more natural looking-appearance are mandatory in the so called "esthetic zone". Usually, soft and hard tissue alterations are seen after tooth loss. This will require bone width and height augmentation procedures, as well as re-establishment of gingival architecture. In this sense, soft tissue esthetics has become an important factor to achieve success in implant-supported restorations.[3] Also, adequate bone and alveolar ridge configuration are essential to common rehabilitation patterns.[4] The knowledge of bone healing process is a key factor regarding the moment of implant placement.[2] Several factors must be considered such as extraction alveolar socket anatomy, surgical procedure, treatment duration, esthetics and osseointegration. The same rationale is necessary for soft tissue management: whether to augment or create a keratinized band, timing of soft tissue management (before, during or after implant placement), regeneration papilla techniques, vestibuloplasty, and root coverage.

Since is not possible to separate soft and hard tissue treatment, both topics will be discussed in the following sections.

Soft Tissue

The importance of keratinized soft tissue

The role and necessity of keratinized soft tissue around osseointegrated implants is unclear.[5] Some studies argue that a keratinized mucosal barrier enhances oral hygiene measures, prevents periimplant infections, protects against traumatic forces, and improves prosthesis appearance.[1,2,3,5,7] Besides, implant thread exposure, subsequent bone loss, and periimplant pocket formation[10] could be avoided when adequate sot tissue thickness is found.

Soft tissue shape and volume can be managed before, during or after implant installation.[5] Some approaches include the connective tissue graft, free gingival graft, coronal or laterally positioned pedicle flap, orthodontic forced eruption, palatal rotated flap, and root reduction below the crest of alveolar bone to cre-

ate adequate gingival thickness. All above techniques will be described to augment the band of keratinized soft tissue. Although not necessary, its presence has several advantages:

❑ gingival margins maintain their positions and became more resistant to recession;
❑ better esthetics due to papilla formation;
❑ oral hygiene is facilitated;
❑ surgical management is improved;
❑ impression making procedures are less aggressive;
❑ periimplant mucosa does not collapse over implant platform;
❑ it creates a mucosal barrier against inflammatory process (less vascularized tissue)[9];
❑ avoids excessive free gingival margin dislocation
❑ offers great resistance to toothbrushing trauma.

A band of keratinized tissue alone does not dictate better outcomes. Gingival thickness is also an important parameter (gingival biotypes).[10] Metallic collar showing through gingival tissues reflects the lack of adequate thickness.

Soft tissue quantity – classification

This approach is necessary before implant placement to optimize achieved results. Surgical intervention depends on the presence, quantity and localization of keratinized gingiva around osseointegrated implants.

CLASSIFICATION ACCORDING TO ONO, NEVINS AND CAPETTA[9]

This classification is based on keratinized tissue around proposed implant site:

❑ **Type I.** More than 5mm of keratinized mucosa overlying the partial or completely edentulous ridge. Flap can be apically positioned to augment thickness of labial tissue (Fig. 11-1).

❑ **Type II**. Less than 5mm of keratinized mucosa is found. This group can be divided into:
Type II, Class 1: minimal keratinized tissue at the alveolar ridge crest, with less or no tissue at the labial area. Also, sufficient attached gingival tissue on the lingual side can be found. A free gingival graft would address deficiencies on the labial side (Fig. 11-2).
Type II, Class 2: the tissue on the lingual side will be excised. A free gingival graft is performed on the labial side and the flap is apically positioned on the lingual side to augment keratinized tissue on both sides (Fig. 11-3).

❑ **Type III.** Keratinized tissue is not found overlying either alveolar crest or labial side. A free gingival graft is indicated to augment the labial side along with apically flap positioned flap (Fig. 11-4).

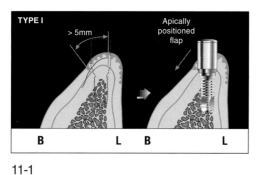

11-1

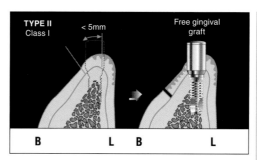

11-2

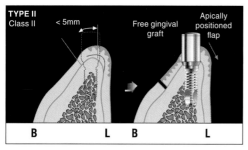

11-3

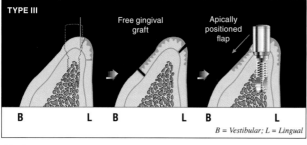

11-4

Fig. 11-1. Type I. Flap can be apically positioned to augment keratinized tissue on the labial side.

Fig. 11-2. Type II, class 1: less or no keratinized tissue is found on labial side. A free gingival graft is recommended.

Fig. 11-3. Type II, class II: Most part of lingual keratinized gingival will be excised. A gingival graft is planned on the labial side along with an apically positioned flap on the lingual side.

Fig. 11-4. Type III. There is no keratinized gingival either on labial or alveolar ridge crest. A gingival graft will be made to augment the area of keratinized tissue on the labial side along with an apically positioned flap.

Esthetic Considerations

A multidisciplinary team is fundamental to achieve success during esthetic planning. In the anterior maxillary region, some considerations can be made:[10]

❏ the proposed edentulous area must have adequate bone volume. This can be provided through alveolar distraction osteogenesis and/or graft techniques, before or during implant placement;

❏ implant insertion must be accurate and planned according to the prosthesis;

❏ the implant-abutment interface must be stable and margin gaps reduced to acceptable parameters;

❏ adequate emergence profile is mandatory;

❏ prosthesis must look like natural tissues.

The esthetic discipline on Implantology aims to create soft tissue harmony without abrupt changes on scalloping, bone crest and papillary height configuration.[10]

During papillary creation, two important anatomic structures must be observed:

❏ bone crest height at interproximal areas
❏ labial cortical plate height and thickness

Tarnow et al.[11] demonstrated that the distance from the crest of bone to the base of contact area could be correlated with the presence or absence of the interproximal papilla in humans. When the distance was 5mm, papilla completely fills the interproximal area. When the distance was 6mm, the papilla was present 56% of time, and when the distance was 7mm or more, the papilla was present 27% of the time or less (Fig. 11-5).

Salama et al.[20] suggested that the presence, contour and thickness of periimplant papilla can be influenced in the same manner. They determined that interpoximal height of bone between tooth and implant would be of 5.5mm, between adjacent implant of 4.5mm, and between adjacent teeth of 5mm (Fig. 11-6).

These authors stated that predictable esthetics can be achieved only when lip line and bone scalloping favors adequate soft and hard tissue contours. Clinical observations suggested a prognostic classification system for the periimplant papillae (PPL). Their classification is based on the available interproximal height of bone (IHB) (Fig. 11-7) for the maxillary anterior sextant.

Biologic Width

Success on the esthetic zone also depends on thorough knowledge of tissue responses, less traumatic management, and good observation of anatomic structures. The arrangement of soft tissue attachment around osseointegrated implants has shown parameters similar to that described for the dentogingival unit[10,11] (Fig. 11-8). Animal model studies reported constant gingival thickness of 3mm. The biologic width of periimplant mucosa comprehends the supracrestal zone, connective tissue (1mm), and the epithelial structure (gingival sulcus and junctional epithelium of 2mm).

Osseous Tissue

Alveolar ridge deformities are due to several factors, such as congenital, developmental, tooth loss, accidents, poor root canal therapy, trauma, advanced periodontal disease, cysts or odontogenic tumors, trauma to the cortical plates during tooth removal, fenestration, dehiscence, and long-term use of removable appliances. Ninety percent of osseous deformities are caused by tooth loss.[12]

The alveolar residual ridge resorption (RRR) has been addressed in the literature. For example, Atwood[21] described six stages of resorption. Clinical observations demonstrated that the ridge resorption is more intense in the first year after tooth extraction when 25% of bone loss is verified, increasing to 40% after three years.

For more than 15 years, several techniques have been used to compensate for alveolar bone loss in the esthetic anterior region: osseous guided regeneration, membrane barriers with or without titanium mesh, onlay bone grafts, block and particulate autologous grafts, bone removed from extra (iliac crest, cranial vault) or intra oral sites, lyophilized bone grafts, and more recently, alveolar distraction osteogenesis.[2,10] However, clinical studies have shown that width augmentation is more favorable than vertical augmentation.[10]

Classification of osseous defects implicated in the soft tissue architecture

There are several classifications for these deformities. In this section we described four that represent most type of defects

SALAMA CLASSIFICATION[24]

According to Salama classification,[22] the tooth to be extracted has two distinct zones: coronal and alveolar defects. In this way, there are three modalities regarding alveolar extraction sockets:

Type I (alveolar) – immediate implant placement is recommended with or without bone guided regeneration.

Type II (alveolar and coronal defect) – implant can be placed

Fig. 11-5. Graphical representations of relationship between osseous crest and gingival papillary tissue.

Fig. 11-6. Class I: optimal prognosis for esthetic restorations; 2mm from cementoenamel junction to contact point areas. IHB is 4 to 5mm.
Class II: guarded prognosis; 4mm from the cementoenamel junction to the contact point areas. IHB is 6 to 7mm.
Class III: poor prognosis; >5mm from the cementoenamel junction to the contact point areas. IHB is >7mm.

Fig. 11-7. A – Contact point area, B – interproximal bone height between natural teeth, C – interproximal bone height between implants.

Fig. 11-8. Biologic width on teeth and implants.

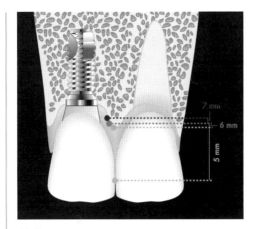

11-5

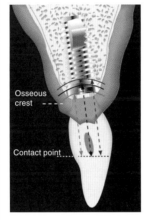

11-6

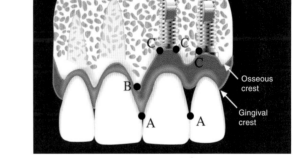

11-7

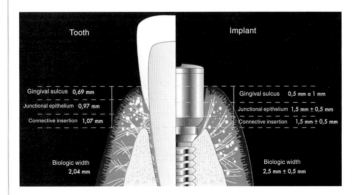

11-8

on facial surface. treatment sequence is orthodontic forced eruption with tooth removal, implant installation, barrier membrane and ridge augmentation.

Type III (coronal defect) – considered problematic, it cannot provide primary implant stability. Tooth extrusion, membrane and ridge augmentation are necessary. The implants must be installed only within 6 to 12 months after bone guided regeneration (BGR).

SEIBERT CLASSIFICATION – RIDGE DEFECTS[23]

Class I: loss of tissue in the buccolingual direction with normal height in the apical-coronal direction;

Class II: loss of tissue in the apical-coronal direction, with normal width in the bucco-lingual direction;

Class III: a combination of Class I and Class II (bone of both height and width).

Seibert[23] introduced this system in 1983, whose treatment options were based on defect type to be restored with a pontic. Width deficiencies had better prognosis than defects in height. With the advent of osseointregrated implants, this classification had to be broadened because other non described defects were found in the dental practice. Several different defects cannot be treated

in the same way. The comprehension of type and defect size extent are necessary for treatment planning, timing, and the need of additional implants Wang & Shammarika[12] proposed a new classification system based on Siebert divisions[14]:

Horizontal, vertical and combined defects: each category was divided into **small** (≤3mm), **medium** (4-6mm) or **large** (≥7mm) (Fig. 11-9).

TINTI AND BENFENATI CLASSIFICATION[24]

Based on the principles of blood clot protection and preservation, these authors classified osseous defects in 5 categories, divided into classes I and II, according to the following situations:

Alveolar bone walls after extrusion

Here, alveolar walls are considered for immediate implant placement or to protect blood clot.

Class I: after tooth removal, intact osseous walls are seen. The implant will be completely surrounded by bone (Figs. 11-10 to 11-12).

Class II: one of the alveolar walls was lost, and some threads will be exposed (Figs. 11-11 and 11-12).

Fig. 11-9. Classification of ridge defects: small – ≤3mm; medium – between 4 and 6mm; large – ≥7mm. (Adapted from Wang HL, Shammarika[12].)

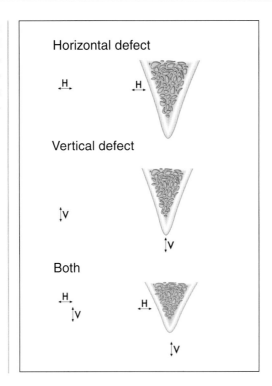

Horizontal defect

Vertical defect

Both

Fenestration

Localized bone loss on the facial or palatal portion (lingual).

Class I: implant is surrounded by less bone but remains inside the alveolar envelope (Fig. 11-13).

Class II: implant is outside the alveolar envelope. There is a convex defect with apical thread exposure (Fig. 11-14).

Bone dehiscence

Bone loss is fewer than 50% from the top to apical portion.

Class I: implant surface is inside the alveolar envelope (Fig. 11-15).

Class II: implant surface is outside the alveolar envelope. (Fig. 11-16)

Horizontal ridge defect

Class I: implant is 50% outside, but inside the alveolar envelope (Fig. 11-17).

Class II: implant is totally on the outer portion. Membrane barriers w/or bone graft are necessary for regeneration (Fig. 11-18).

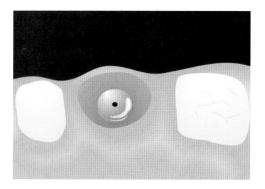

11-10

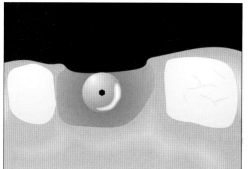

11-11

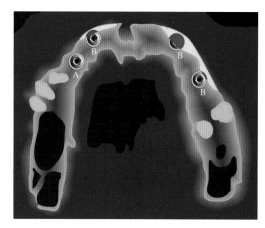

11-12

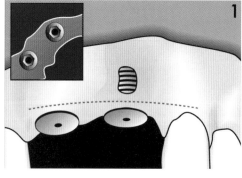

11-13

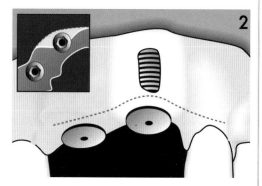

11-14

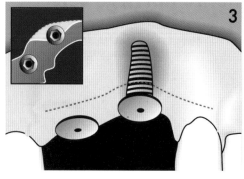

11-15

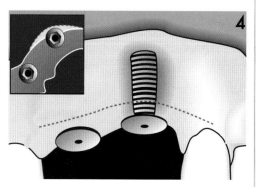

11-16

Fig. 11-10. Class I: the implant is surround by bone.

Fig. 11-11. Class II: some screw threads are exposed.

Fig. 11-12. A – Class I: the implant is completely surrounded by bone walls. B – Class II: the implant is partially involved by bone walls; osseous guided regeneration is necessary.

Fig. 11-13. Fenestration. Class I: the implant is surrounded by less bone, but is inside de alveolar envelope.

Fig. 11-14. Fenestration. Class II: the implant is outside de alveolar envelope. The surgical convexity needs osseous guided regeneration.

Fig. 11-15. Dehiscence. Class I: implant is inside de alveolar envelope.

Fig. 11-16. Dehiscence Class II: implant surface is outside de alveolar envelope and needs osseous guided regeneration.

Vertical ridge defect

Class I: lack of 3mm in bone height. Blood clot itself guarantees osseous regeneration (Fig. 11-19).

Class II: lack of more than 3mm in bone height. Bone grafts are required (Fig 11-20).

PALLACI AND ERICSSON CLASSIFICATION[6]

This classification is based on the amount of vertical and horizontal loss of soft tissue, hard tissue, or both. It is divided into four classes according to the vertical dimension and into four classes according to the horizontal dimension.

Vertical dimension classification for soft and hard tissue defect

Class I: intact or slightly reduced papillae.

Class II: limited loss of papillae.

Class III: severe loss of papillae.

Class IV: absence of the papillae.

Fig. 11-17. Class I: the implant is 50% outside the alveolar ridge, but inside de envelope.

Fig. 11-18. Class II: implant is completely outside de alveolar envelope. Barrier membranes w/or bone graft are necessary.

Fig. 11-19. Class I: vertical deficiency ≤ 3mm. Bone guided regeneration with blood clot protection leads to osseous healing.

Fig. 11-20. Class II: vertical deficiency ≥ 3mm. BGR and grafts are necessary.

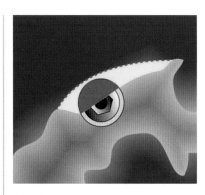

11-17

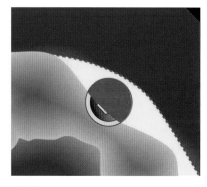

11-18

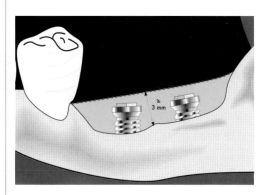

11-19

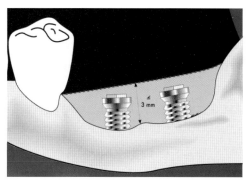

11-20

Horizontal dimension classification for soft and hard tissue defect

Class A: intact or slightly reduced buccal tissue

Class B: limited loss of buccal tissue.

Class C: severe loss of buccal tissue

Class D: extreme loss of buccal tissue, often in combination with a limited amount of attached mucosa. Palacci described a step by step technique to create papilla at the second surgical stage. This will be in further sections.

Soft and hard tissue manipulation

Good esthetic outcomes is a difficult task for surgeons and prosthodontists, specially in cases of large resorptions.[6] The aim of surgical reconstruction for partial or totally edentulous patients, in mild to severe bone resorption cases, is to develop form, height and sufficient volume to avoid esthetic complications and provide functional and physiologic reconstructions.

Soft tissue conditions in the anterior maxilla

Treatment with osseointegrated implants in the anterior maxillary region depends on soft tissue architecture and remaining bone thickness. In this area,

tissue deficiencies results from pathologic or anatomic conditions (Box 11-1).[10]

For years, therapy was aimed toward biomechanical and structural characteristics of bone around implants without considering the natural appearance of implant-supported prosthesis. Pallaci and Ericsson[6] were the first clinicians to address the problem of dental papillae formation in the anterior area.

Factors that Govern Papilla Formation

Soft tissue management before implant insertion

Surgical management will be considered here according to the treatment sequence of hard and soft tissues, implant insertion, and timing for papilla formation (Fig. 11-21).

The first approach is conducted before tooth removal for implant insertion. Surgical maneuvers are used to augment soft and hard tissues, as well as techniques to enhance the recipient bed for implant placement, e.g., orthodontic forced eruption[17], without interfering with mucogingival line position and favors adequate esthetics. The gingival enhancement seen after root sealing only provides primary intention of wound healing.

Box 11-1. Soft tissue management before implant installation

Conditions	Cause and effect
Anatomic deficiency: facial bone loss, narrow alveolar crest	Cause: congenital lost of teeth; effect: large structural bone loss
Pathologic deficiency	
Dental traumatism	Tooth avulsion with fracture of buccal cortical plate
Pos-traumatic conditions	Root anquilosis with infra-occlusion and resorption, root fractures
Acute or chronic infections	Periodontal disease, periodontal-endodontic lesion, periapical lesion
Bone atrophy by disuse	Long-term tooth loss

Modified from Buser et al.,[10] p.44.

Papilla Formation between Implants

Tarnow et al.[11] determined that the presence or absence of interproximal papilla is related to the distance from the crest of the bone to the contact point area (Fig. 11-22).

Their studies showed in 36 patients that considerable bone loss can be seen when the distance between adjacent implants is less than 3mm (Fig. 11-24). Also, mesial and distal bone loss were of 1.34mm and 1.40mm, respectively, whereas 0.45mm of lateral bone loss was seen with more than 3mm between adjacent implants. They concluded that a 3mm distance between adjacent implants or between tooth and implant is necessary to provide space for papilla. Also, crest bone loss is avoided and adequate emergence profile is created to facilitate oral hygiene and esthetics (Fig. 11-23). Besides, this study pointed out that is more difficult to form papilla between adjacent implants than in the tooth-implant situation. Then, it would be beneficial to use implants with reduced diameters in the anterior maxillary region.

First surgical stage

At this time, it is expected that all previous reconstructive procedures have been performed to provide adequate site for implant placement. Otherwise, at

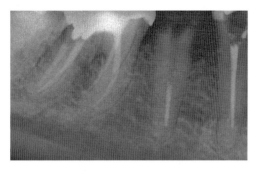

11-21A

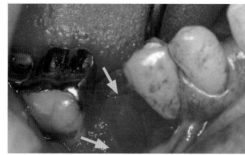

11-21B

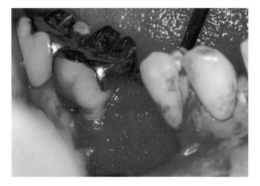

11-21C

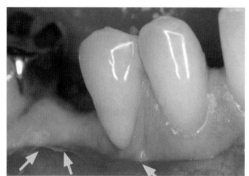

11-21D

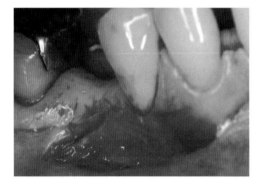

11-21E

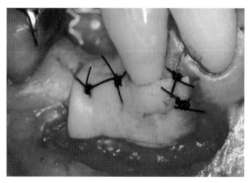

11-21F

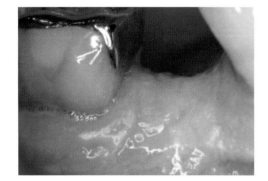

11-21G

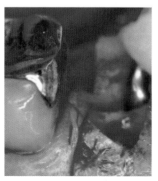

11-21H

Fig. 11-21. Soft tissue conditioning before implant insertion (free gingival graft).

11-21A. Middle third root fracture of tooth 45 (see periapical radiograph).

11-21B. Observe discrepancy between buccal and lingual bone levels after tooth removal and alveolus curettage.

11-21C. A barrier membrane (Resolut) was inserted to protect the alveolar ridge.

11-21D. Clinical situation five months after surgery. Observe the lack of keratinized tissue and buccal fold.

11-21E. Recipient bed preparation for free gingival graft.

11-21F. Graft suturing.

11-21G. Clinical situation three months after surgery. Observe adequate band of keratinized tissue. The buccal fold can be seen.

11-21H. Observe buccal and lingual bone levels due to blood clot protection.

11-21I. Three months after implant insertion. A punch technique was used. Observe papilla integrity. Sutures were not necessary.

11-21J. Observe soft tissue three months after healing abutment connection. Note quality and quantity of keratinized mucosa.

11-21K. Two-year clinical view. Metalloceramic and implant-supported crowns on tooth 44 and 45, respectively. Observe papillary integrity and gingival contours.

11-21L. Five-year clinical view. Observer excellent papillary esthetics.

Fig. 11-22. Papilla formation between adjacent implants. A and B, distance from implant to osseous crest; C, vertical bone loss; D, interimplant distance.

Fig. 11-23. When the distance between adjacent implants is ≥ 3mm, there is papillary formation and adequate height of bone crest.

Fig. 11-24. When the distance between adjacent implants is ≤ 3mm, lack of bone crest height and papilla is observed.

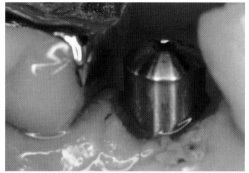
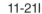
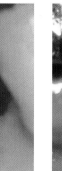

11-21I

11-21J

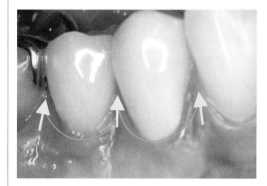
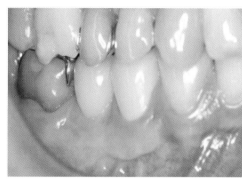

11-21K

11-21L

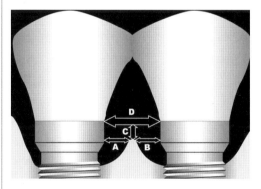
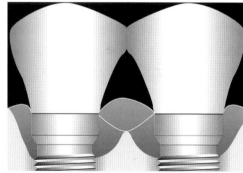

11-22

11-23

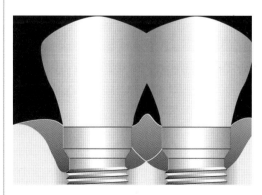

11-24

the implant insertion clinicians can use bone guide generation w/or intra-oral graft procedures (Fig.11-25), as well as maxillary sinus lifting or alveolar crest division/expansion.[13]

The soft tissue can be managed with connective tissue grafts (Fig. 11-26), frenectomy, free gingival graft, coronally positioned flap, and palatal rotated flap. Although many techniques are available, it is very important to achieve a tension-free flap to avoid dehiscence or early graft exposure.

Between first and second surgical stage

At this stage, clinicians can use techniques to augment the band of keratinized mucosa aiming red esthetics, papillae formation and protection against toothbrush trauma.[1]

Possible surgeries include: palatal rotated flap, soft tissue pouch, free gingival graft, connective tissue graft, interpositional or onlay combined grafts[13], and vestibuloplasty[2] (Fig. 11-27).

The use of free gingival grafts and vestibuloplasty to augment attached mucosa has been studied in the literature. Krekeler et al.[26] (1985) installed plasma-sprayed implants on 26 patients. Seventeen patients received previous vestibuloplasty. Half of the implants were installed in non-keratinized tissue. Also, they

concluded that no correlation exists between the attached gingival and plaque level, or with the probing depth. However, in sites with bacterial plaque formation, the lack of attached mucosa contributes to an increase in local inflammation and pocket formation.

Also, concomitant surgical procedures must not disturb osseointegration process. Sometimes, exposed implant threads or fenestration/dehiscence defects are filled with bone particles. Moreover, bone graft performed in the first phase is insufficient or was lost due to postoperative complications, e.g., that occurring after implant placement.[13]

Second surgical stage

Now, the healing abutments are connected. Early protocols aimed to expose the top of implants, evaluate osseointegration condition and to install abutments with enough length to fabricate dental prosthesis. However, this step has received great attention due to the esthetic requirements for the soft tissue in the anterior region. Gingival contour, thickness and the amount of attached tissue can be managed to enhance long-term periimplant performance.

The second surgical stage is directed toward soft tissue management and papilla formation. Available techniques include: use of a circular punch, roll tech-

Fig. 11-25. Bone graft procedure during implant placement.

11-25A. The root fragments in the anterior maxillary area were removed.

11-25B. Flap closure and suturing.

11-25C. Seven titanium fixtures are installed in this region.

11-25D. Implant thread exposure at the region of 24.

11-25E. Autogenous bone graft is placed in the upper left posterior region.

11-25F. A n° 6 Gore-Tex membrane is adapted to the recipient site.

11-25G. Sutures are placed.

11-25H. After membrane removal, good bone regeneration can be seen over the implants.

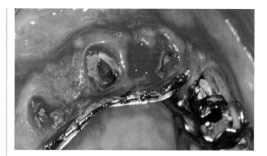

11-25A

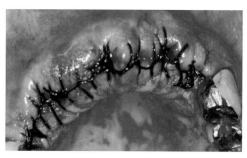

11-25B

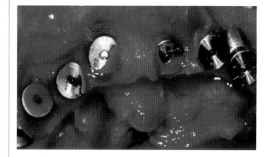

11-25C

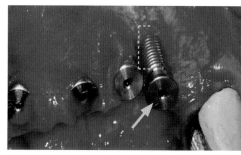

11-25D

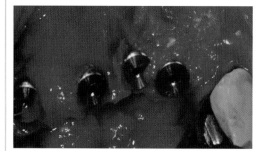

11-25E

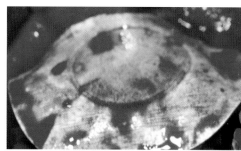

11-25F

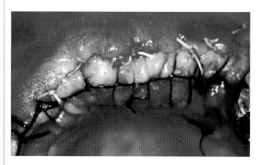

11-25G

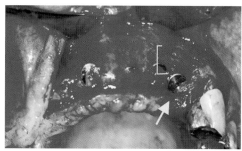

11-25H

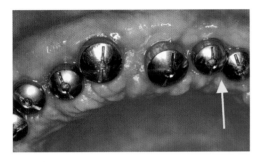

11-25I

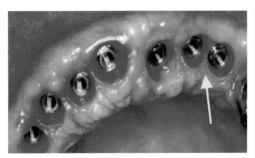

11-25J

Fig. 11-25I. Four months after implant placement. Observe proximity between fixtures. Also, soft tissue healing is adequate.

11-25J. Observe lack of adequate space between implants on regions 23 and 24. this will avoid adequate papilla formation.

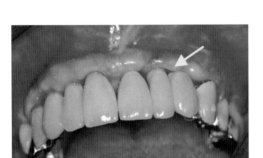

11-25K

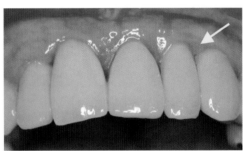

11-25L

11-25K. Metalloceramic units cemented on each implant. There is a generalized lack of papillary formation. Also, some papillae have inverse configuration.

11-25L. Clinical view after seven years. Observe excellent gingival aspect and papilla maturation.

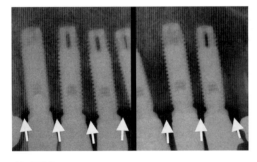

11-25M

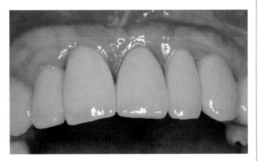

11-25N

11-25M. Periapical radiographs nine years after. Observe good bone quality around implants and interproximal spaces

11-25N. Nine-year postoperative control. Papillae are formed and stabilized.

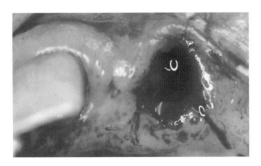

11-26A

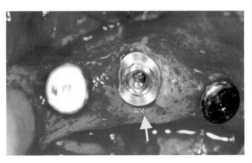

11-26B

Fig. 11-26. Connective tissue graft soon after implant placement.

11-26A. Canine tooth was removed and the implant immediately inserted.

11-26B. Implant occlusal view.

11-26C. Connective tissue graft simultaneous to implant placement.

11-26D. Six months after wound healing. Observe lack of mucosal thickness and labial fold.

11-26E. Apically positioned flap. Incision was placed at 45 degrees angle to augment the amount of keratinized tissue.

11-26F. Soft tissue graft removed from the tuberosity area. The graft was placed between healing abutments to improve tissue aspect.

11-26G. Flap suture. Observe adequate labial tissue volume and graft stabilization.

11-26H. The master cast has the same soft/hard tissue relation.

11-26I. Clinical aspect from canine to the second molar area. After three months, excellent soft tissue quantity and quality has been achieved.

11-26J. Clinical aspect of definitive prosthesis after 5 years. Note the soft tissue quality.

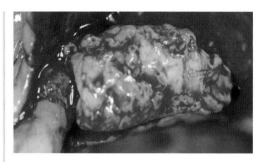

11-26C

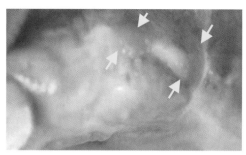

11-26D

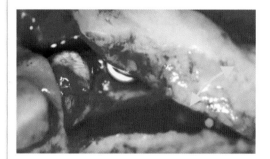

11-26E

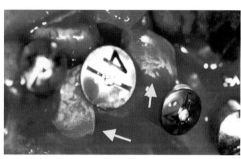

11-26F

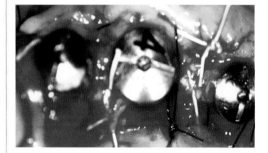

11-26G

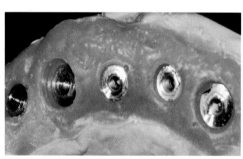

11-26H

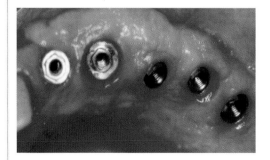

11-26I

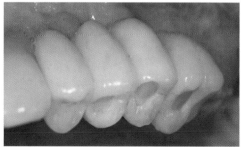

11-26J

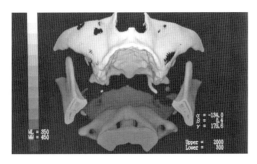

11-27A

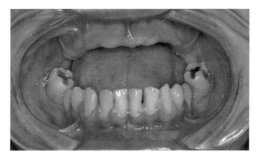

11-27B

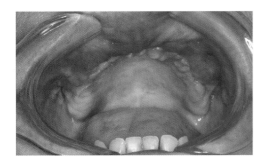

11-27C

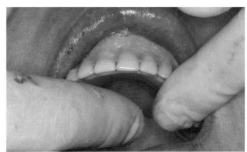

11-27D

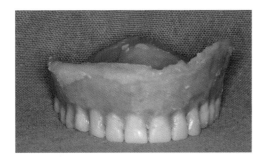

11-27E

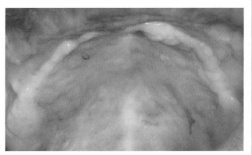

11-27F

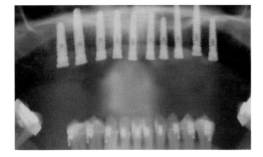

11-27G

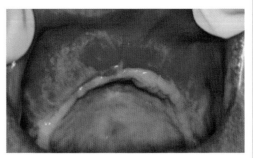

11-27H

Fig. 11-27. Vestibulo-plasty technique.

11-27A. Computerized To-mography scan showing severe maxillary resorp-tion.

11-27B. An iliac crest block graft was inserted. (Cortesy of Dr. Hugo Nary.)

11-27C. Vestibuloplasty six months after graft healing.

11-27D. Total prosthesis relining.

11-27E. Finalized pros-thesis

11-27F. Three months af-ter vestibuloplasty, there is a lack of buccal fold and keratinized mucosa.

11-27G. Panoramic ra-diograph showing 10 implants in the maxillary arch.

11-27H. Observe the lack of keratinized mucosa in the maxilla.

11-27I. Vestibuloplasty was tried again. The flap was apically positioned and sutured. Periosteum was preserved. (Cortesy of Dr. Hugo Nary.)

11-27J. The surgical limits of palatal graft are marked.

11-27K. Palatal graft removed.

11-27L. Graft is positioned along the alveolar crest.

11-27M. Graft sutured.

11-27N. One month later, there is adequate amount of keratinized tissue.

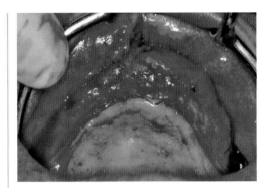

11-27I

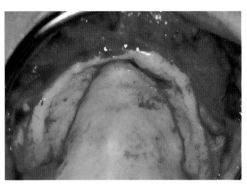

11-27J

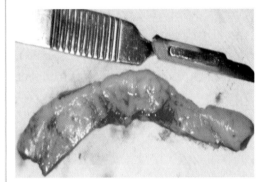

11-27K

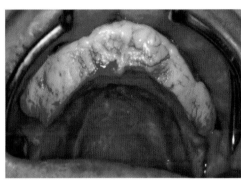

11-27L

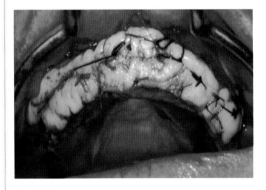

11-27M

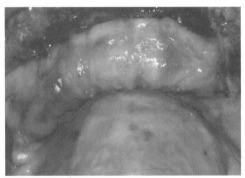

11-27N

nique, apically positioned flap, free gingival graft, and papilla formation strategies.[13]

Treatment possibilities during second surgical phase

❑ Adequate soft tissue thickness to the abutment height contour;

❑ remove bone growth over healing abutment;

❑ bone contouring to enhance emergence profile;

❑ observe direct seating of healing abutments;

❑ to preserve, create or enhance the amount of keratinized mucosa through plastic periodontal periimplant surgeries;

❑ to improve soft tissue adaptation around healing abutment;

❑ improve final esthetics with adequate flap design to create papillary tissue.

Papilla formation on the second surgical stage

Several techniques have been described to minimize tissue recession and improve periimplant healing. An adequate amount of keratinized mucosa around implants could be important to maximize esthetic outcomes, at the same time that prevents in-

flammatory process and trauma to the tissues. These include: the modified roll technique, free gingival grafts, and vestibuloplasty combined with gingival graft.[1]

Nemcovsky et al.[3] technique

A U-shaped incision is made (Fig. 11-28) in the gingival sulcus of adjacent teeth and continues from the facial aspect to the healing abutment localization at the palatal area (Fig. 11-28A and B). A full-thickness flap is elevated. Interproximal papillae are denuded to receive this flap.

The healing abutment is replaced with a new transmucosal component. Now, an incision is placed at the middle of the flap creating two fingers (Fig. 11-28C). Each finger is dislocated to their respective mesial and distal areas (Fig. 11-28D). Each half is placed over the denuded papilla (Fig. 11-28E) and secured with vertical sutures (Fig. 11-28F).

Tinti and Benfenati[15] technique

This technique is indicated when more than two adjacent implants are found (Fig. 11-29). A linear incision is placed 5mm apart from mesial and distal sites. When there is adjacent tooth to implant, intrasulcular incision is made (Fig. 11-29A).

A full-thickness flap is el-

Fig. 11-28. Nemcovsky et al.[3] technique. Indicated for single tooth implants between adjacent teeth with interproximal papilla. Regions with poor keratinized tissue or the need of an apically positioned flap contra-indicates this procedure.

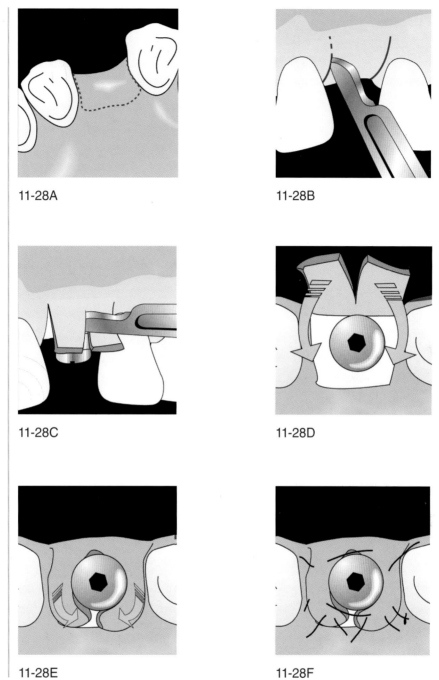

11-28A

11-28B

11-28C

11-28D

11-28E

11-28F

evated, healing abutments are exposed and substituted for transmucosal components (Figs. 11-29B to D).

The flap is rotated to the labial side. Gore-Tex monofilament sutures are placed 5-6mm above the palatal aspect (Fig. 11-29E). After 4-5 weeks, gingivectomy is made at the labial side to provide papilla configuration (Figs. 11-29F to G). When there is insufficient keratinized tissue, flap is extended to the palatal area.

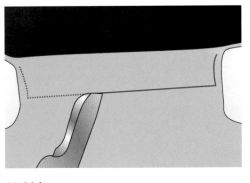

11-29A

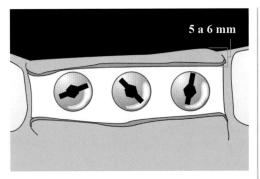

5 a 6 mm

11-29B

Figs. 11-29. Tinti and Benfenati[15] technique. Surgical management for papilla creation.

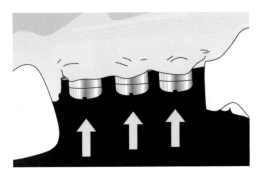

11-29C

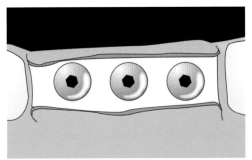

11-29D

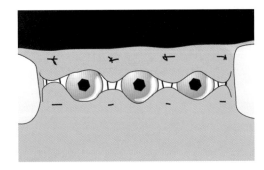

11-29E

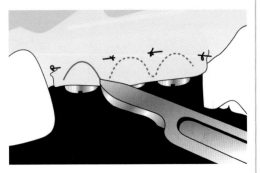

11-29F

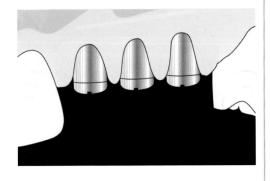

11-29G

Palacci and Ericsson[6] technique

Palacci was the first surgeon to highlight issues on interproximal esthetics for the anterior maxillary region. The papilla regeneration technique (Figs. 11-30 to 11-31) begins with a linear incision placed at the palatal lingual aspect of the cover screws, followed by vertical releasing incisions in a buccal and divergent direction to allow better blood supply to the flap (Fig. 11-30A). It is important to preserve the gingival cuffs at neighboring teeth. A full-thickness flap is elevated in the buccal direction (Fig. 11-30B).

The cover screws are removed and the proper abutments connected to the implants. A semilunar bevel incision is made in the buccal flap toward each abutment (Fig. 11-30C) starting at the distal aspect of the most mesially located implant. The pedicles are disengaged and rotated 90 degrees toward the palatal side to fill in the interimplant space (Fig. 11-30D). This simulates new periimplant papillae (Fig. 11-30E). Tissues are sutured at the interproximal region without tension in the pedicles (Fig. 11-30F).

Healing control after second surgical stage

A second study by Small & Tarnow[19] classified the gingival tissue around implants after surgery to determine its stability. Sixty-three implants in eleven implants were evaluated. The soft tissue characteristics were observed during one and two-stage protocols for osseointegrated implants. Analyses were conducted at one week, 1, 3, 6, 9 months and one-year. Eighty percent of soft tissue sites showed buccal recession. In this way, a 3 month period is recommended before abutment connection or impression making. The results demonstrated recession trends over one year. After 3 months, mesio-buccal recession slightly increased from 0.75mm to 0.85mm, stabilizing after one year. Coronal migration was observed in the first postoperative week due to inflammation and swelling. Thus, impressions taken one week after abutment connection would compromise esthetic results.

Mean mesio-buccal recession value was of 1.05mm (from 0.88mm of coronal migration (first week) to 1.05mm of buccal recession (one year later)). Most recessions were observed three months later second stage surgery. Thus, impression and abutment selection have to be made only three months after soft tissue healing.

After prosthesis delivery

Still, it is possible to retrieve keratinized soft tissue lost after

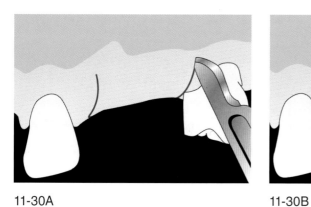

11-30A

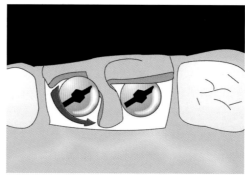

11-30B

Fig. 11-30. Palacci and Ericsson[6] technique for papilla formation.

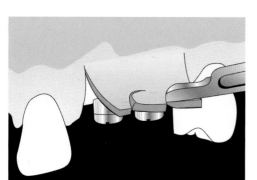

11-30C

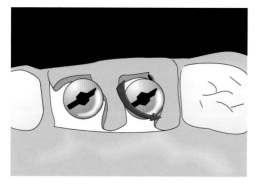

11-30D

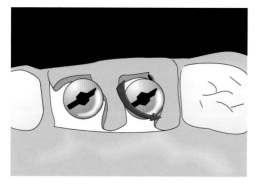

11-30E

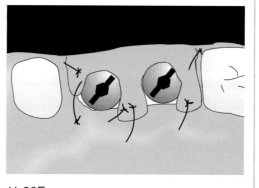

11-30F

prosthesis insertion (Fig. 11-32). A free connective tissue graft and a multidisciplinary interac- tion are necessary to optimize esthetics.

Fig. 11-31. Bone graft and soft tissue management.

11-31A. Shot-gun lesion in the maxillary anterior region.

11-31B. Three months later. Note the total absence of buccal and palatal cortical plates.

11-31C. An iliac crest block bone graft was placed (Cortesy of Dr. Luiz Marinho).

11-31D. Periapical radiograph six months later. Observe bone graft in the graft region.

11-31E. Close view of the anterior area. Observe the lack of keratinized tissue and buccal fold. Also, a lag screw can see through the mucosa.

11-31F. Vestibuloplasty along with lag screw removal.

11-31G. Acrylic stent to guide vestibule configuration.

11-31H. Observe lack of vestibular tissue 3 months after fixture installations.

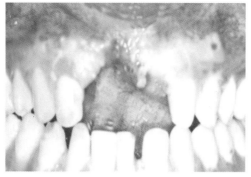

11-31A

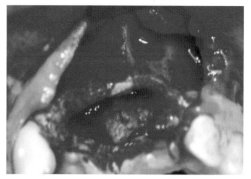

11-31B

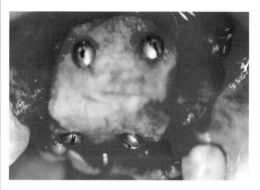

11-31C

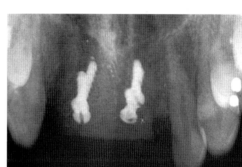

11-31D

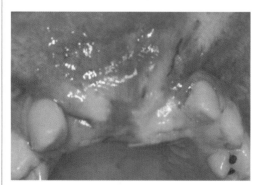

11-31E

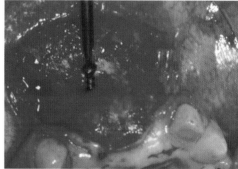

11-31F

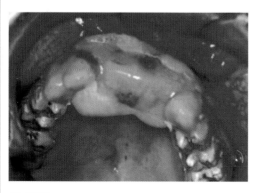

11-31G

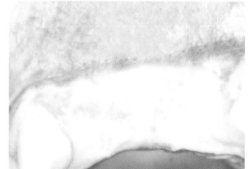

11-31H

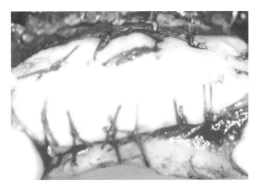

11-31I

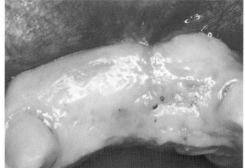

11-31J

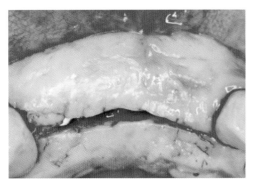

11-31K

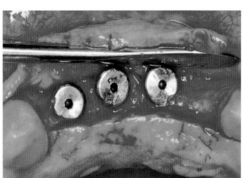

11-31L

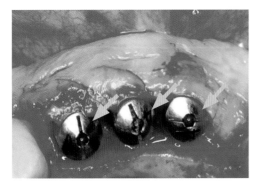

11-31M

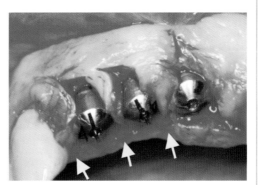

11-31N

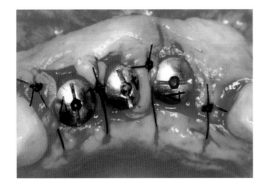

11-31O

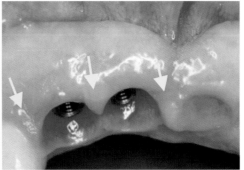

11-31P

11-31I. Free gingival graft and suture.

11-31J. three months after graft surgery observe adequate volume of keratinized tissue and formation of buccal fold.

11-31K. Second surgical stage. A papilla regeneration technique is performed.

11-31L. The implants are osseointegrated.

11-31M. After healing abutment connection, incisions are placed (arrows).

11-31N. Soft tissue pedicles are rotated to interproximal areas.

11-31O. Pedicles are sutured for papilla formation.

11-31P. Observe excellent papillary formation and the quality of soft tissue achieved one year after.

Fig. 11-32. Gingival tissue management after definitive prosthesis installation.

11-32A. Clinical aspect before orthodontic treatment. Observe the congenital absence of superior lateral incisors.

11-32B. Orthodontic finalization (Courtesy of Dr. Onofre Neto) and implants on the region of 12 and 22.

11-32C. Implant exposure. Soft tissue conditioning with provisional acrylic restorations.

11-32D. Observe soft tissue deficiency at mesial aspect of right lateral incisor (arrow).

11-32E. Observe the lack of soft tissue at the mesial aspect of right lateral implant.

11-32F. Excellent papillary configuration on the left lateral implant.

11-32G. Metalloceramic crown in position. Observe that the height of cervical contour of 12 is more apical than cervical contour of 22.

11-32H. Clinical crown lengthening from right premolars to the canine area.

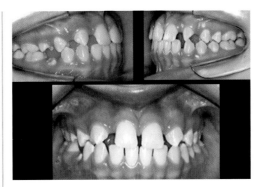

11-32A

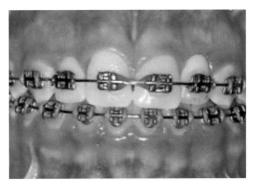
11-32B

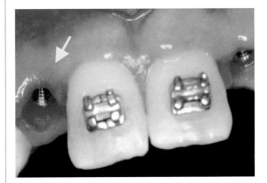

11-32C

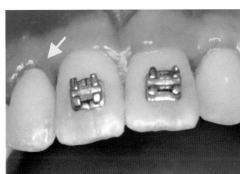
11-32D

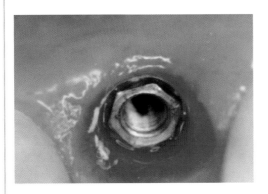
11-32E

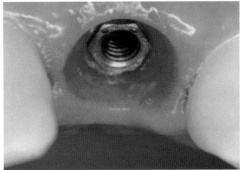
11-32F

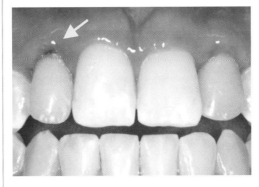

11-32G

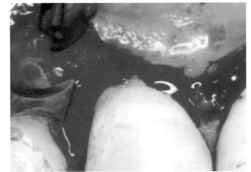
11-32H

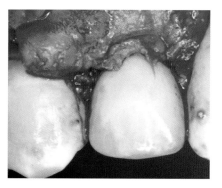

11-32I

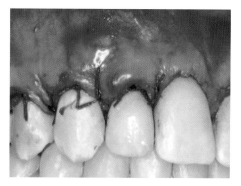

11-32J

11-32I. Connective tissue graft on the left superior lateral incisor area.

11-32J. Free-tension closure is obtained.

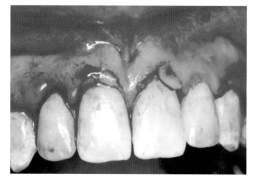

11-32K

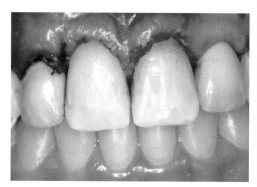

11-32L

11-32K. Clinical crown lengthening in the two central incisors.

11-32L. Observe that papilla between central incisors was maintained.

11-32M. Clinical crown lengthening from left premolars to the canine area.

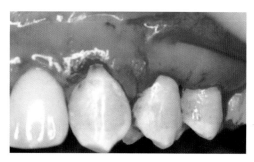

11-32M

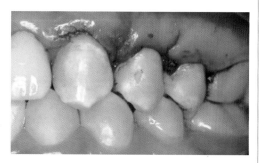

11-32N

11-32N. Again, a free-tension closure must be obtained.

11-32O. Observe papillary formation six months later.

11-32P. Master casts before and after plastic periodontal surgery.

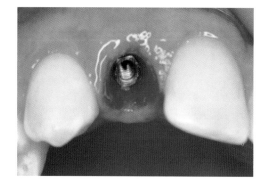

11-32O

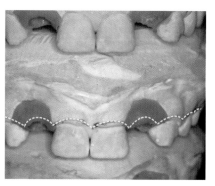

11-32P

11-32Q. Procera abutments were inserted.

11-32R. Procera crown system. Hallogen lamp showing crown translucence.

11-32S. Initial and final clinical aspects.

11-32T. Two-year follow-up. Observe excellent papillary aspect and tissue stability.

11-32U. Patient's smile showing harmony between hard and soft tissues.

11-32V. Four-year follow-up after prosthesis delivery.

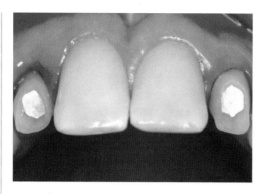

11-32Q

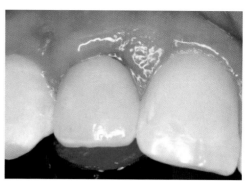

11-32R

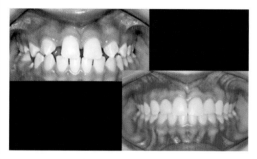

11-32S

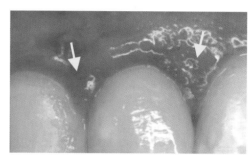

11-32T

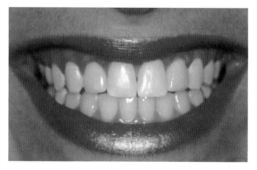

11-32U

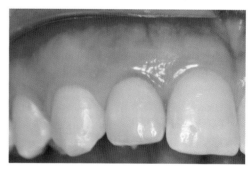

11-32V

References

1. AZZI R, ETIENNE D, TAKEY H, FENECH P. Surgical thickening of existing gingiva and reconstruction of interdental papillae around implant-supported restorations. *Int J Periodontics Rest Dent* 2002; 22: 71-77.

2. NEVES JB. *Implantodontia Oral – Otimização da estética. Uma abordaegem dos tecidos mole e duro.* Belo Horizonte: Ed. Rona, 2001; 6: 125-177.

3. NEMCOVSKY CE, MOSES O, ARTZI Z. Interproximal papillae reconstruction in maxillary implants. *J Periodontol* 2000, 71: 308-314.

4. SCHROPP L, WENZEL A, KOSTOPOULOS L, KARRING T. Bone healing and soft tissue contour changes following single-tooth extraction: a clinical and radiographic 12-month prospective study. *International J Periodontics Rest Dent* 2003; 23: 313-323.

5. NEMCOVSKY CE, MOSES O. Rotated palatal flap. A surgical approach to increase keratinized tissue width in maxillary implant uncovering: technique and clinical evaluation. *Int J Periodontics Rest Dent* 2002; 22(6):607-612.

6. PALACCI P, ERICSSON I. *Esthetic implant dentistry-soft and hard tissue Management.* Chicago: Quintessence, 2001; 2: 33-45

7. HOELSCHER DC, SIMONS AM. The rationale for soft-tissue grafting and vestibuloplasty in association with endosseous implants: a literature review. *J Oral Implantology* 1994; 20: 282-291.

8. KAN JY, SHIOTSU G, RUNGCHARASSAENG K, LOZADA JL. Maintaining and attenuating periodontal tissue for aesthetic implant placement. *J Implantology* 2000; 26: 35-41.

9. MELLONING JT, NEVINS M. *Implantoterapia – abordagens clínicas e evidências de sucesso.* São Paulo: Quintessence, 2003; 5: 56-81, 7: 98-110.

10. BUSER D, MARTIN W, BELSER UC. Optimizing esthetics for implant restoration in the anterior maxilla: anatomic and surgical considerations. *Int J Oral Maxillofac Implants,* 2004; 19: 43-61.

11. TARNOW DP, CHO SC, WALLACE SS. The effect of inter-implant distance on the height of inter-implant bone crest. *J Periodontol* 2000; 71: 546-549.

12. WANG GHL, AL-SHAMMARI K. HVC ridge deficiency classification: a therapeutically oriented classification. *Int J Periodontics Restorative Dent,* 2002; 22: 335-343.

13. SCARSO JF, BARRETO MA, TUNES UR. *Planejamento Estético cirúrgico e protético em implantodontia.* São Paulo: Artes Médicas, 2001; 3: 57-61, 7: 111-155.

14. JOVANOVIC SA. Bone rehabilitation to achieve optimal aesthetics. *Pract Periodontics Aesthet Dent* 1997; 9: 41-51.

15. TINTI C, BENFENATI SP. The ramp mattress suture: a new suturing technique combined with a surgical procedure to obtain papillae between implants in the buccal area. *Int J Periodontics Restorative Dent* 2002; 22(1): 63-69.

16. SAADOUN AP, LeGALL M, TOUATI B. Selection and ideal tridimensional implant position for soft tissue aesthetics. *Pract Periodontics Aesthet Dent* 1999; 11: 1063-1072.

17. JEMT T. Regeneration of gingival papillae after single-implant treatment. *Int J Periodontics Restorative Dent,* 1997; 17: 327-333.

18. MULLER HP, EGER T. Masticatory mucosa and periodontal phenotype: a review. *Int J Periodontics*

Restorative Dent 2002; 22: 173-183.

19. SMALL PN, TARNOW DP. Gingival recession around implants: a 1-year longitudinal prospective study. *Int J Oral Maxillofac Implants,* 2000; 15: 527-32.

20. SALAMA H, SALAMA MA, GARBER D, ADAR P. The interproximal height of bone: A guidepost to predictable aesthetic strategies and soft tissue contours in anterior tooth replacement. *Pract Periodontics Aesthetic Dent* 1998; 10: 1131-1141.

21. ATWOOD DA. Reduction of residual ridges: a major oral disease entity. *J Prosthet Dent* 1971; 26: 266-279.

22. SALAMA H, SALAMA M. The role of orthodontic extrusive remodeling in the enhancement of soft and hard tissue profiles prior to implant placement: a systematic approach to the management of extraction site defects. *Int J Periodontics Restorative Dent* 1993;13:312-333.

23. SEIBERT JS. Reconstruction of deformed partially edentulous ridges, using full thickness onlay grafts. Part I Technique and wound healing. *Compend Contin Educ Dent* 1983; 4: 437-453.

24. TINTI C, PARMA-BENFENATI S. Clinical classification of bone defects concerning the placement of dental implants. *Int J Periodontics Restorative Dent* 2003;23:147-155.

25. KREKELER G, SCHILLI W, DIEMER J. Should the exit of the artificial abutment tooth be positioned in the region of the attached gingiva? *Int J Oral Surg* 1985;14:504-508.

12

RECONSTRUCTION OF CRANIOFACIAL FUNCTION USING OSSEOINTEGRATED IMPLANTS IN PATIENTS WITH MANDIBULAR DEFECTS

Maria B. Papageorge
Robert J. Chapman

Introduction

Damage from major diseases of the jaws or anatomic defects resulting from surgical resection of benign or malignant diseases, can be devastating. Disfigurement, masticatory and speech disorders, and discomfort from hypo or hyper sensation, often dictates that a patient must experience a poorer quality of life. Well conceived surgical and prosthetic reconstruction however, can not only result in successful rehabilitation, but can enhance the patient's self esteem and quality of life. There are many conditions for which extensive surgery and subsequent surgical and prosthodontic reconstruction are necessary. Without an accurate diagnosis and comprehensive treatment plan, the outcome will be unsatisfactory.

Interdisciplinary treatment involving members of the oncology team is necessary for a successful outcome in craniofacial reconstruction. Removal of disease, surgical reconstruction of missing anatomical structures, and prosthetic restoration of esthetics and function requires close collaboration between surgeon and prosthodontist. When possible, the ultimate goal of replacing and reconstructing the dentition should be considered along with surgical planning for restoration of form. Once anatomical form has been re-established, insertion of osseointegrated implants provides optimal foundation for occlusal reconstruction.

A thorough discussion of the specifics of diagnoses of diseases requiring extensive treatment, and the varying treatment options based on co-existing problems or concerns, is an extensive subject. The objective of this chapter is to describe the overall direction for the surgical and prosthodontic reconstruction of patients with mandibular defects rather than attempting to detail the diagnoses and treatment options of specific disease entities.

Craniofacial function though, must be achieved, and therefore understanding the craniofacial complex and its relationship to the dentition is necessary to achieve rehabilitation of these patients.

Craniofacial Complex

The craniofacial complex encompasses the lower third of the face and the muscles of the neck to C5 (Fig. 12-1A and B). Its primary functions are eating and social communication. A less realized function is keeping the head balanced on the spinal column. In most animals, the head is cantilevered from the spine and primarily held in place by the nuchal ligament. However, the dentition appears to be an important element in maintaining head position. When posterior teeth are lost in hamsters, head drop occurs rapidly and is followed shortly by death.[1] In humans, the anterior and posterior muscles of the neck keep the head from tipping. These muscles have an intimate relationship with the muscles of mastication. If the masticatory muscles are not working harmoniously, the muscles of the neck

may be affected[a]. When the dentition is damaged or lost, the complex, interdependent, masticatory and neck muscles are likewise often affected. In-coordination of this muscular interdependence can lead to tempero-mandibular dysfunction.[3] Teeth provide the normal stop – vertical dimension of occlusion - for contraction of the muscles of mastication. However, if all teeth are lost, these muscles over close the jaws. This may result in hyper tonicity of the posterior, and stretching of the anterior neck muscles. Such overcompensation can lead to muscle tenderness, spasm, or fatigue. With the dentition limiting muscle contraction, masticatory muscles help maintain normal tonicity of the muscles of the neck to keep the head balanced properly on the spine[b]. Removal of a quadrant of teeth unilaterally or bilaterally, results in a loss in muscular stop on one or both sides. The medial pterygoid, masseter, and temporalis muscles may become hypertonic and relocate the condyle or condyles superior and posterior, invading the retro-discal space.

Animal studies have shown that muscle damage can be temporary or permanent depending on duration of tooth loss.[5] Muscle "imbalances" from complete or partial tooth loss, or possible disc space inflammation, have been implicated in the etiology of tempero-mandibular disorders.[4] A healthy dentition maintains the antero-posterior and medio-lateral vertical dimension[6] needed for muscular balance and is the foun-

Fig. 12-1A and B. The craniofacial complex is roughly bounded by the nose and hyoid bone, structures between the ears, muscles of mastication, and muscles of the neck to the 5th cervical vertebra.

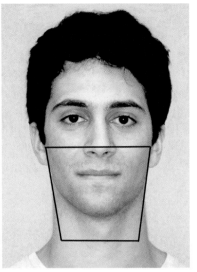

12-1A

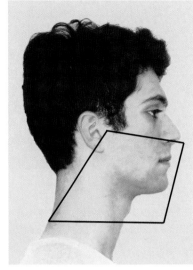

12-1B

dation for healthy craniofacial function. Healthy posture, gait,[7-9] and even acuity of sight have been attributed to proper dental occlusion.

The craniofacial complex is one of the first organ complexes, and arguably, all other systems evolved to support and enhance its primary function of eating. Approximately one quarter of the entire external surface of the brain's sensory cortex is dedicated to the teeth, lips, and tongue.[11]

As evolution proceeded, the teeth and tongue, ancient organs for grasping and manipulating food, morphed in shape and position to become integral to clear speech and social cooperation.

Teeth or their replacements, are important for producing the complex sounds that make up speech. Vowels are shaped when the tongue's borders are support-ed by the palatal surfaces of the maxillary posterior teeth and its tip is braced on the lingual surfaces of the mandibular anterior teeth. The fricative "F" and "V" sounds are expressed as air is forced between the incisal edges of the maxillary anterior teeth and the lower lip (Fig. 2). Sibilants, the hissing "S", "Sh", "Ch", and "Z", are produced when air is compressed between the palatal-incisal edges of the maxillary anterior teeth, and the facial-incisal edges of the mandibular anterior teeth (Fig. 12-3). Clear and distinct pronunciation is a hallmark of an intact dentition.

When teeth are well positioned, well shaped, and appropriately shaded, social acceptance is simply better (Fig. 12-4A, B, C). In today's world, teeth or their replacements are a social necessity (Fig. 12-5A, B and Fig. 12-6A, B).

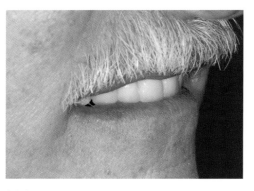

12-2

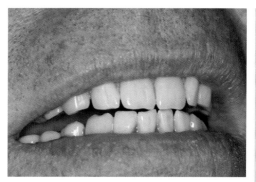

12-3

Fig. 12-2. The fricative "F" and "V" sounds are made with the maxillary anterior teeth touching the wet/dry border of the lower lip.

Fig. 12-3. The sibilant "S", "Sh", Ch" and "Z" sounds are produced when air hisses between the almost-touching incisal edges of the maxillary and mandibular anterior teeth.

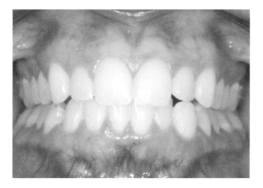

12-4A

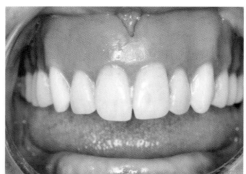

12-4B

Fig. 12-4

12-4A. Healthy, well shaped, positioned, and shaded teeth in a healthy periodontal environment are esthetic.

12-4B. The esthetics of the maxillary denture is unsatisfactory and the patient could not wear the poorly extended mandibular denture.

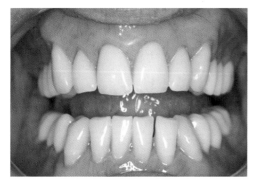

12-4C

12-4C. New complete dentures provided satisfactory esthetics and comfort for this patient.

Fig. 12-5

12-5A. A thirty-six year old woman whose teeth were extracted at 18 years of age shows considerable loss of midface shape and vertical dimension.

12-5B. New complete dentures have reconstructed the midface and vertical dimension of her craniofacial complex.

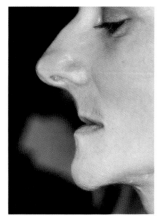

12-5A

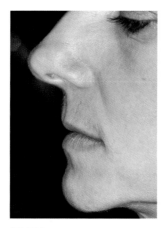

12-5B

Fig. 12-6A and B. This 50 year old woman suffered from generalized severe periodontal disease and full mouth extractions were indicated. She did not want to wear removable prosthetics even temporarily and thus her treatment was staged. Initially she underwent extraction of the most diseased posterior and anterior teeth and placement of a temporary fixed prosthesis on the remaining teeth. After two months of healing, implants were placed strategically to eventually support fixed maxillary and mandibular implant reconstructions. After appropriate healing for osseointegration, the remaining teeth were removed and the existing temporary bridges were modified to fit the interim implant abutments. Additional implants were placed after the last extraction sites had healed. All implants integrated well and the prosthesis has satisfied all OHR QOL indices. The patient is functioning well for the past 6 years (photographs courtesy of Dr. Nopsaran Chaimattayompol).

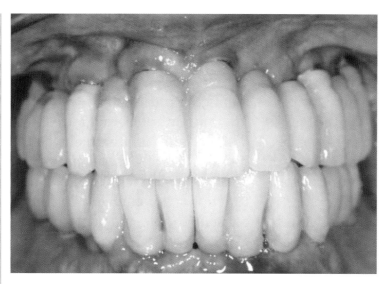

12-6A

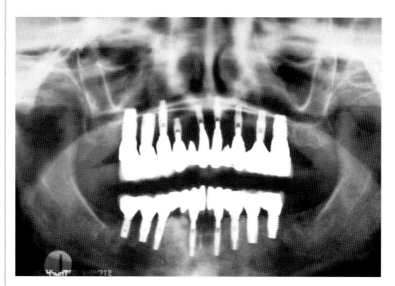

12-6B

Oral Health Related Quality of Life

Well-being, or quality of life, has been investigated considerably over the past two decades and is the short and long-term goal of medical and dental treatment.[12,13] The quality of life indicators in dentistry (Oral Health Related Quality of Life – OHR QOL) have been identified as esthetics, comfort, function and biologic health of the craniofacial complex.[14-16]

Pleasing esthetics is a social phenomenon, and disfigurement is not accepted well by individuals or societies. Speech, eating, chewing, and swallowing, are functions necessary for social interaction and nourishment. Comfortable communication requires a lower third of the face that appears reasonably normal, and speech that is minimally comprehensible.

Discomfort can be *disease* (not feeling "good" or "just right"), and may be physical and/or psychological. A loose denture is often uncomfortable and may cause inflammation and pain, yet a bulky crown may be uncomfortable but not necessarily painful. Psychological discomfort can be as debilitating as chronic pain and long-term discomfort can be a social problem as well as a personal one.

In addition to an individuals desire to enjoy good health, craniofacial diseases that negatively affect OHR QOL will affect economic productivity.[17]

Oral health related quality of life indicators can be used to communicate treatment goals to the patient. Successfully achieving these indicators depends on the amount of damage to the craniofacial complex. When implants are used to restore missing teeth, the parameters are easier to accomplish and quality of life is enhanced.[18] Osseointegrated dental implants create reconstructions that result in a quality of life that approaches pre-surgical levels. However it is important all patients understand that the limiting factor in restoring reasonable quality of life satisfaction depends on the extent of the damage from disease.[16]

Informed Consent

As with any surgical and/or prosthetic procedure, it is extremely important to obtain informed consent. It is generally impossible to recreate with the best surgical or prosthodontic procedures the identical pre-existing anatomy. The amount of damage from the disease, and/or treatment of the disease, largely determines the level of esthetics, comfort and function obtainable. Informed consent should include whatever OHR QOL level is realistically achievable.[21] Facing possible disfigurement often shuts down the patient's ability to listen, as fear becomes the prominent emotion. A written informed consent for both surgical and prosthodontic phases of treatment provides information for patient study after verbal communication. Trust is established with communication and, if subsequent problems occur or the final result is not what was hoped for, patient fear and anger are mitigated. Disappointments in treatment are generally accepted well if there is communication of realistic results.

Restoration of Anatomic Form

The primary goal for treatment of patients with diseases of the jaw is to render them disease free. However, to achieve a reasonable quality of life, anatomic and functional reconstruction should follow. Indications for reconstruction of mandibular defects include surgical resection for neoplastic disease, trauma, infection, osteoradionecrosis, and congenital deformities. The most common indication however is surgery for neoplastic disease of the oral cavity and oropharynx. Reconstruction of these often complex three dimensional composite bony and soft tissue defects is often difficult but is paramount for rehabilitation of the patient.

The esthetic deformity and functional losses that occur with mandibular defects depend on the size and location of the segmental defect. Defects in the posterior body or ramus are better tolerated by the patient and usually easier to reconstruct. Defects of the anterior body or symphysis of the mandible often result in poor tongue function and a greater cosmetic defect, thus presenting greater challenges for reconstruction and rehabilitation. However, regardless of the size or location of the discontinuity defect, malocclusions will result if the defect is not restored, as the remaining mandibular segments collapse due to muscle pull.

There are numerous surgical techniques for reconstruction of anatomical form, but not all permit optimal occlusal reconstruction and oral function. Techniques for mandibular reconstruction include grafting with autogenous vascularized and free bone grafts, cadaveric irradiated bone, alloplastic materials acting as spacers such as polyvinyl plastics, hydroxylapatite or metal, a combination of alloplastic and autogenous bone[22,23] and transport distraction osteogenesis.[24] The technique chosen should depend upon the complexity of the case, extent of defect, treatment of malignant or benign disease, surgical expertise, and general health and age of the patient. Each of these techniques has its indications, benefits, and limitations. The ultimate goal for any graft is to support endosseous implants in a favorable position and relationship to the opposing arch for restoration of occlusal and craniofacial function.

Autogenous bone grafts

Of these surgical techniques, autogenous bone grafting plays a primary role in mandibular reconstruction, and allows for a more favorable outcome in regards to oral function. Indications for the use of vascularized versus non-vascularized grafts are controversial. Vascularized bone grafts are advocated when reconstructing defects resulting from malignant disease, in patients who have received prior radiation therapy, and in reconstruction of longer bony defects. Non-vascularized free grafts are used more frequently for patients with benign disease, no prior radiation therapy and for reconstruction of shorter defects.[25,26] Since surgical treatment of malignant disease usually requires more extensive resection of not only bone but also surrounding soft tissue, and these patients often receive postoperative radiation therapy and/or chemotherapy, tissue transfer reconstruction with microvascular anastomosis provides reliable repair of the resultant defect.

The most commonly used vascularized grafts for mandibular reconstruction are from the fibula, iliac crest, scapula and radius.[27,31] Each of these grafts has its benefits and limitations when restoring the relationship of the mandible to its surrounding anatomy.

Of these vascularized grafts, the fibula can be used to repair bony defects as long as 30 cm with a vascular pedicle 6-10 cm in length (Fig. 7A to H). It can be easily contoured along with a reconstruction plate for restoring anatomic form. Inadequate or poor contouring of the reconstruction plate and thus the fibula graft itself, or fracture of a miniplate, will result in malocclusion.[32] Bone height of this graft is preserved allowing for placement of osseointegrated implants.[33]

The iliac crest graft is a good reconstructive option for patients with bony as well as significant soft-tissue defects. The natural contour of the ipsilateral iliac crest is helpful in reconstructing lateral and hemi-mandibulectomy defects.[29]

The scapular graft is not usually the first choice for mandibular reconstruction. It is used more for composite defects involving facial skin, bone, and mucosac because of its generally good flexibility of the soft tissue in relation to the bone.[29]

In both the iliac crest and scapula grafts, once microvascular anastomosis occurs the bone will accept osseointegrated implants as well as the fibula graft. The radial forearm graft is the least frequently used microvascular graft for mandibular reconstruction. It is suitable only for small mandibular defects and the bone stock is not as favorable for osseointegrated dental implants as the other vascular grafts.[29,35] Donor site morbidity can include limited range of motion, grip strength, and supination.

Non-vascularized free grafts such as autogenous block or particulate cancellous bone marrow from the iliac crest have been used extensively for mandibular reconstruction.[26,36] Particulate cancellous bone marrow often requires additional structural support or scaffolding for anatomic contouring (Fig. 8A to D). Freeze-dried irradiated cadaveric rib or mandible (Fig. 9A and B), and bone plates or titanium mesh trays have been used to add rigidity and better establish the form (Fig. 10A and B).

All non-vascularized free grafts must undergo a process of maturation. Particulate cancellous bone marrow provides transplanted cells necessary for proliferation and formation of new osteoid for a successful phase I of the 2-phase process of osteogenesis.[37] This phase I dictates the quantity of bone that the graft will form. Particulate cancellous bone marrow can be mixed with particulate freeze dried bone, however, this combination reduces the number of osteocompetent cells forming new osteoid and in turn compromises the quantity of bone that is formed.[26]

Fig. 12-7

12-7A. Intra-oral photo-graph of a patient with an extensive ameloblastoma of the mandible. The tumor had caused sig-nificant destruction and expansion of the jaw.

12-7B. Frontal view of the same patient showing the enlargement of the man-dible.

12-7C. Profile view of the patient also reveals the extensive nature of the tumor.

12-7D. The 3D CT scan shows the growth of the tumor extending from the right mandibular angle to the left parasymphysis.

12-7E. The fibular graft contoured prior to vascu-lar anastamosis.

12-7F. The panoramic radiograph shows the re-constructed mandible.

12-7G. Frontal view of the patient one year after re-construction shows good symmetry of the lower third of the face.

12-7H. The profile view also shows an acceptable esthetic result.

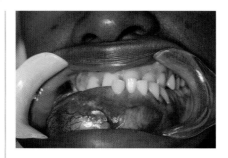

12-7A

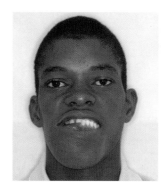

12-7B

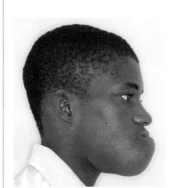

12-7C

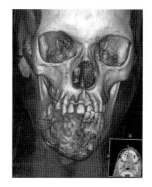

12-7D

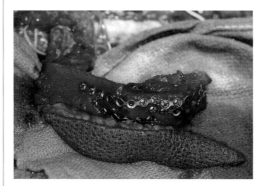

12-7E

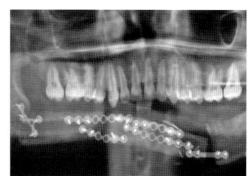

12-7F

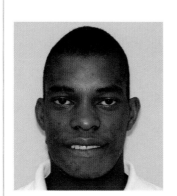

12-7G

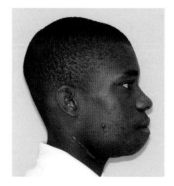

12-7H

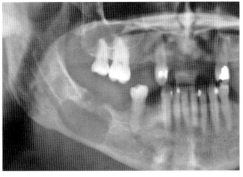

12-8A

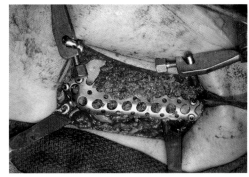

12-8B

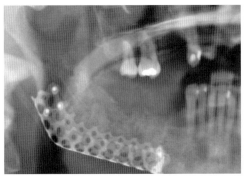

12-8C

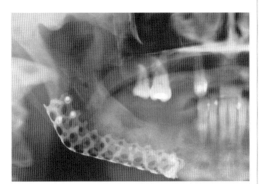

12-8D

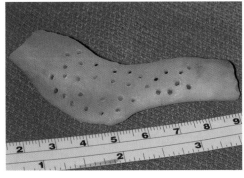

12-9A

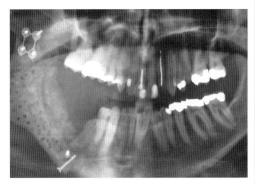

12-9B

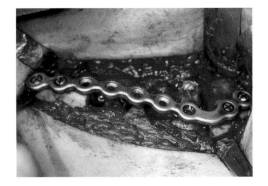

12-10A

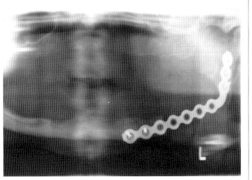

12-10B

Fig. 12-8

12-8A. The panoramic radiograph shows a radiolucency in the mandible which when biopsied was consistent with an odontogenic keratocyst.

12-8B. The resected mandible was reconstructed with autogenous cancellous bone. A titanium mesh tray was used for support and anatomic contour.

12-8C. The panoramic radiograph shows the newly reconstructed mandible. The grafted bone is less dense than the surrounding host bone soon after surgery.

12-8D. Six months after reconstruction the grafted bone has matured and is indistinguishable from the surrounding host bone.

Fig. 12-9

12-9A. A cadaveric freeze-dried mandible is perforated prior to use for reconstruction to allow for vascular ingrowth of the bone graft.

12-9B. The panoramic radiograph shows the cadaveric mandible used for structural support for the autogenous particulate cancellous bone graft used for reconstruction of a resected mandible.

Fig. 12-10

12-10A. A reconstruction plate allows for temporary replacement of anatomic form and maintenance of the position of the remaining mandibular segments.

12-10B. The reconstruction plate can be contoured to better simulate the resected mandible.

Particulate cancellous bone marrow provides a large phase I cell population and can be packed and contoured for more predictable esthetic results. Once the transplanted cells have survived and phase II osteogenesis, in which the recipient bed dictates the resorption and remodeling of the immature bone to mature bone, is complete, the new bone can be used for insertion of osseointegrated implants and support of a prosthesis.

Block grafts may provide better structure and support, but the cell population transplanted in these grafts is relatively small, decreasing the phase I component of osteogenesis and making vascular ingrowth difficult. These grafts are approximately 50% weaker than normal bone for 6 weeks to 6 months following transplantation and exhibit greater resorption.[36] Complications with non-vascularized grafts include bone resorption and infection, especially in patients requiring adjuvant radiation therapy.[29]

Regardless of whether vascularized or non-vascularized grafts are used, the result of reconstruction is usually more favorable if the resection and the reconstruction are performed during the same surgical procedure. This allows for more accurate contouring of the graft to better simulate the contour of the contra lateral side and avoids having to recreate a bed for the graft, often through scarred tissue. When the resection of the mandible necessitates an intra-oral/extra-oral communication, which is inevitable when teeth are present in the planned resection, there is a greater risk of infection with non-vascularized free grafts. For benign disease, with slow growth potential, treatment can be staged. Teeth can be extracted and a primary closure of the intraoral soft tissue achieved initially. The resection and reconstruction can then be performed 3-4 weeks later via an extra-oral approach, after mucosal healing has taken place. This minimizes oral contamination of the grafted bone.

With any technique for mandibular reconstruction, a critical factor in restoring form and function is maintaining the correct preoperative three-dimensional relationships of the bony and soft-tissue components. It is important also to maintain the position of the preserved mandibular segments. This is commonly accomplished with a bridging reconstruction bar (Fig. 10B), external rigid fixation (Fig. 11) or the use of arch bars and intermaxillary fixation (Fig. 12). Accurately restoring the mandibular segments to their original preoperative alignment after surgery is crucial.

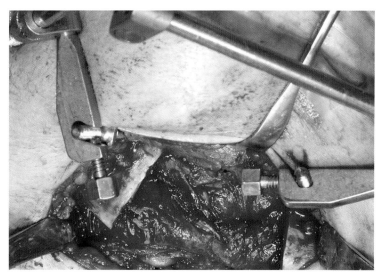

12-11

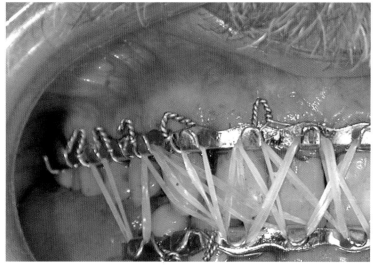

12-12

Alloplastic material

The most commonly used alloplastic materials for mandibular reconstruction are bone plates and screws.[38] This technique is generally indicated when the soft tissue defect is more extensive than the bony defect.[39] Although this technique may present with significant delayed complications such as hardware extrusion and infection, it is a reasonable option for patients with a poor prognosis or poor general health. Long and complex reconstructions involving microvascular procedures and autogenous bone harvesting entail high risk. Other complications of alloplastic materials include plate fractures, and delayed wound healing making it necessary for secondary reconstructive procedures with vascularized grafts.[40]

It is important to remember that use of reconstruction bone plates without bone grafts, only bridges the anatomic defect. It does not reconstruct anatomic form nor restore adequate function. This type of reconstruction infrequently provides adequate support for even conventional prosthetic reconstruction with removable prostheses making it difficult to restore craniofacial function.

More recently, the potential use of bioresorbable bone graft substitutes for mandibular reconstruction has been explored. The use of a porous, biodegradable biopolymer scaffold for mandibular defects in a rat model showed enhanced *in vivo* new bone formation.[41] As the field of tissue engineering advances, new techniques for skeletal reconstruction will continue to be developed.

Distraction Osteogenesis

The technique of distraction osteogenesis was originally developed by Dr. G. A. Ilizarov for orthopedic application to lengthen long bones. He also demonstrated the scientific basis and clinical efficacy of this technique.[42] Over the past decade, distraction osteogenesis has also been applied to craniofacial deformities. It has been especially useful for congenital deformities of the mandible such as in hemifacial microsomia, severe micrognathia and other craniofacial syndromes.[43,44] The first step involves a mandibular oste-

otomy and insertion of the distraction device. The distraction device allows for progressive separation or distraction of the bony surfaces over several days resulting in bone elongation and soft tissue regeneration. This makes distraction ostegenesis a good treatment option in treating composite mandibular defects.

Using the same principle, transport distraction has been used to reconstruct larger discontinuity defects by regenerating bone and soft tissue. In this technique, an osteotomy is performed to create a bone transport segment. The distraction process continues transporting this segment under mechanical guidance until it reaches the opposing bone or sufficient bone and soft tissue are reconstructed for oral rehabilitation.[45] The guidance of the transport segment is necessary to achieve the desired contour of the mandibular anatomy being reconstructed. The new bone that is generated behaves identically to the host bone and thus can accept osseointegrated implants[d]. The challenge in this technique is to maintain the correct vector during the distraction process. Also, the distraction period is lengthy, taking several weeks to accomplish the desired bone length.

Factors increasing wound healing

There is great interest in enhancing wound healing with the use of growth factors. Platelet-rich plasma (PRP) extracted from autologous whole blood is known to contain high concentrations of a number of different growth factors. Specifically, the growth factors transforming growth factor-beta (TGF-beta) and platelet derived growth factor (PDGF) have profound effects on bone healing. Studies have shown that PRP enhances osteoconduction, improves adhesion of cancellous marrow during graft delivery and advances the rate and amount of newly regenerated bone.[47] The addition of PRP to bone grafts produces a quantifiably enhanced result in comparison with grafts performed without it.[47] The addition of PRP to autologous iliac cancellous bone for repair of alveolar clefts shows an increased volume of regenerated bone in these patients when compared to the group who underwent alveolar bone grafting without PRP.[48]

Another growth factor used for increased healing is recombinant human bone morphogenetic protein BMP7. It is an osteoinductive factor that initiates conversion of undifferentiated precursor stem cells into osteoprogenitor cells, which produce mature bone.[49]

Prefabrication of bone grafts for reconstruction after tumor surgery has also become a possibility. Recently an extensive mandibular discontinuity defect was repaired by growth of a custom bone transplant using iliac crest bone marrow to provide undifferentiated precursor cells as a target for recombinant human BMP inside the latissimus dorsi muscle of an adult male patient.[50] The use of

BMP7 also has been shown to accelerate the regenerate ossification during distraction osteogenesis.[51]

As the evolution of novel regenerative procedures continues, advances in tissue engineering will play an important role and reduce extensive surgical procedures necessary for graft harvesting.

Osseointegrated Implants

Osseointegrated implants have become a standard approach for prosthodontic treatment in dentistry.[52-54] The application of implants in combination with bone grafting, has become more important in jaw reconstruction over the last decade, and has allowed for improved esthetic and functional results. Implants have been inserted either simultaneously with bone grafts[55-56] or at a later stage after the bone grafts have healed.[57,58] Implant placement requires a minimum bone height of approximately 6 to 7 mm and a minimum width of 4 mm. These criteria can easily be met in reconstruction with either vascularized or non-vascularized bone grafts.

Once the reconstructed bone is viable – anastomosis in vascularized grafts or matured in non-vascularized grafts – it behaves like any other viable bone and implants placed and loaded in reconstructed bone perform identically to implants placed in native bone.[26,59] A comparison of implant success in vascularized and non-vascularized bone grafts revealed a 99% osseointegration in vascularized versus 82% in non-vascularized grafts,[25] although it is possible these results may be related to factors other than the grafting technique. Our clinical experience with titanium screw-type implants in reconstructed mandibles using non-vascularized particulate cancellous bone marrow revealed an 85% osseointegration[26] but we are experiencing a higher rate of osseointegration with increasing number of patients and change in technique. Osseointegration of 91% has been reported in patients reconstructed with non-vascularized free corticocancellous iliac crest block grafts.[58]

The rate of osseointegration has been compared in immediate implants placed in cortical block and particulate grafts. After one month, the implants in cortical block demonstrated a greater percentage of osseointegration than those placed immediately in particulate grafts.[37] Immediate versus delayed implant placement has also been compared in autogenous iliac bone grafts which revealed more predictable bone formation around implants that were placed 90 to 180 days after bone grafting.[56] Osseointegration of implants placed in vascularized bone grafts in the early stage after graft transplantation is compromised. This is due to the fact that vascularized bone grafts do not have both intact medullary and periosteal blood supply, but only intact periosteal supply.[55]

Osseointegration of implants in irradiated bone has also been examined.[56,60-62] There is a statistically significant higher failure rate in implants inserted in irradiated bone than implants inserted in non-irradiated tissue.[62] Irradiated tissue provides a hypoxic, hypovascular, hypocellular recipient bed,[63] which compromises phase II of osteogenesis. Hyperbaric oxygen therapy prior to and after implantation, has been shown to improve the integration of implants.[44,64]

Even though placement of implants in the reconstructed mandible poses unique challenges, some of the limitations or restrictions such as the position of the inferior alveolar nerve, does not exist in most of these patients. The number of implants that can be placed is determined by the three dimensional location and bone quantity available. From a prosthetic reconstruction point of view, two implants is the minimum desired number.

Soft tissue considerations

The condition of the intraoral soft tissue after reconstruction is of concern and can place restrictions on implant placement. Patients who have had intra-oral soft tissue reconstruction with a myocutaneous flap often require debulking of the soft tissue prior to implant placement. Other soft tissue problems in these patients include soft tissue scarring, fibrosis, and banding of the mucosal tissue.

This often necessitates soft tissue plasty to reduce tissue thickness aound the prosthetic abutments and to allow for easier restoration. Multiple surgical procedures may be necessary for proper and successful implant placement in these patients.

However, despite the challenges and restrictions for implant placement in reconstructed bone, the osseointegration rate in grafted and in irradiated bone is high enough to warrant their use in reconstructed patients, especially since the anatomic alterations following surgery often prohibits fabrication of any conventional prosthesis.

Prosthetic Reconstruction

Morphologic Information: Mounted Study Casts

Preoperative study casts when available can provide valuable information on the patient's preoperative occlusion, tooth position, tissue contours, and esthetics. All casts should be mounted with a face bow as a facebow transfer shows right and left antero-posterior and medio-lateral occlusal plane inclinations (Fig. 12-13). A centric relation intermaxillary record is advised as it provides information on what inclined plane contacts may occur during closure on the side or sides to be restored. Although the reconstruction may not be made

in centric relation, the record serves diagnostically to assess preoperative contacts. It is also important to obtain an habitual occlusal record especially when casts do not provide an easily identifiable or stable habitual occlusal position. Obtaining centric and habitual preoperative information ensures easier reconstruction of tooth contacts at appropriate vertical dimension.

Post-surgical casts are the most important morphologic information for planning the prosthetic reconstructive phase. Surgical reconstruction generally cannot replace all the hard and soft tissues removed, and in most instances only a very narrow bucco-lingual space will remain between the tongue, cheek and lips. Realistically, this narrow zone usually means replacement teeth will be narrower bucco-lingual and with a narrower occlusal table. Additionally, as placement and positioning of implants is mostly influenced by height, width, and quality of bone, prosthetic compromises of tooth position often will occur in these reconstructions. Thus adaptation to the overall damage will have to take place and some degree of relearning on how to comfortably eat, speak, and swallow will be necessary.

A wax-up/set-up on the post-surgical cast is done and becomes the blueprint for the reconstruction. Implant placement is optimized with a surgical

Fig. 12-13. A face bow transfer orients the maxilla to the rotation of the condyles.

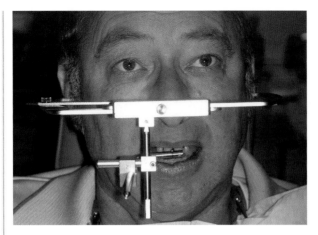

12-13

template made from the wax/set-up. When implant placement is closely related to the planned prosthodontic result the ease of achieving realistic OHR QOL parameters is enhanced.

Prosthodontic techniques: fixed prosthesis is most likely to achieve optimal OHR QOL, and when possible is the prosthetic reconstruction goal for these patients.

PROSTHODONTIC MATERIALS

Acrylic, composite, and porcelain are currently the most common veneering materials on a cast metal framework for implant supported fixed prostheses. Acrylic, though simple to apply and initially esthetic and functional, stains easily, wears and fractures away more than do any other materials, and thus it is not a good choice.[66,67] Composite materials wear better than acrylic, but not significantly, and composite wears and stains more than does porcelain. Gold

occlusal surfaces wear about the same as the natural dentition, but are unaesthetic to most. Porcelain wears better than acrylic and composite and looks better than gold. But once porcelain glaze wears off, the relative roughness of unglazed porcelain compared to enamel will wear the opposing natural dentition. There is no perfect material to use in a restoration, and determining what material is used results from communicating their pros and cons to the patient. Generally, porcelain is better accepted by patients because of esthetics, better wear, and less maintenance. Along with gold it is the preferred material to maintain occlusal contacts and appropriate vertical dimension.

IMPRESSION MATERIALS

Any polymerizing electrometric impression material is adequate. Polyether materials have great accuracy and are generally more rigid, although polyvinyl siloxane materials do not stain clothing, and casts are easier to remove from impressions made with polyvinyl materials.[68] However, accuracy of the impression material does not guarantee accurate fit of the prosthesis to abutments. Stabilizing the position of the inter-implant distance before the impression is made is equally important. Luting square impression copings to each other with the open tray technique produces a more accurate cast[69] (Fig. 12-14A and B). The accuracy of inter-implant spacing in the cast reduces the need for cutting and soldering the framework, and framework accuracy reduces screw loosening.[70]

IMPRESSIONS

Local anesthesia to the tissues may be needed, especially on the lingual, as manipulating the tissue around the implants is painful when nervous innervation of any kind remains. Impression at the fixture level is a better approach than choosing and placing abutments. An open tray technique is preferred even though access to the impression copings is sometimes difficult. But, attaching the impression copings together with acrylic reduces cutting and soldering the framework. However if there is limited opening as a result of surgical treatments, it may be necessary to use a closed-tray technique. Regardless of the impression technique, before the impression is made, a radiograph to assure copings are completely seated on fixtures is required.

Fixture impressions also allow choosing abutments long enough to completely traverse the mucosa. Notwithstanding attempts to surgically debulk these tissues, they generally often remain thick and not bound down. A smooth, machined titanium surface is generally kinder to the mucosa and easier to clean than a cast-metal or porcelain surface. When pouring the impression, tissue analog materials give the prosthodontist

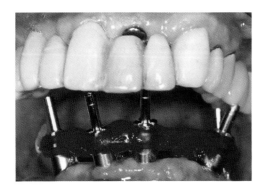

12-14A

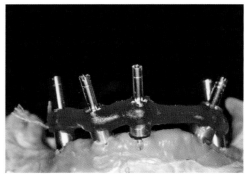

12-14B

Fig. 12-14A and B. Square impression copings luted together with auto polymerizing resin provide greater reliability of fixture analog orientation in the master cast. This is a particularly valuable approach when implants are inserted off-angle *(photographs courtesy of Dr. Nopsaran Chaimattayompol).*

the ability to determine the appropriate length of the abutments. Two to three millimeters above the mucosa is optimal. Fixture impressions also make it easier to determine if an angled abutment is required.

INTERMAXILLARY RELATIONSHIPS

A centric relation record, when possible, is most likely to assure simultaneous contact of both the natural dentition and reconstructed sides. A centric relation record is preferable as it provides a starting, or reference, position that is generally reproducible. However, the musculature is affected by removal of the disease and reconstruction of jaw form. Muscles on the surgical side often tend to pull the jaw to that side, making a centric relation record and therefore subsequent reconstruction of a centric relation functioning position difficult if not impossible to accomplish. When a new, well functioning closure pattern has developed after the surgery, reconstruction in this new habituated occlusal position is quite acceptable. The technique of making the record depends on the preference of the prosthodontist.

If the replacement and natural teeth come together harmoniously, most patients' function and comfort are accomplished. The mediolateral and antero-posterior components of vertical dimension are also achieved when simultaneous contact and equal force distribution occur bilaterally.

Because of the long-term surgical treatments, and often severe occlusal contact changes, the opposing teeth will shift and new opposing casts and facebow transfer must be made. When the final prosthesis cast framework is tried in, a new interocclusal record also must be made to assure final proper occlusion.

PROVISIONALIZATION

As mentioned previously, surgical reconstruction often results in a narrow zone between the tongue and cheek. Testing patient adaptation to the occlusal reconstruction with a provisional prosthesis can provide information on tooth position and shape for the final prosthesis. A week or two for assessing and making needed modifications on the provisional prosthesis before sending the mounted final casts to the laboratory enhances the final result. Testing esthetics, chewing, speaking, and comfort can be accomplished before the final prosthesis is completed. The diagnostic set-up/wax-up can be used as a template for the provisional.

If temporization is decided upon, a laboratory processed provisional may be relined on temporary abutment cylinders on the mounted master casts. The major problem with making a provisional restoration intraorally in these patients is access to the implants; the top of the fixtures may be inferior to adjacent teeth if present. Another problem is tissue depth. Once a healing abutment is removed the tissue immediately collapses, and placing and preparing temporary cylinders intraorally is difficult.

A provisional restoration can be either temporarily cemented or screwed into the implants. Either approach is acceptable, although screwing in the provisional avoids cement being caught in the mucosal sulcus. If the provisional meets all or most of the QOL parameters, a study impression is made, and this cast is sent with mounted final casts to the dental laboratory to help develop the final restoration.

THE FRAMEWORK CASTINGS

The longer the casting, the poorer the fit.[71] A length of four units almost always fits accurately. If longer, it is best cast in two sections and a solder index made when the sections are tried-in.

For long span castings, especially those that turn the corner in the canine region, an internal key and keyway attachment can be used to connect segments of the framework together for passive fit of castings to abutments. Using attachments also reduces metal warping when fusing porcelain. Implant prostheses are frequently large containing a great deal of metal, so porcelain cracking is reduced if the length of the castings is kept to three to four units. Two implants as abutments for each casting segment are needed for best prosthesis stability.

PROSTHETIC RETENTION TO IMPLANTS

There is increasing desire to cement prosthetics to custom or preparable abutments for esthetic reasons, but this should be done with caution. Since there is no periodontal ligament around implants, occlusal forces are undampened and these forces can create problems with screw loosening. Almost inevitably when screws loosen they break. When prosthesis and abutments are screw retained and screws are easily accessible, retightening is easy. Proper torqueing has substantially reduced abutment and/ or prosthesis screw loosening, but it still occurs and access to the screws is easier if the prosthesis is not cemented. Although there is less porcelain fracture with a cement-retained design because there is no screw access hole, any porcelain failure is almost impossible to repair if the prosthesis is cemented permanently. Cement is also very difficult to remove from the peri-implant sulcus, and can result in chronic discomfort if not removed. If abutment screws loosen under a permanently cemented prosthesis, there is no access to tighten them and the prosthesis would have to be cut off. While large implant castings may fit better on abutments if cement rather than screw retained, there is no difference in success of the implants using either technique.[72] However, there are ways to unite the advantages of both cement and screw retention. A technique that combines screw stability with a weak luting agent has been studied and found reliable.[73] A framework is cast to cementable abutments and a lateral set screw in one or more abutment is used for stability. This provides for relatively easy removal of the prosthesis as needed for maintenance, screw tightening, or repair.

Screw retention for most implant-supported prosthetics is reliable and remains the standard. However, two implants per prosthetic segment reduce the overall force to retentive components and reduce the chance of screw loosening.

INSERTION OF THE PROSTHESIS

Three factors influencing OHR QOL indicators should be evaluated at prosthetic insertion: occlusal contacts, esthetics, and comfort. As long as occlusal contacts are bilateral and simultaneous with a generally even distribution on each side, it is best to avoid the temptation to adjust the occlusion to completion. As the patient will not have had occlusion on at least one side for a long time, muscles will require some adaptation to the newly restored tooth contacts.[74] Seeing the patient the day after insertion to begin refinement of the contacts and adjusting them

over one to four weeks until stable is advised.[75]

The loss of a large section of the jaw means that major neural innervation to that area will be destroyed, but this does not mean that there is a total lack of sensation. Osseoperception[76] provides feedback to the CNS to redevelop adequate muscular function.[77] Patients can identify stress applied to dental implants similarly to the forces applied to the natural dentition.[78] The physiology of osseoperception is not completely understood, but evidence strongly suggests that the CNS processes jaw stress information and relates it to habituated patterns of muscular function.[77] Indeed muscle function is not dependant on proprioception from the periodontal ligament alone.[79] The relative success of complete dentures is an example.[80] Control of jaw function seems to be similar with the natural dentition or with prosthetic reconstructions on dental implants.[81,82]

All patients are concerned with esthetic and functional loss, and it is no exaggeration these patients are devastated by their loss. Psychologically they suffer from greater or lesser degrees of depression. However within a few days or weeks, the majority of patients have adapted to the prosthesis.

Patient Cases

Patient 1 – This patient is a 58 year old male who was diagnosed with squamous cell carcinoma of the anterior floor of the mouth and mandible. He was treated with extensive mandibular and soft tissue resection and bilateral neck dissections, followed by radiation therapy. He underwent a secondary procedure for reconstruction with an iliac crest and musculo-cutaneous graft (Fig. 12-15A). A reconstruction plate was used for rigidity and to help contour the bone graft. After radiation therapy was completed, he received hyberbaric oxygen prior to placement of 6 osseointegrated implants (Fig. 12-15B). The musculo-cutanous graft was debulked at the same time. Four of the implants were placed in the graft and 2 in the pre-existing host bone. Five of the implants integrated and were used to support a removable denture (Fig. 12-15C and D). The patient was very satisfied with the retention of a removable denture on the healing abutments and elected not to have a fixed prosthesis or a bar retained removable denture made. The restoration of this patient's function enabled him to maintain his nutrition and regain his social and psychological self esteem (Fig. 12-15E).

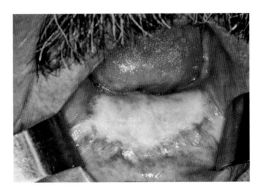

12-15A

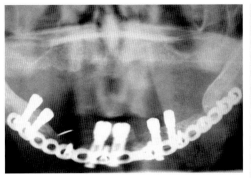

12-15B

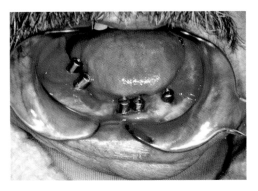

12-15C

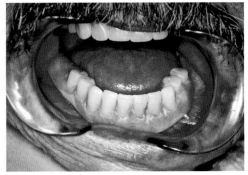

12-15D

Fig. 12-15

12-15A. This patient underwent extensive mandibular resection followed by reconstruction with a free iliac crest block graft and musculo-cutaneous graft to replace the intra-oral soft tissue.

12-15B. Four osseointegrated implants were inserted in the reconstructed bone and two in the pre-existing mandible.

12-15C. The soft tissue was debulked before implants were placed. One of the implants in the grafted bone failed to integrate.

12-15D. The patient's occlusion was restored with an implant supported denture.

12-15E. The restoration of the patient's function and esthetics restored his self esteem and quality of life.

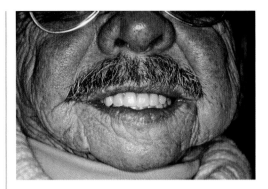

12-15E

Patient 2 – This 41 year old male was diagnosed with squamous cell carcinoma in a non-healing third molar socket (Fig. 12-16A). He was treated with a segmental resection of the mandible followed by secondary reconstruction with autogenous non-vascularized particulate cancellous bone graft from the iliac crest. A cadaveric rib was used for structural support of the bone graft (Fig. 12-16B and C). Six months after reconstruction, three osseointegrated implants were inserted in the reconstructed mandible for support of a fixed prosthesis (Fig. 16D and E). The tissue on the reconstructed ridge was thick and moveable, so 5.0 mm standard abutments were used. Movement of the tissue around the polished titanium abutments is comfortable, and cleaning of these surfaces is very easy. Prosthetic esthetics was not a concern of the patient. He is disease free and functioning well with excellent facial form and OHR QOL 15 years later (Fig. 12-16F).

Patient 3 – This 11 year old girl

was diagnosed with a plexiform ameloblastoma of the right mandibular parasymphysis (Fig. 12-17A). This was treated with mandibular en-bloc resection (preserving the inferior border) and reconstruction with autogenous non-vascularized particulate cancellous bone graft from the iliac crest (Fig. 12-17B). Six months after reconstruction, three osseointegrated implants were inserted for support of a fixed prosthesis (Fig. 12-17C). Although with normal speech and facial expressions the prosthetic reconstruction cannot be seen, esthetics relating to shape and contour of the hard and soft tissues was a major concern for the patient. Thus it was elected to construct the prosthesis at the fixture level to minimize the possibility of any part of the titanium abutments showing. Pink porcelain placed to mimic the shade of the soft tissue on the prosthesis. The patient was very pleased with the result notwithstanding the light pink shade of the porcelain at the gingiva. The patient is disease free and functioning well 10 years later (Fig. 12-17D).

Fig. 12-16

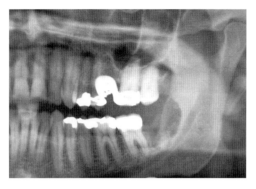
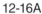

12-16A

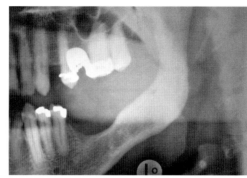

12-16B

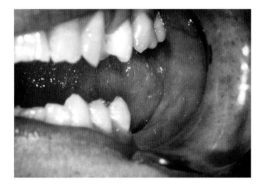

12-16C

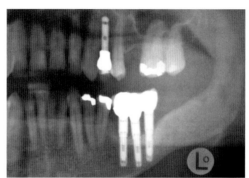

12-16D

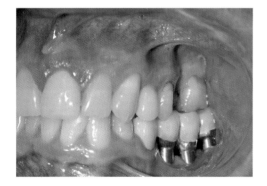

12-16E

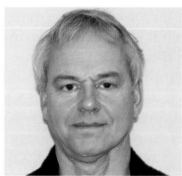

12-16F

12-16A. The panoramic radiograph shows a radiolucency extending from the left mandibular second molar superiorly along the ascending ramus. This radiograph was taken two months after removal of a symptomatic third molar. A biopsy revealed squamous cell carcinoma.

12-16B. The panoramic radiograph shows the reconstructed mandible. The angle of the mandible was preserved in this patient and there is good cortical and cancellous definition of the grafted site.

12-16C. There is a lack of attached mucosa on the reconstructed alveolar ridge because the initial resection necessitated excision of intra-oral soft tissue along with the diseased mandible. There is good bone height for prosthetic reconstruction.

12-16D. Implants in the reconstructed mandible have good bone support.

12-16E. Prosthetic reconstruction was accomplished with a fixed implant supported prosthesis. Because of the lack of attached mucosa in this case, long abutments were used to traverse the movable tissue. This prosthetic design allows for good oral hygiene and comfort.

12-16F. The patient is disease free 15 years later and has an excellent functional and cosmetic result.

Fig. 12-17

12-17A. The panoramic radiograph reveals a mixed radiolucent-radio-opaque lesion involving the mandibular right canine and bicuspids.

12-17B. The panoramic radiograph shows the newly reconstructed mandible. The borders of the osteotomy are evident and the grafted bone appears less dense than the surrounding pre-existing bone. The inferior border was retained in this patient, thus preserving the continuity of the mandible.

12-17C. The panoramic radiograph shows the integrated implants used to support a fixed prosthesis.

12-17D. The design of the prosthesis allows for good hygiene and esthetics in an area with limited attached mucosa. The patient is functioning well 10 years later.

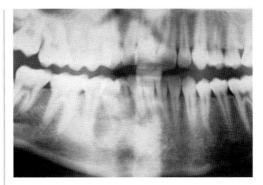

12-17A

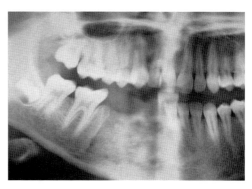

12-17B

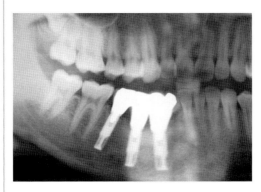

12-17C

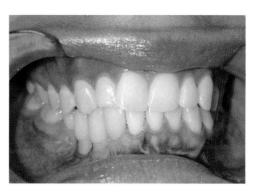

12-17D

Patient 4 – This 51 year old woman was diagnosed with ameloblastoma of the right mandible (Fig. 12-18A to C). She was treated with en-bloc mandibular resection along with excision of overlying soft tissue followed by immediate reconstruction with autogenous non-vascularized particulate cancellous bone graft from the iliac crest. Six months after reconstruction four osseointegrated implants were inserted in the grafted mandible for restoration with fixed prosthetics (Fig. 12-18D and E). The patient's function and esthetics have been restored and she is disease free 4 years later (Fig. 12-18F and G).

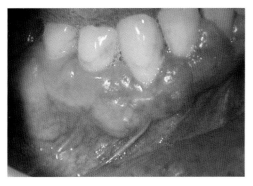

12-18A

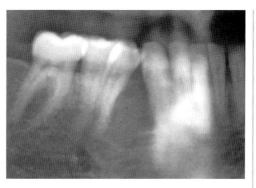

12-18B

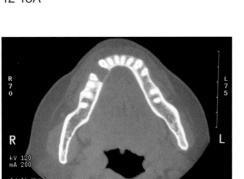

12-18C

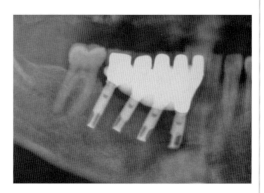

12-18D

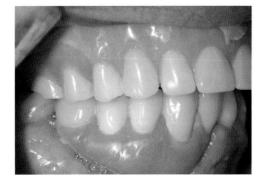

12-18E

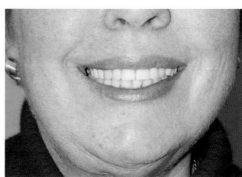

12-18F

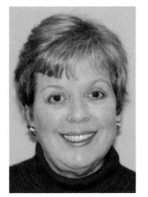

12-18G

Fig. 12-18

12-18A. This clinical photograph shows a soft tissue mass between the canine and the first premolar.

12-18B. The panoramic radiograph shows a radiolucency between the canine and first premolar. The lesion is causing divergence of the root of these teeth.

12-18C. The CT scan shows the complete erosion of the buccal and thinning of the lingual cortex caused by the ameloblastoma.

12-18D. Four osseointegrated implants were inserted in the reconstructed mandible for support of a fixed prosthesis.

12-18E. Functional reconstruction was achieved with fixed implant supported hybrid prosthesis restoring the dentition and the soft tissue.

12-18F. The prosthetic reconstruction has restored this patient's occlusion and smile.

12-18G. The reconstruction of her occlusion provides support of her lower lip and cheek thus resulting in a favorable cosmetic result.

Patient 5 – This 24 year old woman was diagnosed with fibrous dysplasia of her right mandible when she was 9 years old. She had undergone three previous surgeries for reducing the diseased mandible. The fibrous dysplasia continued to spread affecting more of her mandible (Fig. 12-19A to C). She eventually complained of pain and numbness of the distribution of the right inferior alveolar nerve. Because of the chronicity, extent of disease and the patient's symptoms, this was treated with partial resection of the right mandible, followed by immediate reconstruction with autogenous non-vascularized particulate cancellous bone graft from the iliac crest with the addition of platelet rich plasma. A titanium tray was used as structural support and to define the contour of the mandibular angle (Fig. 12-19D). The use of cancellous bone allowed for shaping and molding of the bone graft to create an alveolar ridge in a favorable relationship to the opposing arch, contralateral side and remaining dentition (Fig. 12-19E). Also, extraction of teeth prior to resection and reconstruction allowed for healing of the intra-oral soft tissue, thereby preserving much of the attached mucosa. This bound-down tissue minimized possible intra-oral communication during the reconstruction. Six months after reconstruction, 4 osseointegrated implants were inserted for support of fixed restorations (Fig. 12-19F and G). The existing attached mucosa allowed for easier placement and contour of the restorations. Esthetics was satisfactory to the patient. Although the need for such surgery was initially devastating for this patient, the surgical and prosthodontic restoration of craniofacial function, dental and facial esthetics has restored her self esteem and social acceptance (Fig. 12-19H and I).

Fig. 12-19

12-19A. The panoramic radiograph shows a dense radiopaque lesion involving the four posterior teeth and inferior alveolar nerve. The second bicuspid and first molar had undergone endodontic treatment in an attempt to resolve the patient's symptoms.

12-19B. Despite the progressive nature of the disease there was little expansion of the mandible on the buccal aspect.

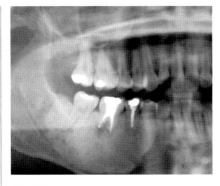
12-19A

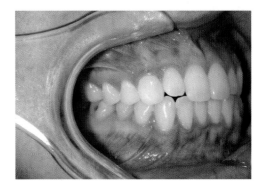
12-19B

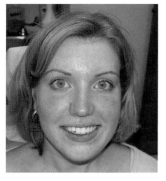

12-19C

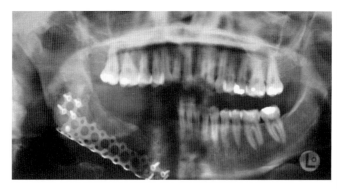

12-19D

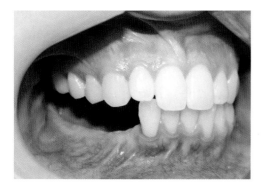

12-19E

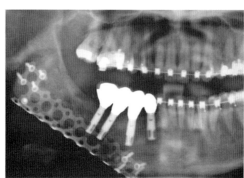

12-19F

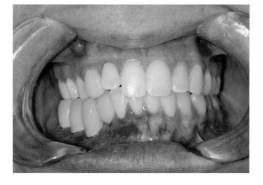

12-19G

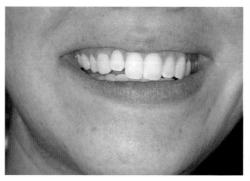

12-19H

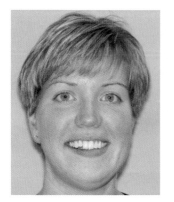

12-19I

12-19C. There was no evidence of facial asymmetry.

12-19D. The panoramic radiograph shows the reconstructed mandible. The titanium tray was used for structural support of the particulate cancellous bone graft and to provide anatomical contour of the mandibular angle.

12-19E. Six months after reconstruction, the resultant alveolar ridge had excellent height and relationship with the adjacent anatomy. There was also preservation of the attached mucosa.

12-19F. Four osseointegrated implants were inserted in the reconstructed mandible with no appreciable bone loss around the implants two years later.

12-19G. Occlusal reconstruction was accomplished with implant supported fixed prosthetics. The prosthetic design allows for good oral hygiene.

12-19H. The prosthetic reconstruction provides support of the lip and cheek.

12-19I. The anatomical reconstruction replaced the resected mandible and restored the facial contour and esthetics.

Conclusions

The loss of any facial part decreases one's ability to function socially or biologically. Even the loss of a single tooth can alter self perception and one's place in society. Loss of large segments of the craniofacial complex requires not only anatomical restoration, but also considerable emotional support. Sympathetic, encouraging, yet very realistic appraisal for the short and long term outcomes is strongly advised. Even with today's surgical and prosthodontic reconstruction techniques, it is still impossible to restore complete functionality, esthetics, and comfort lost from large resections. Osseointegrated implant reconstructions dramatically increase the quality of life of patients, and that alone is cause for encouraging patients to realize a positive outcome of their treatment.

We believe it is very important to know the craniofacial complex's role in biologic and psychological health. Combined with understanding oral health related quality of life parameters, patient care is greatly improved. A process is inevitably created that focuses on overall treatment rather than the linear, segmental approach of eliminating disease, and surgical reconstruction followed by prosthetic reconstruction.

To successfully reconstruct and rehabilitate the patient, the treatment team must:

❑ understand the craniofacial complex and OHR QOL

❑ diagnose the disease and its extent

❑ plan surgical removal and any other treatment of the disease

❑ plan surgical and prosthetic reconstruction together

❑ inform the patient of treatment options and consequences of treatment

❑ anatomically restore, within the limits of damage from disease, the oral health related quality of life parameters of esthetics, comfort, function, and biologic and psychological health.

If all this is taken into consideration, the patient will be returned as a functional member of society with regained self esteem and quality of life.

References

1. AZUMA, Y.; MAEHARA, K.; TOKUNAGA, T.; HASHIMOTO, M.; IEOKA, K.; SAKAGAMI, H. *Systemic affects of the occlusal destruction in guinea pigs.* In Vivo. 1999; 13:519-24.

2. GILLIES, G.T.; CHRISTY, D.W.; STENGER, J.M.; BROADDUS, W.C. Equilibrium and non-equilibrium dynamics of the cranio-mandibular complex and cervical spine. *J Med Eng Technol* 2003; 27:32-40.

3. SHIMAZAKI, T.; MOTOYOSHI, M.; HOSOI, K.; NAMURA, S. The effect of occlusal alteration and masticatory imbalance on the cervical spine. *Eur J Orthod* 2003; 25:457-63.

4. SLAVICEK, R. The *Masticatory Organ: Functions and Dysfunctions.* Klosterneuburg, Áustria 2002; Gamma Med-wiss. Fortbildungs-AG.

5. BANI, D.; BANI, T.; BERGAMINI, M. Morphologic and biochemical changes of the masseter muscles induced by occlusal wear: studies in a rat model. *J Dent Res* 1999; 778:1735-44.

6. MEHTA, NR. Understanding the influence of occlusal modifiers as they affect occlusal diagnosis. *KMC Dent J* 1995; 6:69-78.

7. MILANI, R.S.; DEPERIERE, D.D.; LAPEYRE, L.; POURREYRON, L. Relationship between dental occlusion and posture. *Cranio* 2000; 18:127-34.

8. WATANABE, I. Influence of wearing complete denture on body balance in edentulous elderly. *Kokubyo Gakkai Zasshi.* 1999; 66:8-14.

9. FUJIMOTO, M.; HAYAKAWA, L.; WATANABE, I. Changes in gait stability induced by alteration of mandibular position. *J Med Dent Sci* 2001; 48:131-6.

10. GANGLOFF, P.; LOUIS, J.P.; PERRIN, P.P. Dental occlusion modifies gaze and posture stabilization in human subjects. *Neurosci Lett* 2000; 3:203-6.

11. PENFIELD, W.; RASMUSSEN, T. *The Cerebral Cortex of Man.* New York 1950; Macmillan.

12. FALLOWFIELD, L. *The Quality of Life: The missing measurement in health care.* London 1990; Souvenir Press.

13. INGLEHART, M.R.; BAGRAMIAN, R.A. Eds: *Oral Health-Related Quality of Life.* Chicago 2002; Quintessence Pub Co Inc.

14. NORDENRAM, G.; RONNBERG, L.; WINBLAD, B. The perceived importance of appearance and oral function, comfort and health for severely demented persons rated by relatives, nursing staff and hospital dentists. *Gerodontology* 1994; 11:18-24.

15. KRESSIN, N.; SPIRO, A. 3RD, BOSSE, R.; KAZIS, L. Assessing oral health-related quality of life: findings from the normative aging study. *Med Care* 1996; 34:416-27.

16. STANDARDS OF CARE: Delta Dental of Massachusetts. Medford, MA 1996; Delta Dental Plan of Massachusetts.

17. HOLLISTER, M.C.; WEINTRAUB, J.A. The association of oral status with systemic health, quality of life, and economic productivity. *J Dent Educ* 1999;57:901-12.

18. AWAD, M.A.; LOCKER, D.; KORNER-BITENSKY, N.; FEINE, J.S. Measuring the effect of intra-oral implant rehabilitation on health-related quality of life in a randomized controlled clinical trial. *J Dent Res* 2000; 79:1659-63.

19. UEDA, M.; HIBINO, Y.; NIIMI, A. Usefulness of dental implants in maxillofacial reconstruction. *J Long Term Eff Med Implants* 1999; 9:349-66.

20. LEUNG, A.C.; CHEUNG, L.K. Dental Implants in reconstructed jaws: patients' evaluation of functional quality-of-life outcomes. *Int J Oral Maxillofac Implants* 2003; 18:127-34.

21. SLOAN, J.A.; TOLMAN, D.E.; SUGAR, A.W.; WOLFAARDT, J.F.; NOVOTNY, P. Patients with reconstruction of craniofacial or Intraoral

defects: development of instruments to measure quality of life. *Int J Oral Maxillofac Implants* 2001; 16:225-45.

22. MILITSAKH, O.N.; WALLACE, D.I.; KRIET, J.D.; GIROD, D.A.; OLVERA, M.S.; TSUE, T.T. Use of the 2.0-mm locking reconstruction plate in primary oromandibular reconstruction after composite resection. *Otolangol Head Neck Surg* 2004; 131:660-5.

23. ROSELLI, R.; MUSCATELLO, L.; VALDATTA, L.; PAVA, G.; SPRIANO, G. Mandibular reconstruction with frozen autologous mandibular bone and radial periosteal fasciocutaneous free flap: preliminary report. *Ann Otol Rhinol Laryngol* 2004; 113:956-60.

24. WHITESIDES, L.M.; WUNDERLE, R.C.; GUERRERO, C. Mandible reconstruction using a 2-phase transport disc distraction osteogenesis: a case report. *J Oral Maxillofac Surg* 2005; 63:261-6.

25. FOSTER, R.D.; ANTHONY, J.P.; SHARMA, A.; POGREL, M.A. Vascularized bone flaps versus nonvascularized bone grafts for mandibular reconstruction: an outcome analysis of primary bony union and endosseous implant success. *Head Neck* 1999; 21:66-71.

26. PAPAGEORGE, M.B.; KARABETOU, S.M.; NORRIS, L;H. Rehabilitation of patients using osseointegrated implants: clinical report. *Int J Oral and Maxillofac Implants* 1999; 14:118-26.

27. PELED, M.; EL-NAAJ, I.A.; LIPIN, Y.; ARDEKIAN, L. The use of free fibular flap for functional mandibular reconstruction. *J Oral Maxillofac Surg* 2005; 63:220-4.

28. BILKAY, U.; TOKAT, C.; HELVACI, E.; OZEK, C.; ALPER, M. Free fibular flap mandible reconstruction in benign mandibular lesions. *J Craniofac Surg* 2004; 15:1002-9.

29. GENDEN, E.; HAUGHEY, B.H. Mandibular reconstruction by vascularized free tissue transfer. *Am J Otolaryngol* 1996; 17: 219-27.

30. URKEN, M.L.; WEINBERG, H.; VICKERY, C.; BUCHBINDER, D.; LAWSON, W.; BILLER, H.F. Oromandibular reconstruction using microvascular composite free flaps. Report of 71 cases and a new classification scheme for bony, soft-tissue, and neurologic defects. *Arch Otolaryngol Head Neck Surg* 1991; 117:733-44.

31. DAVID, J.D.; TAN, E.; KATSAROS, J.; SHEEN, R. Mandibular reconstruction with vascularized iliac crest: A 10-year experience. *Plast Reconstr Surg* 1988; 82:792-801.

32. CHANG, Y.M.; CHANA, J.S.; WEI, F.C.; SHEN, Y.F.; CHAN, C.P.; TSAI, C.Y. Osteotomy to treat malocclusion following reconstruction of the mandible with the free fibular flap. *Plast Reconstr Surg* 2003; 112:31-6.

33. HIDALGO, D.A.; PUSIC, A.L. Free-flap mandibular reconstruction: a 10-year follow-up study. *Plast Reconstr Surg* 2002; 110:438-49.

34. DESCHLER, D.G.; HAYDEN, R.E. The optimum method for reconstruction of complex lateral oromandibular-cutaneous defects. *Head Neck* 2000; 22:674-9.

35. WERLE, A.H.; TSUE, T.T.; TOBY, E.B.; GIROD, D.A. Osteocutaneous radial forearm free flap: its use without significant donor site morbidity. *Otolaryngol Head Neck Surg* 2000; 123:711–17

36. FERRARO, N.F.; AUGUST, M. Reconstruction following resection of maxillofacial tumors. *Oral Maxillofac Surg Clin North Am* 1993; 5:355-83.

37. AXHAUSEN, W. The osteogenic phases of regeneration of bone, a historical and experimental study. *J Bone Joint Surg Am* 1956; 38-A:593-600.

38. KOCH, W.M.; YOO, G.H.; GOODSTEIN, M.L.; EISELE, D.W.; RICHTSMEIER, W.J. Advantages of mandibular reconstruction with the titanium hollow screw osseointegrating reconstruction plate (THORP). *Laryngoscope* 1994; 104:545-52.

39. POLI, T.; FERRARI, S.; BIANCHA,

B.; SESENNA, E. Primary oromandibular reconstruction using free flaps and THORP plates in cancer patients: a 5 year experience. *Head and Neck* 2003; 25:15-23.

40. WEI, F.C.; CELIK, N.; YANG, W.G.; CHEN, I.H.; CHANG, Y.M.; CHEN, H.C. Complications after reconstruction by plate and soft tissue free flap in composite mandibular defects and secondary salvage reconstruction with osteocutaneous flap. *Plast Reconstr Surg* 2003; 112:37-42.

41. TRANTOLO, D.J.; SONIS, S.T.; THOMPSON, B.M.; WISE, D.L.; LEWANDROWSKI, K.U.; HILE, D.D. Evaluation of a porous, biodegradable biopolymer scaffold for mandibular reconstruction. *Int J Oral Maxillofac Implants* 2003; 18:182-8.

42. ILIZAROV, G.A. The principles of the Ilizarov method. *Bull Hosp Jt Dis Orthop Inst* 1988; 48:1-11.

43. MCCARTHY, J.G.; SCHREIBER, J.; KARP, N.; THORNE, C.H.; GRAYSON, B.H. Lengthening of the human mandible by gradual distraction. *Plast Recons Surg* 1992; 89:1-8.

44. KABAN, L.B.; MOSES, M.H.; MULLIKEN, J.B. Surgical correction of hemifacial microstomia in the growing child. *Plast Reconstr Surg* 1988; 82:9-19.

45. HERFORD, A. Use of a plate-guided distraction device for transport distraction osteogenesis of the mandible. *J Oral Maxillofac Surg* 2004; 62: 412-20.

46. FUKUDA, M.; IINO, M.; YAMAOKA, K.; OHNUKI, T.; NAGAI, H.; TAKAHASHI, T. Two-stage Distraction Osteogenesis for mandibular segmental defect. *J Oral Maxillofac Surg* 2004; 62:1164-8.

47. MARX, R.E.; CARLSON, E.R.; EICHSTAEDT, R.M.; SCHIMMELE, S.R.; STRAUSS, J.E.; GEORGEFF, K.R. Platelet-rich plasma: Growth factor enhancement for bone grafts. *Oral Surg Oral Med Oral Pathol Oral Radiol Endod* 1998; 85:638-46.

48. OYAMA, T.; NISHIMOTO, S.; TSUGAWA, T.; SHIMIZU, F. Efficacy of platelet-rich plasma in alveolar bone grafting. *J Oral Maxillofac Surg* 2004; 62:555-58.

49. ROLDAN, J.C.; JEPSEN, S.; SCHMIDT, C.; KNUPPEL, H.; RUEGER, D.C.; ACIL, Y. Sinus Floor augmentation with simultaneous placement of dental implants in the presence of platelet-rich plasma or recombinant human bone morphogenic protein-7. *Clin Oral Implants Res* 2004; 15:716-23.

50. WARNKE, P.H.; SPRINGER, I.N.; WILTFANG, J.; ACIL, Y.; EUFINGER, H.; WEHMOLLER, M.; RUSSO, P.A.; BOLTE, H.; SHERRY, E.; BEHRENS, E.; TERHEYDEN, H. Growth and transplantation of a custom vascularized bone graft in man. *The Lancet* 2004; 364:766-70.

51. MIZUMOTO, Y.; MOSELEY, T.; DREWS, M.; COOPER, V.; REDDI, H. Acceleration of regenerative ossification during distraction osteogenesis with recombinant human bone morphogenetic protein-7. *J Bone Joint Surg* 2003; 85-A-Suppl3: 124-30.

52. ADELL, R.; ERIKSSON, B.; LEKHOLM, U.; BRANEMARK, P-I; JEMT, T. Long-term follow-up study of osseointegrated implants in the treatment of totally edentulous jaws. *Int J Oral Maxillofac Implants* 1990; 5:347-59.

53. ATTARD, N.J.; ZARB, G.A. Long-term treatment outcomes in edentulous patients with implant-fixed prostheses: the Toronto study. *Int J Prosthodont* 2004; 17:417-24.

54. ATTARD, N.J.; ZARB, G.A. Long-term treatment outcomes in edentulous patients with implant overdentures: the Toronto study. *Int J Prosthodont* 2004; 17:425-33.

55. SHIROTA, T.; SCHMELZEISEN, R.; NEUKAM, F.; MATSUI, Y.; OHNO, K.; MICHI, K. Immediate insertion of two types of implants into vascularized bone grafts used for man-

dibular reconstruction in miniature pigs. *Oral Surg Oral Med Oral Pathol* 1994; 77:222-31.

56. SHIROTA, T.; OHNO, K.; MICHI, K.; TACHIKAWA, T. An experimental study of healing around hydroxylapatite implants installed with autogenous iliac bone grafts for Jaw reconstruction. *J Oral Maxillofac Surg* 1991; 49:1310-15.

57. MOUNSY, R.A.; BOYD, J.B. Mandibular reconstruction with osseointegrated implants into the free vascularized radius. *Plast Reconstr Surg* 1994; 94:457-64.

58. HOTZ, G. Reconstruction of mandibular discontinuity defects with delayed nonvascularized free iliac crest bone grafts and endosseous implants. A clinical report. *J Prosthet Dent* 1996; 76:350-5.

59. NEVINS, M. Treatment of the atrophic mandibular ridge. *Int J Oral Maxillofac Implants* 2003; 18:765.

60. KOMISAR, A. The functional result of mandibular reconstruction. *Laryngoscope* 1990; 100:364-74.

61. TAYLOR, T.D.; WORTHINGTON, P. Osseointegrated implant rehabilitation of the previously irradiated mandible: Results of a limited trial at 3 to 7 years. *J Prosthet Dent* 1993; 69:60-9.

62. GRANSTOM, G.; TJELLSTROM, A.; BRÅNEMARK, PI. Osseointegrated implants in irradiated bone: A case-controlled study using adjunctive hyperbaric oxygen therapy. *J Oral Maxillofac Surg* 1999; 57:493-9.

63. MARX, R.E. Osteoradionecrosis: A new concept of its pathophysiology. *J Oral Maxillofac Surg* 1983; 41:283-8.

64. MARX, R.E. A new concept in the treatment of osteoradionecrosis. *J Oral Maxillofac Surg* 1983; 41:351-7.

65. JACOB, R.F.; REECE, G.P.; TAYLOR, T.D.; MILLER, M.J. Mandibular reconstruction in the cancer patient: Microvascular surgery and implant prostheses. *Tex Dent J* 1992; 123-6.

66. JOHANSSON, G.; PALMQVIST, S. Complications, supplementary treatment, and maintenance in edentulous arches with implant-supported fixed prostheses. *Int J Prosthodont* 1990; 3:89-92.

67. CARLSON, B.; CARLSSON, G.E. Prosthodontic complications in osseointegrated dental implant treatment. *Int J Oral Maxillofac Implants* 1994; 9:990-4.

68. WEE, A.G. Comparison of impression materials for direct multi-implant impressions. *J Prosthet Dent* 2000; 83:323-31.

69. VIGOLO, P.; MAJZOUB, Z.; CORDIOLI, G. Evaluation of the accuracy of three techniques used for multiple implant abutment impressions. *J Prosthet Dent* 2003; 89:186-92.

70. KALLUS, T.; BESSING, C. Loose gold screws frequently occur in full-arch fixed prostheses supported by Osseointegrated implants after 5 years. *Int J Oral Maxillofac Implants.* 1994; 9:169-78.

71. SCHIFFLEGER, B.E.; ZIEBERT, G.J.; DHURU, V.B.; BRANTLEY, W.A.; SIGAROUDI, K. Comparison of accuracy of multiunit one-piece casting. *J Prosthet Dent* 1965; 54:770-6.

72. VIGOLO, P.; GIVANI, A.; MAJZOUB, Z.; CORDIOLI, G. Cemented versus screw-retained implant-supported single-tooth crowns: a four year prospective study. *Int J Maxillofac Implants* 2004; 19:260-5.

73. PREISKEL, H.W.; TSOLKA, P. Cement and screw-retained implant-supported prostheses: up to 10 years of follow-up of a new design. *Int J Oral Maxillofac Implants* 2004; 19:87-91.

74. LUNDQVIST, S.; HARALDSON, T. Oral function in patients wearing fixed prosthesis on osseointegrated implants in the maxilla: 3-year follow-up study. *Scand J Dent Res* 1992; 100:279-83.

75. KILIARIDIS, S.; TZAKIS, M.G.; CARLSSON, G.E. Short-term and

long-term effects of chewing training on occlusal perception of thickness. *Scand J Dent Res* 1990; 98:159-66.

76. KLINEBERG, I.; MURRAY, G. Osseoperception: sensory function and proprioception. *Adv Dent Res* 1999; 13:120-9.

77. WILLIAMS, E.; RYDEVIK, B.; JOHNS, R.; BRÅNEMARK, P-I, Eds: *Osseoperception and Muscolu-skeletal Function*. Goteborg, Sweden 1999; The Institute for Applied Biotechnology.

78. MATTES, S.; ULRICH, R.; MUHL-BRADT, L. Detection times of natural teeth and endosseous implants revealed by the method of reaction time. *Int J Oral Maxillofac Implants* 1997; 12:399-402.

79. WILLIS, R.D.; DICOSIMO, C.J. The absence of proprioceptive nerve endings in the human periodontal ligament: the role of periodontal mechanoreceptors in the reflex control of mastication. *Oral Surg Oral Med Oral Pathol* 1979; 48:108-15.

80. MERICSKE-STERN, R.; HOFMANN, J.; WEDIG, A.; GEERING, A.H. In vivo measurements of maximal occlusal force and minimal pressure threshold on overdentures supported by implants or natural roots: a comparative study, Part I. *Int J Oral Maxillofac Implants* 1993; 8:641-9.

81. LEUNG, T.; LAI, V.F. Control of jaw closing forces: a comparison between natural tooth and osseointegrated implant. *Eur J Prosthodont Restor Dent* 2000; 8:113-6.

82. MERICSKE-STERN, R.; ASSAL, P.; MERICSKE, E.; BURGIN, W. Occlusal force and oral tactile sensibility measured in partially edentulous patients with ITI implants. *Int J Oral Maxillofac Implants* 1995; 10:345-53.

13

Oral Fixed Rehabilitation of Atrophic Jaws

Paulo Malo
Isabel Lopes
Raul Costa

Introduction

Demographics of edentulism

As mentioned in the World Health Organization Report (WHO[1]) the number of edentulous patients is growing and there is a continuous increase in the incidence of edentulism among the world population. These findings are explained by the increase of the population's life expectancy.

In fact, it is expected that in the United States the number of edentulous increases up to 38 million in the year 2020, corresponding to a 5% increase during 20 years. In the period from 1991 to 2000 there was an increase of about 2 million cases of edentulism.[1, 2] In Europe, similar numbers were achieved. The WHO estimates that 6 to 10% of the worldwide population is edentulous.

These numbers do not enter the cases of patients with refractory periodontal disease to treatment, a condition that affects a considerable percentage of the worldwide population. The absence of a healthy and adequate periodontal support of the remaining teeth makes them not viable. Treatment of these patients will include the extraction of all the remaining teeth and rehabilitation as edentulous patients. Therefore, the amount of edentulous persons is even higher as the patients with periodontal disease are not mentioned in the statistics.

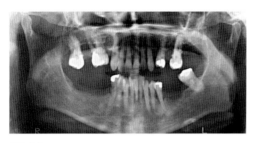 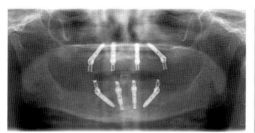

13-1A   13-1B

Fig. 13-1A and B. Pre and postoperative ortho-pantomographies of a periodontal patient that was treated with all-on-4 bimaxillary surgeries.

Table 13-1

Country	% Edentulous	Age Group
Europe	42%	65-74 years
USA	26%	65-69 years
Canada	58%	65+ years
Japan	20%	65 years

2000 data.

The impact of edentulism – associated problems

The majority of the edentulous patients report severe to moderate discomfort with their removable prosthesis. There are quite numerous cases mentioning intolerance to the use of removable prosthesis due to vomit reflex complaints. On the other hand, the globalization of the pattern "beautiful and perpetual young" increases aesthetic and beauty requirements, as the total number of edentulous patients become a weak link in the society.

Therefore, the impact of edentulism is not only functional (compromised phonetic and mastigatory functions), but also psychosocial due to the aesthetic deformation associated.

The widely accepted definition of health from the WHO, states that "health is a state of complete physical, mental and social well-being and not merely the absence of disease or infirmity. This helps us to conclude that edentulous patients need particular attention by the medical community in this demanding society for high quality life.

If we, as health professionals, try to imitate Nature in our practice, it is easy to conclude that the ideal treatment for an edentulous patient is a fixed "third dentition".

Even with the latest bio-engineering advances, only the use of

Fig. 13-2. Edentulous patients pictures after All-on-4 and Malo bridge rehabilitation at Malo clinic Lisbon.

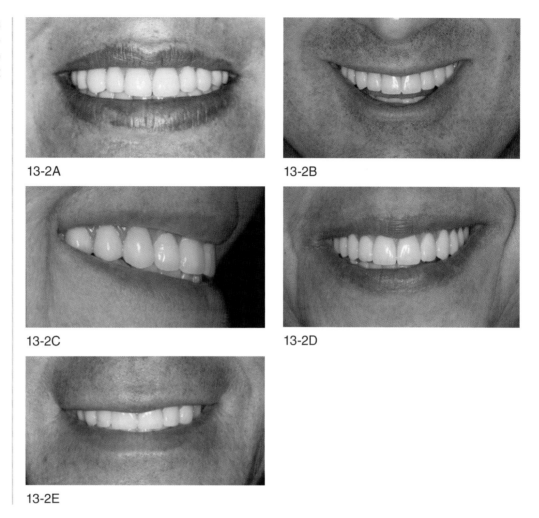

13-2A

13-2B

13-2C

13-2D

13-2E

innovative surgical approaches and top quality materials that mimic lost oral tissues allow the rehabilitation of the edentulous patient with significant improvement in his quality of life and self-confidence.

Malo Clinic has been pioneer in the development and implementation of high success surgical and prosthetic techniques for patients and oral health professionals worldwide. This chapter intends to contribute for spreading the Malo Clinic multidisciplinary teamwork, which undoubtedly improved totally edentulous health.

Edentulous patient rehabilitation – surgical and prosthetic Malo Clinic protocol

Definition and statistic data

The All-on-4 is a simple surgical technique, developed in the beginning of the 90´s by Dr. Paulo Malo at Malo Clinic with the co-operation of Professor Bo Rangert in order to rehabilitate the edentulous maxilla and mandible with fixed prosthesis. This concept allows the edentulous rehabilitation avoiding the need of complex, debilitating and costly procedures of maxillary reconstruction with bone grafting. In this technique 4 implants are placed in the anterior region of the jaws, which has the highest bone density and also present the highest success rate, allowing the fitting of a fixed prosthesis with 12 teeth in immediate function with minimum cantilever.

The loss of posterior teeth, usually in an earlier age, leads to the loss of alveolar bone with pneumatization of the maxillary sinus and surfacing of the mandibular nerve in the mandibular arch, disabling the immediate placement of implants in the posterior regions.

In each quadrant two implants are placed, an anterior straight implant, ideally in the lateral incisor region and a posterior implant tilted 45º with the head of the implant located in the region between the first premolar and first molar, making a total of 4 implants per arch.

The tilting of the posterior implant allows maximum use of the existing bone with maximum bone anchorage and at the same time the placement of posterior fixed teeth, in a region where the bone height would not allow immediate load.

The placement of these tilted implants is done using a surgical guide- Malo edentulous guide [a], which guides the placement of the tilted implants, or using the computer guided surgical technique (NobelGuide™).

The follow-up studies started in 1999 reveal a high success rates: 98.5% for implants in the All-on-4 rehabilitation of the upper jaw and 99.86% for the lower jaw. Interesting results were obtained comparing the use of 4 implants with the use of a superior number of implants in the maxillary rehabilitation. It was verified through statistical analyses that diminishing the number of implants increases the success rates significantly. In part, this can be explained by the easier way each patient can perform the hygiene of the rehabilitations with few implants. Moreover, in the majority of the cases, there is not enough remaining maxillary bone to correctly place more than 4 implants.

Advantages

The definition of this technique implies a revolutionary treatment of the edentulous patient, allowing the immediate rehabilitation of all cases without the need of debilitating maxillary reconstruction surgeries. Through this technique the rehabilitation of aesthetics and function can be achieved, with high success rates, in minutes or in a few hours after surgery. Furthermore, the use of fewer implants simplifies and speeds up the surgical and prosthetic procedures, such as taking impressions, achieving passivity

Fig. 13-3. All-on-4 and Malo Bridge scheme. In Nobelbiocare™ All-on-4 catalogue.

Fig. 13-4. Surgical guide scheme- Malo edentulous guide[a]. In Nobelbiocare™ All-on-4 catalogue.

Fig. 13-5. Surgical guide picture – Malo edentulous guide[a]. Maxillary All-on-4 surgery: 30° Multi-unit abutment[d] connection.

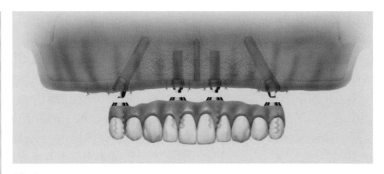

13-3

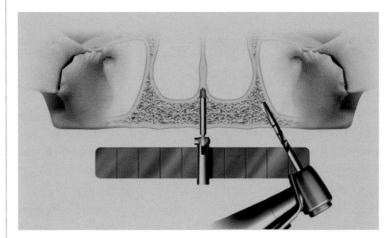

13-4

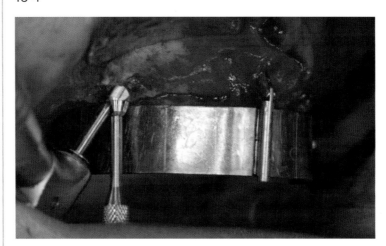

13-5

Products References – In NobelBiocare™ Catalogue	
References	**Product**
32068	[a] Malo edentulous guide
25028	[b] Round bur
32299	[c] Twist drill
29192 / 29193	[d] 30° Multi-unit abutments
32112	[e] Direction Indicator
29196-29206	[f] Straight Multi-unit abutments
29187-29191	[g] 17° Multi-unit abutments
29089	[h] Impression copings

between implants and prosthetic structure and allows high aesthetic outcomes. Hygienic maintenance is also favored, which increases the longevity of the rehabilitation.

The All-on-4 surgery, due to its simple surgical protocol, can be performed in patients of any age and even in patient with previous systemic compromise could not be submitted to implant rehabilitation because this would involve maxillary reconstruction with bone graft. Nevertheless, the All-on-4 technique is still not indicated in patients undergoing radiotherapy in the maxillary region. Bone graft surgeries generally are too invasive, present a high morbidity and delay the rehabilitation due to the healing period for bone graft integration. In old or debilitated patients this kind of procedure is contraindicated. Now these patients can have fixed teeth trough an All-on-4 surgery.

The All-on-4 technique allowed the simplification and standardization of the edentulous rehabilitation, thus resulting in drastic reduction of costs for the patient. Therefore more people can benefit from this treatment and stop suffering from physical and psychological consequences of not having teeth.

All-on-4 Standard, All-on-4 Hybrid and All-on-4 Zygoma

To plan an All-on-4 Surgery a careful clinical examination with a pre-operative orthopantomography and a CT scan is needed. The height and width of the residual crest bone available between the anterior walls of the maxillary sinus, and between the mental foramina for the mandible, will establish the type of All-on-4 surgery approach: All-on-4 Standard, All-on-4 Standard High Skilled, All-on-4 Hybrid or All-on-4 Zygoma. To place the 4 implants in these regions, for the maxilla All-on-4 standard surgery an ideal of 5mm of width and 10 mm of height of bone is needed. For the mandibular all-on-4 surgeries the ideal amount of bone is 5mm of width and 8 mm of height.

The mandibular bone between canines represents the mandibular symphysis, which is kept even in the total edentulous jaw. Thus, it is always possible to perform the standard All-on-4.

In the maxilla, the maxillary sinus and the nasal fossae tend to occupy a crucial amount of volume leaving the inter-canine area with less than 5 mm of width and 10 mm of height in a significant percentage of patients. In several cases only an extremely thin layer of cortical bone is left between the floor of the maxillary sinus, nasal fossae and oral cavity. These extreme atrophic situations used to be rehabilitated with autogenous bone grafts, using for example the iliac crest bone as a donor site. The Malo Clinic protocol avoids these uncomfortable and complex surgeries by using zygomatic implants through a new surgical technique that does not have the

Fig. 13-6. Surgical Maxila All-on-4 (ortho-pantomographics) Malo Clinic Protocol. Clinical cases examples. (A) All-on-4 Standard; (B) All-on-4 Hybrid; (C) All-on-4 Zygoma.

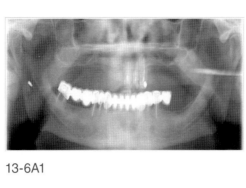

13-6A1

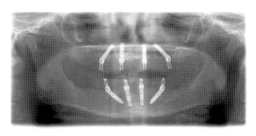

13-6A2

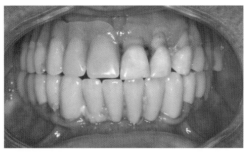

13-6A3

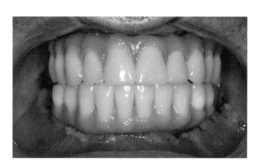

13-6A4

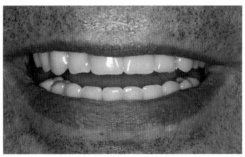
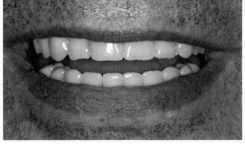

13-6A5

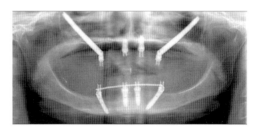

13-6B1

13-6B2

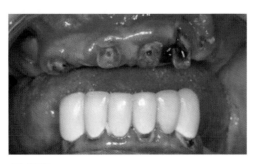

13-6B3

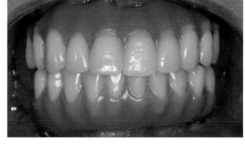

13-6B4

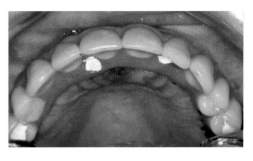

13-6B5

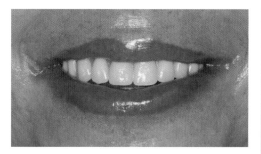

13-6B6

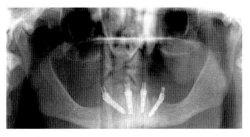

13-6C1

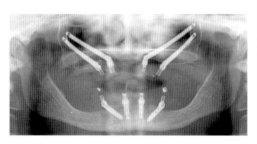

13-6C2

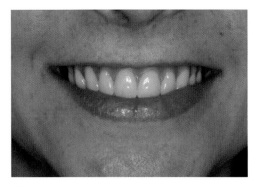

13-6C3

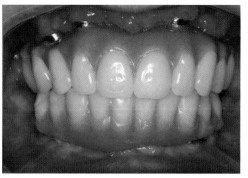

13-6C4

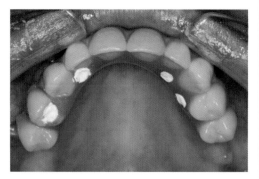

13-6C5

Fig. 13-6. Continuation.

prosthetic and hygienic limitations of a regular zygomatic implant surgery: as Dr. Paulo Malo and Dr. Reginaldo Migliorança developed. In the All-on-4 hybrid are used implants with maxillary and zygomatic anchorage, whereas in All-on-4 Zygoma exclusively this bone is used, in a total of 4 implants. In both All-on-4 Hybrid and Zygoma techniques, the foreseen screw exits are the same as for the Standard All-on-4, that is, on the occlusal surfaces of teeth or on the internal wall of the bridge on it's artificial gingiva.

Surgical approaches for the All-on-4 technique

Flap approach

The first all-on-4 surgeries were performed in 1995 in the mandible with the flap technique. The official follow-up started in 1999. After 4 years, in 2003, this innovative surgical concept was presented to the scientific community. Flapless All-on-4 surgery became possible with the appliance of the NobelGuide™ technology to the all-on-4 concept, with maximum comfort to the patient.

In the maxillary flap approach, the surgery starts with a mucoperiosteal incision along the crest of the ridge, slightly palatal, with extension between the first molars and two vertical-releasing incisions in each posterior end. After mucoperiosteal flap reflection, the periapical region should be carefully curetted to remove any periapical lesions. Depending on the degree of irregularity of the alveolar ridge, recontouring can be accomplished with a rounger or a bone bur in a handpiece, alone or in combination. Following bone recontouring the Malo edentulous guide[a] is positioned throughout osteotomy with a round bur[b] and a 2 mm twist drill[c]. This guide will aid in the correct placement of the posterior tilted implants at 45 degrees. The tilted distal fixtures should be the first to be delivered. Their position and inclination is determined by the anterior wall of the maxillary sinus. This wall anatomy is accessed by drilling a small opening on the lateral wall of the maxilla where the anterior wall should be inspected with a periodontal probe. The position of the anterior sinus wall can be marked with a surgical marker. The site preparation for the distal fixture must be performed as posterior as possible allowing approximately 3 to 4 mm from the sinus wall. Bone site preparation must be adjusted to bone density in order to achieve primary implant stability equal or higher to a 30 Ncm insertion torque. The "osteotome" capacity of the NobelSpeedy™ implant makes this implant the ideal for immediate function, due to the following characteristics: 1. higher primary anchorage, as this unique fixture has threads all the "way up" allowing maximum contact with bone surface; 2. maximum crest expansion related to the shape of the apex. To compensate the inclination of the tilted implants and screw-retained prosthesis passive fit attainment it is placed a 30º Multi-unit abutment[d].When both distal implants are delivered and respective angulated abutments screwed, the Malo edentulous guide is removed and replace by a direction indicator pin[e] to anterior implants preparation. The anterior straight implants are supposed to be as far apart from each other as possible. To the straight implants are screwed straight[f], 17[g] or 30[d] degrees angulated Multi-unit abutments depending on the predicted foreseen screw exists from the fixed screwed prosthesis. To obtain a hygienic and mechanically resistant prosthesis the 4 abutments should be at the same height. After copious irrigation, the edges of the flaps can be trimmed to remove excess tissue and sutured with interrupted sutures. Whenever possible buccal, keratinized gingiva should be preserved, especially around the implants.

After suturing, the open tray impression copings[h] are screwed and joined together with orthodontic wire and acrylic resin, and an impression with putty material is taken in a custom open tray. Lighter impression materials are not used since they enter trough the suture and can cause postoperative infections. The remaining steps for a screwed implant-retained prosthesis are subsequently performed.

In the mandible, the flap approach protocol is similar to the one described for the maxilla apart from the incision and the identification of the mental foramina. Vertical-releasing incisions are not performed along with the lower incision, since they are not necessary for adequate exposure and flap flexible reflection. Therefore the healing delay caused by the blood supply compromise is prevented. Nevertheless, in extremely resorbed mandibles where the mental foramina are superficial, a vertical-releasing incision is done at the middle line allowing proper flap pulling and easy mental nerve identification preventing nerve damage. The final position of the distal tilted implants should be 4 mm in front of the anterior loop of the mental nerve, which is explored with a periodontal probe.

Fig. 13-7. Operative view of a maxillary All-on-4 flap surgery. Preparation of the distal tilted fixture with round bur[b] after exploration and marking sinus anterior wall.

Fig. 13-8. Operative view of a maxillary all-on-4 impression taking.

Fig. 13-9. Operative view of a mandibular All-on-4 flap surgery. Distal implant placement, Malo edentulous guide[a], mental nerve and foramen.

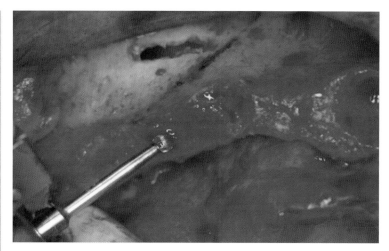

13-7

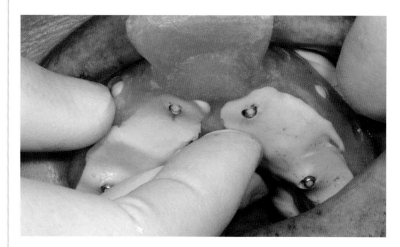

13-8

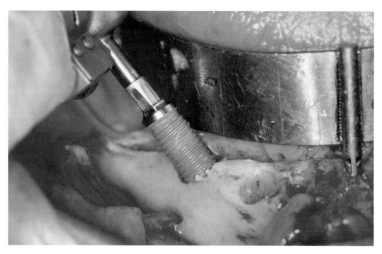

13-9

Flapless approach (NobelGuide™ concept)

The Nobelguide™ technology adapted to the All-on-4 concept made possible the total edentulous rehabilitation without the need of incision and flap raising. The basis of this approach is a computer planning of the surgical procedure and implant placement in a 3D bone model of the patient that is obtained from the axial cuts of a jaw Ct-Scan. From the planning is manufactured a surgical template that is used as a guide to fixture delivery. The knowledge of the exact implant localization before surgery permits the dentist to have a pre-made customized fixed bridge before the surgical procedure takes place. Thus, the patient surgery ends with the immediate placement of the bridge saving the patient from the time consumed at the laboratory for prosthesis manufacture. Since no flap is reflected, the postoperative period is much comfortable with less swelling and no hematoma. However, this approach has the same selection criteria, namely: goad mouth opening capability, absence of teeth that interfere with surgical template placement and no osteotomy or bone trimming needed.

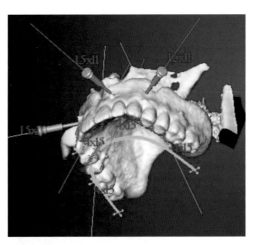

13-10A

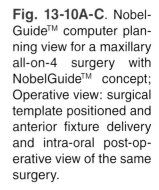

Fig. 13-10A-C. Nobel-Guide™ computer planning view for a maxillary all-on-4 surgery with NobelGuide™ concept; Operative view: surgical template positioned and anterior fixture delivery and intra-oral post-operative view of the same surgery.

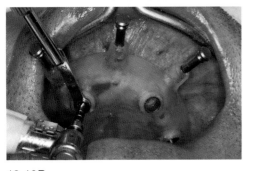

13-10B

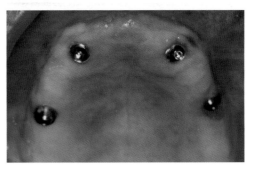

13-10C

Malo Clinic Prosthetic Protocol: Malo Bridge

Concept definition

The prosthesis screwed onto the implants placed during the All-on-4 surgery is called Malo Bridge. There are 3 types of Malo Bridge: Ceramic, Acrylic and All-Acrylic.

The Malo Bridge replaces not only hard tissues (teeth and bone) but also soft tissues (gingival with maximum aesthetics and function, allowing the rehabilitation of the lip support and the height of the inferior third of the face, decreased due to teeth loss. One verifies the immediate smoothing of nasolabial wrinkles and corrects repositioning of the labial commisures, providing a younger appearance to the total edentulous patient.

Ceramic or Acrylic Malo Bridge has a customized titanium infrastructure (Procera® system) that supports acrylic or ceramic teeth and customized acrylic gingiva, allowing a perfect reproduction of the patient's mucosa. A high quality resin cured at a high pressure is used to guarantee the absence of micropores. The advantage of an acrylic gingiva lies on the possibility of individual characterization, which is not possible with a

Fig. 13-11. Postoperative lateral skull radiograph from a edentulous patient with an all-on-4 and CM Bridge Rehabilitation. Note the reposition of the upper lip soft tissue with this procedure.

Fig. 13-12. Extra-oral view of Lip support before and after Malo All-acrylic Bridge.

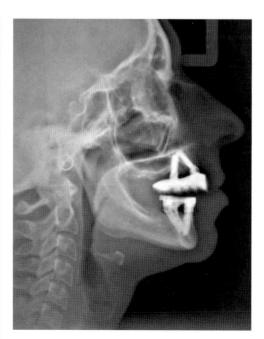

13-11

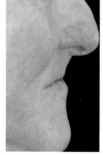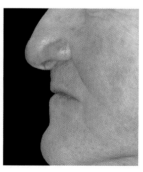

13-12

ceramic gingiva, and on the easiness of repair.

The part of the Malo Bridge, which is to be in close contact with the mucosa and with the abutments, is planned so that it slightly pressures the soft tissues. In this way, a gap between the prosthesis and the mucosa is avoided improving oral hygiene and word pronunciation. This part is bullet shaped (convex) and, as the rest of the prosthetic structure, is highly polished.

Malo bridge All-Acrylic

The All-Acrylic Bridge corresponds to the immediate prosthesis made in the day of the surgery, but can be used as a final prosthesis whenever the amount of false gengiva ensures mechanical resistance. It has acrylic teeth and gum and it is reinforced with laser-welded titanium bars. This structure has good mechanical properties and excellent clinical results, as it is evidenced by the clinical follow-up of the cases rehabilitated since 1995.

In the immediate bridge, cantilevers can be avoided and occlusal contacts are stronger within anterior teeth, where smaller forces occur due to a longer distance from the hinge axis. Canine and anterior guidance are preferred. Sixteen to 24 weeks later, this prosthesis should be adjusted in order to have the same occlusion criteria as for the dentate patient

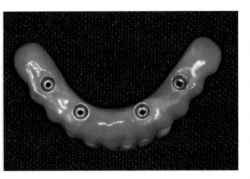

13-13

Fig. 13-13. Malo bridge All-Acrylic inferior view.

Fig. 13-14. Titanium CAD/CAM – Procera System® substructure from a Malo Bridge Ceramic, and the prosthesis finished.

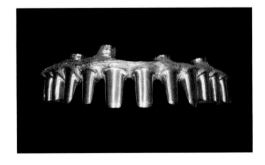

13-14A

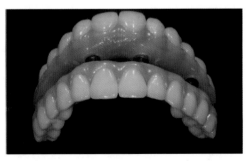

13-14B

and to have first molars: cantilevers are not avoided.

The All-acrylic Bridge is easy and quick to fabricate making it possible to deliverer it in the day of the surgery, thus it is a high aesthetic and low cost option.

Malo bridge ceramic

The Malo Bridge Ceramic is the result of several years of clinical and laboratorial investigation. It is a high aesthetic screwed prosthesis, unique in biofunctional, mechanical and hygienic characteristics.

Both the Malo Bridge Ceramic and the Malo Bridge Acrylic have a Titanium CAD/CAM – Procera System® substructure. With this system the occurrence of a human error in the prosthesis confection is probably reduces because it is not necessary to wax, muffle or weld the structure and to use materials with dimensional shrinkage. This titanium substructure (Procera System®) allows the prosthetic component to have high mechanical resistance and due to its precision confection system, it has a passive fitting over the abutments-implants.

The Malo Bridge Ceramic and the Malo Bridge Acrylic slightly diverge in their substructure. The first one has retentive preparations similar in shape to crown preparations made in natural teeth. Over these preparations, individualized Procera® crowns are cemented, imitating the natural dentition. After crown cementation, a high quality and individual characterized acrylic resin is applied over the titanium structure to imitate gingiva and mucosa. Being individualized crowns replace them, in case of fracture, is a fast and easy procedure without the need of removing the bridge. But if it is needed, the screw bridge is easily removed.

The clinical procedure requires: a definitive impression with an open custom tray using putty and a light addition silicone materials, and splinting the impression copings. This is a fundamental step to obtain a precise model and as a consequence a totally adjust and passive fitting bridge. Then the acrylic provisional prosthesis will be duplicated but only if it fulfills all the aesthetic and functional requisites. Otherwise, another Malo Bridge Acrylic must be done.

Today the Malo Bridge Ceramic is the prosthesis that best imitates natural dentition, with the highest degree of aesthetics and repair capacity.

Malo bridge acrylic

In bimaxillary clinical cases, the Malo Bridge Acrylic is a good solution to rehabilitate the mandible while the superior maxillary arc is rehabilitated with a ceramic bridge. A bimaxillary ceramic prosthesis is not recommended, especially in patients with parafunctional habits, due to the risk of ceramic fracture. Although ceramic is extremely durable and

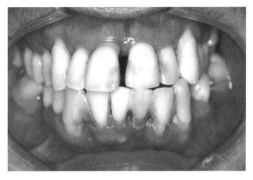

13-15

Fig. 13-15. Pre-operative intra-oral view.

Fig. 13-16. Extra-oral views of a Malo Bridge Ceramic.

Fig. 13-17. Extra and Intra-oral view of a Malo bridge acrylic.

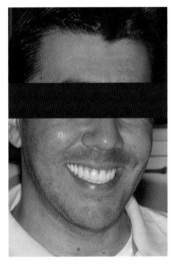

13-16A

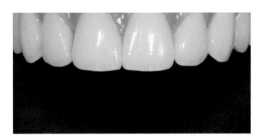

13-16B

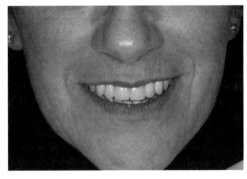

13-17A

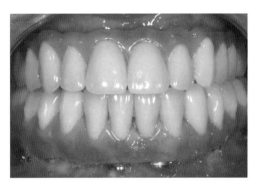

13-17B

aesthetic, it is also a brittle material which brings limitations to its use. The rehabilitation of the superior maxillae with ceramic permits to get excellent aesthetic results without the risk of wearing that occurs with acrylic prosthesis after years of constant use. If the inferior acrylic prosthesis is worn after some years of use it can be more easily replaced without compromising the patient smile and self-esteem.

Hygienic Maintenance for Patients With All-on-4 Rehabilitation – Malo Clinic Hygienic Protocol

The hygienic maintenance for patients with All-on-4 rehabilitation has two phases: 1st phase, encloses the functional osseointegration period, and 2nd phase the long-term maintenance.

The aim of the 1st phase, which lasts between 16 to 24 weeks, is to induce bone and tissue healing, reducing patient discomfort and preventing infection. The cases of non-osseointegrating implants occur during this initial period. In the 2nd phase, the purpose is to keep the implants in excellent conditions of oral hygiene, for

Table 13-2. Malo Clinic protocol of the 1st phase hygienic maintenance for rehabilitation with immediate function implants- clinic appointments

Appointment Day pos-op	Clinic acts
10th	• Panoramic X-ray; • Periapical X-ray; • Removal of the prosthesis for disinfection and cleaning; • Check for any fracture or loosening of prosthetic components; • Check the torque of the prosthetic abutments; • Removal of suture; • Application of a chlorhexidine gel; • Application of a hyaluronic acid gel (0.2%); • Control of suppuration by finger pressure; • Control of occlusion; • Information that should not overload the structure.
60th	• Oral Hygiene with Jet-clean; • Application of a chlorhexidine gel; • Control of suppuration by finger pressure; • Control of occlusion; • Check for any fracture or loosening of prosthetic components.
120th day	• Oral hygiene with pressure jet • Periapical x-ray • Prosthesis removal for hygiene and disinfection • Clorohexidine gel appliance • Occlusion checking • Prosthesis exam (search for possible factures) • Prosthetic screws' torque checking • Search of possible infection and/or inflammation existence

maximum rehabilitation longevity. Both phases rely on the patient's home care (hygiene), with rigorous instructions from the dental hygienist and regular dental hygiene appointments. In the first phase of the hygienic maintenance, the first appointment takes place 10 to 15 days after the surgery, the second appointment 60 days after, and the third 120 days after.

In the last appointment of the 1st phase, before beginning the final Malo Bridge, the oral hygienist performs periapical x-rays. The x-rays are preformed with a radiographic support for a precise paralelometric technique, ideal to evaluate implant-bone continuity (osseointegration).

Hygienic instructions and motivation of the patient rehabilitated with an All-on-4 are essential for the rehabilitation longevity. Totally edentulous patients lost their teeth, in the majority of the cases, due to the lack of efficient hygienic care. This factor also predisposes to implant failure and must be eliminated.

The Malo Clinic's oral hygiene protocol is adapted to the several healing phases. Therefore, in the first ten days, the patient is informed to perform his oral hygiene twice a day (morning and evening), with a soft surgical toothbrush and hyaluronic acid gel followed by hyaluronic acid mouthwash. It should be focused the importance of cleaning the transition region between the prosthesis and the gingiva. Between 10th and 60th post-operative day, the patient is taught to use additional means of plaque removal such as dental floss and interdental brushes. After 60th day, the gingival tissue should be completed healed and capable of tolerate the change for a soft toothbrush. The water jet is also added to the oral hygienic procedures. In the 2nd phase of hygienic maintenance the professional should adapt the frequency of the oral hygiene appointments to the needs of each patient.

SPECIAL THANKS TO:

All members of the surgical, prosthetic and research and development Malo Cinic departments and to Malo Ceramics.

References

Articles that contribute to the development of the All-on-4 concept

1 BRÅNEMARK, P-I.; HANSSON, B.O.; ADELL, R et al. *Osseointegrated implants in the treatment of edentulous jaw. Experience from a 10-year period.* Sweden:Almqvist &Wiksell, 1977.
2 ADELL, R.; ERICSSON, B.; LEKHOLM, U.; BRÅNEMARK, PI.; JEMT, T. A long-term follow-up study of osseointegrated implants in the treatment of totally edentulous jaws. *Int J Oral Maxillofac Implants* 1990; 5:347-359.

Articles that corroborate the All-on-4 approach

3. SCHNITMAN, P.A.; WÖHRLE, P.S.; RUBENSTEIN, J.E.; DASILVA, J.D.;

WANG, N.H. Tem-year results for Brånemark implants immediately loaded with fixed prosteses at implant placement. *Int J Oral Maxillofac Implants* 1997; 12:495-503.

4. CHIAPASCO M, GATTI C, ROSSI E, HAEFLIGER W, MARKWALDER TH. Implant-retained mandibular overdentures with immediate loading. A retrospective multicenter study on 226 consecutive cases. Clin Oral Impl Res 1997; 8:48-57.

5. TARNOW, D.P.; EMTIAZ, S.; CLASSI, A. Immediate loading of threaded implants as stage-1 surgery in edentulous arches: ten consecutive case reports with 1- to 5-year data. *Int J Oral Maxillof Impl* 1997; 12:319-324.

6. ESPOSITO, M.; HIRSCH, J.M.; LEKHOLM, U.; THOMSEN, P. Failure patterns of four osseointegrated oral implant systems. *J. Materials Science in Medicine* 1997; Suppl 8:843-847.

7. BALSHI, T.J.; WOLFINGER, G.J. Immediate loading of Brånemark implants in edentulous mandibles. A preliminary report. *Implant Dent* 1997; 6:83-88.

8. RANDOW, K.; ERICSSON, I.; NILNER, K.; PETERSON, A.; GLANTZ, P.O. Immediate functional loading of Brånemark dental implants. An 18month clinical follow-up study. *Clin Oral Implants Res* 1999;10:8-15.

9. BRÅNEMARK, P-I.; ENGSTTRAND, P.; ÖHRNELL, L.O. et al. A new treatment concept for rehabilitation of edentulous mandible. Preliminary results from a prospective clinical follow-up study. *Clin Implant Dent Relat Res* 1999; 1:2-16.

10. FRIBERG, B.; SENNERBY, L.; LINDÉN, B.; GRÖNDAHL, K.; LEKHOLM, U. Stability measuements of one-stage Brånemark implants during healing in mandibles, a clinical resonance frequency analysis study. *Int J Oral Maxillofac Surg* 1999; 28:266-272.

11. BRUNSKI, J. In vivo bone response to biomechanical loading at the bone-dental interface. *Adv Dent Res* 1999, 13:99-119.

12. ERICSSON, I.; RANDOW, K.; PETERSON, A. Early funtional loading of Brånemark dental implants: 5-year clinical follow-up study. *Clin Implant Dent Relat Res* 2000; 2:70-77.

13. MALO, P.; RANGERT, B.; DVARSATER, L. Immediate function of Brånemark implants in the esthetic zone: A retrospective clinical study with 6 months to 4 years of follow-up. *CIDRR* 2000; Vol. 2, N. 3: 138-145.

14. DUYCK, J.; VAN OOSTERWYCK, H.; VANDER SLOTEN, J.; DE COOMAN, M.; PUERS, R.; NAERT, I. Magnitude and distribution of occlusal forces on oral implants supporting fixed prostheses: an in vivo study. *Clin Oral Implants Res* 2000; 11:465-475.

15. KREKMANOV, L.; KAHN, M.; RANGERT, B.; LINDSTROM, H. Tilting os posterior mandibular and maxillary implants of improved prosthesis support. *Int J Oral Maxillofac Implants* 2000; 15:405-414.

16. APARICIO, C.; PERALES, P.; RANGERT, B. Tilted implants as an alternative to maxillary sinus grafting: A clincal, radiologic, and periotest study. *Clin Implant Dent Relat Res* 2001; 3: 39-49.

17. CHAUSHU, G.; CHAUSHU, S.; TZOHAR, A.; DAYAN, D. Immediate loading of single tooth implants: immediate versus non-immediate implantation. A clinical report. *Int J Oral Maxillofac Implants* 2001; 3:79-86.

18. CHOW, J.; HUI, E.; LIU, J. et al. The Hong Kong Bridge protocol. Immediate loading of mandibular Brånemark fixtures using a fixed provisional prosthesis: preliminary results. Clin Implant Dent Relat Res 2001; 3:166-174.

19. BALSHI, T.J.; WOLFINGER, G.J.

Teeth in a day. Implant Dent 2001; 10:231-33.

20. PETERSON, A.; RANGERT, B.; RANDOW, K.; ERICSSON, I. Marginal boné resorption at different treatment concepts using Brånemark dental implants in anterior mandibles. *Clin Impl Dent Relat Res* 2001; 3:142-147.

21. CHIAPASCO, M.; GATTI, C.; GOTTLOW, J.; LUNDGREN, A.; MALO, P.; MEREDITH, N.; POLIZZI, G.; SENNERBY, L. *Osteointegrazione e carico immediato. Fondamenti biologici e applicazioni cliniche*. Milano, Itália: Masson, Spa, 2002: 60-102.

22. ÖRTORP, A.; JEMT, T. Clinical experience of CNC-milled titanium frameworks supported by implants in the edentuolous jaw: a 3-year interim report. *Clin Implant Relat Res* 2002; 4:104-109.

23. MALO, P.; RANGERT, B.; NOBRE M. "All-on-4" Immediate function concept with Brånemark system implants for completely edentulous mandibles: a 3 year retrospective clinical study. *CIDRR* 2003; vol. 5, Suppl. 1: 2-20.

24. APARICIO, C.; AREVALO, X.; OUZZANI, W.; GRANADOS, C. A retrospective clinical and radiographic evaluation of tilted implants used in the treatment of severely resorbed edentulous maxilla. *Appl Osseointegrat Res* 2003; 1:17-21.

25. MALO, P. Carga inmediata en pacientes con maxilar superior totalmente edéntulo. In: JIMENEZ-LÓPEZ, V.; BEJARANO, S.D.; GONZÁLEZ, R.F.; ALONSO, J.M.N. *Carga o Función Inmediata en Implantología. Aspectos quirúrgicos, protéticos, oclusales y de laboratorio*. Barcelona: Editorial Quintessence, S.L., 2004: 22, 23, 187-221.

26. MALO, P.; RANGERT, B.; NOBRE, M. All-on-4 Immediate-Function Concept with Brånemark System® Implants for Completely Edentulous Maxillae: A 1-Year Retrospective Clinical Study. *CIDRR* 2005; vol. 7, supplement.

27. MALO, P.; RANGERT, B.; NOBRE, M. Mise en function immediate d'implants Brånemark pour la restauration d'édentements unitaires et de faible étendue maxillaries et mandibulaires. Étude clinique retrospective de 6 mois à 8 ans. *Implant* 2005; Vol. 11, n.1: 23-32.

Other sources

28. GLOBAL HEALTH Data Bank and WHO Oral Health. *Country/Area Profile Programme, 2000*, Poul Erik Petersen, World Health Organization.

29. DOUGLASS, C.W.; WATSON, A.J. Future needs for fixed and removable partial dentures in the United States. *J Prosthet Dent*. 2002 Jan; 87(1):9-14

30. PETERSON, L.J. *Contemporary Oral Maxillofacial Surgery*. 4th Edition; Mosby; St. Louis, Missouri 2003.

14

SURGICAL TECHNIQUES FOR ZYGOMATIC IMPLANT PLACEMENT IN ATROPHIED MAXILLARY ARCHES

Reginaldo Mario Migliorança

Gisseli Bertozzi Ávila

Marcelo de Sá Zamperlini

Thiago Martins de Mayo

Anchorage of implants into the zygomatic bone[2-5,8,14,16] is an alternative to bone graft reconstructions for the rehabilitation of severely atrophied maxillae (Figs. 14-1 and 14-2). There are three reconstruction techniques: original Brånemark Technique, Stella's Technique and Migliorança Exteriorized Technique. Thus, zygomatic anchorage technique is indicated in the following occasions:

❑ severe posterior maxillary bone resorption with subsequent pneumatization of maxillary sinus: the maxillary anterior region still possess adequate bone height to receive conventional fixtures. Also, zygomatic implants are placed in the posterior region (Fig. 14-3);

❑ severe bone resorption on the posterior and anterior regions, along with pneumatization of maxillary sinus: no implants can be placed in the anterior region. In this case, four zygomatic fixations are installed (Fig. 14-4).

A surgical planning is fundamental for the success of zygomatic fixations. Also, long-term prosthetic follow-up is mandatory. The following conditions must be assessed:

❑ patient's facial profile;
❑ parafunctional habits;
❑ maxilomandibular relationships;
❑ occlusal plane orientation;
❑ occlusal conditions of the opposing arch.

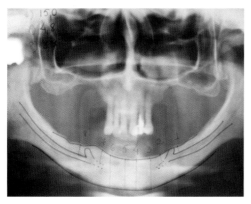

14-1

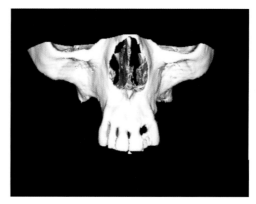

14-2

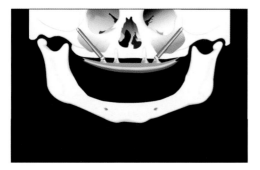

14-3

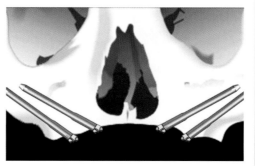

14-4

Fig. 14-1. Panoramic radiograph showing the atrophic maxilla with pneumatization of the maxillary sinus

Fig. 14-2. A prototype is made after computerized tomography confirming the radiographic findings. Also, the anterior part was preserved.

Fig. 14-3. Schematic drawing of zygomatic installment technique (All-on-Four Hybrid).

Fig. 14-4. Schematic representation. All-O-Four technique.

The reverse planning is fundamental for adequate esthetics and function during prosthetic rehabilitation.[1,4,5,20] This is achieved by duplication and wax-up of the existing complete prosthesis. Thus, the surgeon now has a clear idea of precise implant position, which in turn will favorable prosthetic and biomechanical relationships.

In the zygomatic anchorage technique, attention must be driven to bending force moments.[1,3,6] These must be counteracted with the following measures:

❑ cross-arch implant stabilization;

❑ reduction of distal and buccal cantilevers;

❑ harmonious occlusion, according to the principles of ADO's Factors (see Chapter 15).

When compared to conventional fixtures, zygomatic fixations show a tendency of deformation under horizontal loads; this can be related to (1) implant length and (2) limited bone support on the alveolar bone crest.

Thus, this implies that complete maxillary rehabilitation must be provided with two zygomatic fixations and at least to standard fixtures in the anterior maxillary region. To guarantee long-term stability, prostheses must be rigid to avoid bending or deformation moments that lead to further implant loss or screw loosening at the implant-prosthesis interface.[9,10,15,18]

The pre-surgical routine for zygomatic fixations is similar to other surgical intra-oral procedures. Also, general anesthesia is highly recommended due to increased time exposure and surgical complexities.

Brånemark's original technique

The original Brånemark technique[4,5] is shown on figures 14-5 to 14-12. The patients are selected according to rigid protocols. After, pre-prosthetic and surgical steps are performed, already described throughout this book.

An incision is placed along the bone crest, with buccal and lingual flaps raised. Care must be taken to avoid the parotid gland duct and exposure of the infra-orbital foramen. An 5-10mm aperture at the buccal wall of the maxillary sinus is made to visualize and elevate the sinus membrane. At this point, osteotomies will allow a square/round window at the posterior aspect, with its main axis in the vertical direction and parallel to the pterygomaxillary fissure, enhancing the surgical field.

In this technique, the implants must pass through the maxillary sinus to end at the zygoma crest, perforating its upper cortical plate. This is necessary because the implant platform will emerge in the palatal area. Drilling sequence (Fig. 14-15) begins with a round bur to delimitate the implant emergence in the palatal region. The drilling course toward the zygomatic bone is checked by direct visualization at the lateral window created in the maxillary sinus. Now, a 2.9mm twist bur is used to perforate the cortical layer of the zygomatic bone. After, the depth gauge is inserted to determine the implant length.

After, the bone site is prepared with the following sequential burs: 3.5mm Pilot Bur, 3.5mm twist bur, and 4.0mm twist bur. The 4.0mm bur has two different lengths depending on implant size. It is important to bear in mind that a thin, delicate palatal bone must no receive a 4.0mm twist bur.

Now, the implant is loaded in position with a 45Ncm torque. The implant platform is driven to an ideal occlusal position. Then, the Unigrip key is used to remove de insertion implant component. After installing the two zygomatic fixtures, the standard implants are positioned in the pre-maxilla region (Fig. 14-3). Herein, the surgeon has to decide whether to immediately load or allow the osseo-integration period. Of course, the clinical decision depends on primary implant stability achieved during surgery.[6,7,10,11,18]

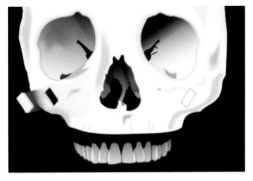

14-5

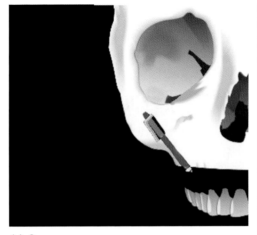

14-6

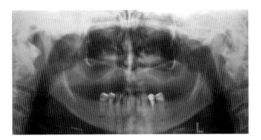

14-7

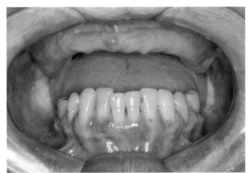

14-8

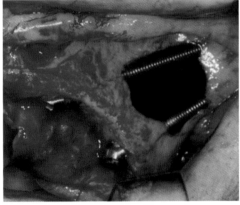

14-9

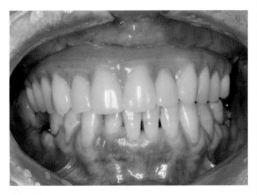

14-10

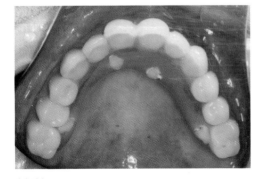

14-11

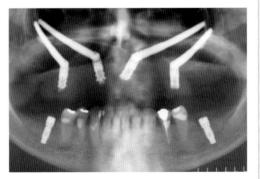

14-12

Fig. 14-5. Schematic representation. Original Brånemark technique.

Fig. 14-6. (continued) Schematic representation. Original Brånemark technique.

Fig. 14-7. Initial panoramic radiograph.

Fig. 14-8. Initial clinical aspect.

Fig. 14-9. Clinical aspect of already installed zygomatic fixtures according to the original Brånemark technique.

Fig. 14-10. The correspondent upper complete dental prosthesis.

Fig. 14-11. Occlusal view of the complete dental prosthesis.

Fig. 14-12. Final panoramic radiograph.

Fig. 14-13. A depth gauge is used to measure the implant length.

Fig. 14-14. The depth has been determined for implant installation.

Fig. 14-15. Drilling sequence of the Zygoma Fixtures System kit (Nobel Biocare).

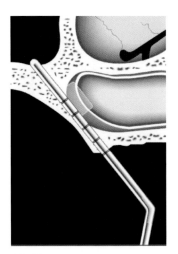

14-13

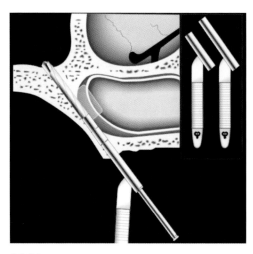

14-14

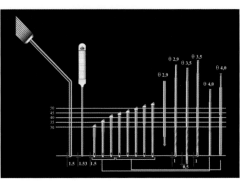

14-15

Fig. 14-13. A depth gauge is used to measure the implant length.

Fig. 14-14. The depth has been determined for implant installation.

Fig. 14-15. Drilling sequence of the Zygoma Fixtures System kit (Nobel Biocare).

Stella's Technique

As mentioned in the previous section, the Stella's technique begins with patient selection and indication, pre-prosthetic management, and finally, implant placement.[19] In addition, surgical procedures (eg, incision, flap rising, and visual contact with the zygomatic bone) are performed according to the Brånemark protocol.

After flap elevation, the alveolar bone crest is exposed including de palatal area. A round bur creates perforations on the lateral sinus wall, which will be joined together with transversal cuts, re-gardless of the integrity of sinus membrane (Figs. 14-16 and 14-17). Perforations are placed 5mm apart from the bone crest and toward the zygomatic bone base.[17] Later, these perforations are joined, creating a bony buccal channel that servers a dual purpose: first, it provides an insertion path for the surgeon; second, it creates an irrigation access area to the zygomatic implant (Figs. 14-18 to 14-19). Now, the drilling sequence is initiated with the Zygoma Fixtures System burs (Nobel Biocare) (Fig. 14-20).

In this technique, the implant platform can be placed more occlusal than in the original Brånemark technique.

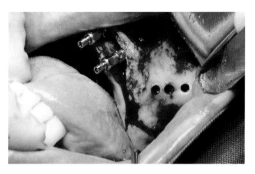

14-16

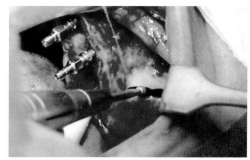

14-17

Fig. 14-16. Serial perforations are made with a round bur.

Fig. 14-17. A buccal bony channel is performed joining the perforations together.

Fig. 14-18. Drilling is initiated following the channel path.

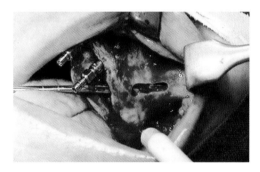

14-18

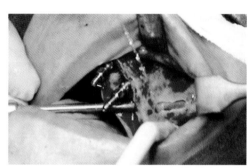

14-19

Fig. 14-19. The zygomatic implant has been over the alveolar bone crest.

Fig. 14-20.

Fig. 14-21.

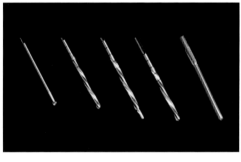

14-20

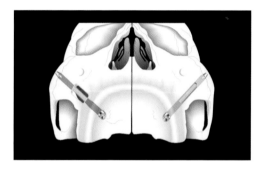

14-21

Exteriorized Migliorança's technique

Again, surgical protocols are performed according to the previous sections in this chapter.[13] Two zygomatic implants are placed, and the pre-maxilla receives either 2 or four implants (classic tech-

nique). Also, the All-On-Four-Zygoma prosthetic resolution can be employed.[12] The later is indicated for completely edentulous patients with severely atrophied maxillae and oftentimes for patients with Combination syndrome. (Figs. 14-4 and 14-29).

First, the standard implants are placed in the anterior region. After, the zygomatic fixtures are placed bilaterally. When there is extreme bone resorption in the pre-maxillary area, four zygomatic implants are inserted. In the Exteriorized technique, the zygomatic fixtures are positioned in the premolar and molar regions (Figs. 14-22 and 14-23), avoiding sinus lifting and the bony buccal channel procedures. The drilling sequence is initiated with a round bur (Fig. 14-24), creating an insertion path for the 2.9mm bur. This bur enters the palatal area, further emerging at the buccal side of the maxillary sinus and towards the zygomatic bone (Fig. 14-25). The cortical layer of the zygomatic incisure is trespassed and the depth gauge is inserted to determine the most appropriate zygomatic implant length. The bone site is prepared with the following sequential burs: 2.9m Twist bur, 3.5mm Pilot bur, and 3.5mm Twist bur. Figures 24 to 32 illustrate the placement of zygomatic implants according to the Exteriorized Migliorança's technique.

Final implant positioning is achieved near the alveolar crest in the molar region; it is important to highlight that the middle portion of the fixture remains exteriorized to the maxillary sinus (Figs. 14-26 to 14-28). Figures 14-29 to 14-39 represent the Exteriorized technique with four zygomatic fixations.

Fig. 14-22. The zygomatic implant can be placed between the upper first premolar and molar regions.

Fig. 14-23. Another option is to positioning the zygomatic implant also between the upper lateral incisor and canine

Fig. 14-24. Drilling with the round bur.

Fig. 14-25. The 2.9mm bur has entered the palatal area and emerges externally to the maxillary sinus toward the zygomatic body.

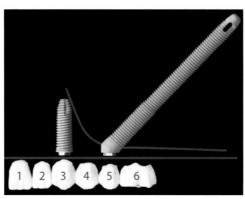

14-22

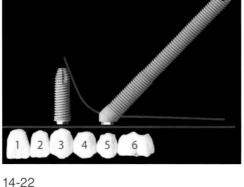

14-23

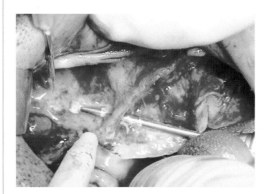

14-24

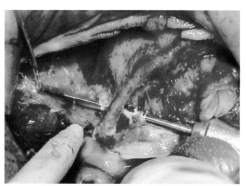

14-25

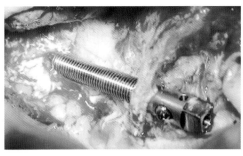

14-26

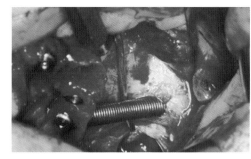

14-27

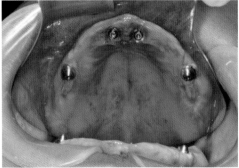

14-28

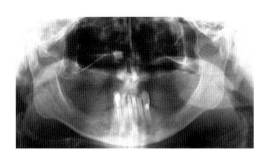

14-29

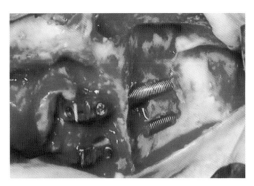

14-30

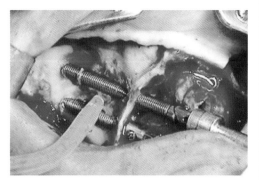

14-31

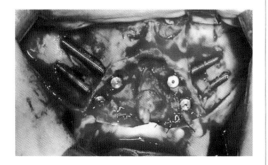

14-32

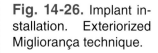

Fig. 14-26. Implant installation. Exteriorized Migliorança technique.

Fig. 14-27. The zygomatic implants are installed according to exteriorized technique.

Fig. 14-28. Final implant position into the mouth.

Fig. 14-29. Initial panoramic radiograph.

Fig. 14-30. Four zygomatic implants Exteriorized Migliorança technique.

Fig. 14-31. Occusal view of the same technique.

Fig. 14-32. Detailed occlusal of view of the same technique on figure 31.

Fig. 14-33. Metallic infra-structure try-in over the four zygomatic installed implants.

Fig. 14-34. The new complete prosthesis: metallic infra-structure try-in.

Fig. 14-35. Intaglio view of the definite prosthesis.

Fig. 14-36. Finalized prosthesis.

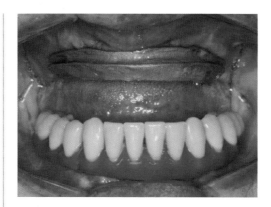

14-33A

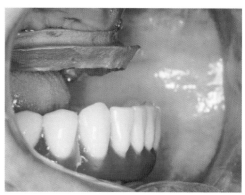

14-33B

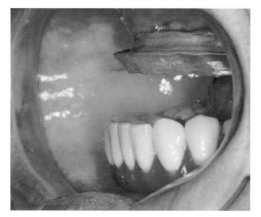

14-33C

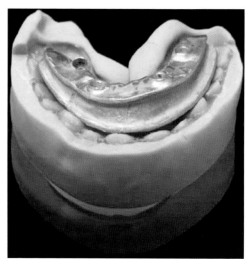

14-34

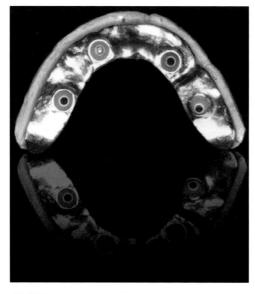

14-35

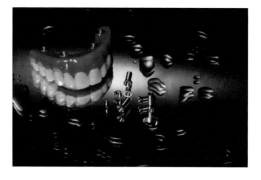

14-36

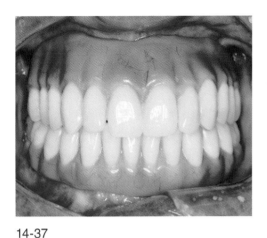

14-37

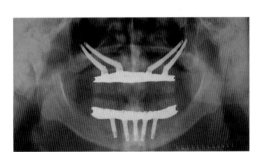

14-38

Fig. 14-37. Prosthesis into the mouth.

Fig. 14-38. Final radiographic exam.

Fig. 14-39.

Fig. 14-40. The zygomatic implantation techniques are compared one by one.

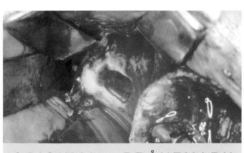

14-39

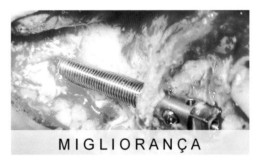

ORIGINAL – BRÅNEMARK

14-40A

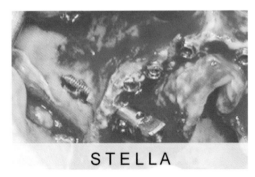

STELLA

14-40B

MIGLIORANÇA

14-40C

Clinical follow-up

On zygomatic implant cases conducted by Dr. Reginaldo Migliorança et al., between 1999 to 2007, with 982 fixations installed. Of these, 25 were lost, resulting in a cumulative sucess rate of 97.45%. Details can be seen on the table 14.1.

Table 14-1

Year	Implant/ Year	Original Technique (Brånemark)	Simplified Technique (Stella)	Exteriorized Technique (Migliorança)	Sucess Rate	Failure Rate
1999	12	12	–	–	12 (100%)	0 (0%)
2000	21	21	–	–	20 (95.24%)	1 (4.76%)
2001	31	31	–	–	30 (96.77%)	1 (3.23%)
2002	104	32	72	–	100 (96.15%)	4 (3.85%)
2003	165	–	96	69	161 (97.58%)	4 (2.42%)
2004	152	–	40	112	148 (97.30%)	4 (2.63%)
2005	147	–	–	147	142 (96.60%)	5 (3.40%)
2006	168	–	–	168	162 (96.43%)	6 (3.57%)
2007	182	–	–	182	177 (97.25%)	5 (2.75%)
Total	**982**	**96**	**208**	**678**	**957 (97.45%)**	**25 (2.55%)**

Final considerations

The exteriorized technique is more user-friendly due to the facilitated surgical access, thus reducing the chair time, with a less invasive procedure, providing a more controlled postoperative process. Other positive aspect is the final positioning of the proposed implants: the screw access holes will be found near the alveolar bone crest (occlusal surface of prosthetic teeth or slightly palatal to the bone crest area.

References

1. BALSHI, S.F.; WOLFINGER, G.J.; BASHI, T.J. A prospective study of immediate functional loading, following the Teeth in a Day protocol: a case series of 55 consecutive edentulous maxillas. *Clin Implant Dent Relat Res* 2005;7(1):24-31.

2. Bedrossian, E.; Stumpel, L.J. 3rd. Immediate stabilization at stage II of zygomatic implants: rationale and technique. *J Prosthet Dent* 2001 Jul;86(1):10-4.

3. BOYES-VARLEY, J.G.; HOWES, D.G.; LOWNIE, J.F. The zygomaticus implant protocol in the treatment of the severely resorbed maxilla. *SADJ.* 2003 Apr;58(3):106-9, 113-4.

4. BRÅNEMARK, P.-I.; GRONDAHL, K.; WORTHINGTON, B. *Osseointegration and Autogenous Onlay Bone Grafts: Reconstruction of the Edentulous Atrophic Maxilla.* Chicago: Quintessence; 2001.

5. BRÅNEMARK, P.-I. *Zygoma fixture: clinical procedures.* Götemborg, Sweden: Nobel Biocare, 2000.

6. CHOW, J.; HUI, E.; LEE, P.K.; LI, W. Zygomatic implants-protocol for immediate occlusal loading: a preliminary report. *J Oral Maxillofac Surg* 2006 May;64(5):804-11.

7. DUARTE, L.R.; PEREDO, L.G.; NARY, H.F.; FRANCISCHONE, C.E.; BRÅNEMARK, P.-I. Reabilitação da Maxila Atrófica Utilizando Quatro Fixações Zigomáticas em Sistema de Carga Imediata. *Implant News* 2004 Jan-Fev; 1(1):45-50.

8. DUARTE, L.R.; NARY, H.F.; FRANCISCHONE JR., C.E.; VIANA, A. Fixações Zigomáticas: Uma excelente cirurgia para a maxila severamente reabsorvida. Revisão de literatura e estágio científico atual. *Implant News* 2004; Nov-Dez;1(6):477-86.

9. HIGUCHI, K.W. The zygomaticus fixture: an alternative approach for implant anchorage in the posterior maxilla. *Ann R Autralas Coll Dent Surg* 2000 Oct;15:28-33

10. HIRSCH, J.M.; OHRNELL, L.O.; HENRY, P.J.; ANDREASSON, L.; BRÅNEMARK, P.-I.; CHIAPASCO, M.; GYNTHER, G.; FINNE, K.; HIGUCHI, K.W.; ISAKSSON, S.; KAHNBERG, K.E.; MALEVEZ, C.; NEUKAM, F.W.; SEVETZ, E.; URGELL, J.P.; WIDMARK, G.; BOLIND, P. A clinical evaluation of the Zygoma fixture: one year of follow-up at 16 clinics. *J Oral Maxillofac Surg* 2004 Sep;62(9 Suppl 2):22.

11. JENSEN, O.T.; SHULMAN, L.B.; BLOCK, M.S.; LACONO, V.J. Report of the Sinus Consensus Conference of 1996. *Int J Oral Maxillofac Implants* 1998;13 Suppl:11-45.

12. MALO, P.; RANGERT, B.; NOBRE, M. All-on-4 Immediate-function concept With Branemark System implants for completely edentulous maxillae: a 1-year retrospective clinical study. *Clin Implant Dent Relat Res* 2005;7 Suppl 1:S88-94.

13. MIGLIORANÇA, R.M.; ILG, J.P.; SERRANO, A.S.; SOUZA, R.P.; ZAMPERLINI, M.S. Exteriorização de Fixações Zigomáticas em Relação ao Seio Maxilar: Uma nova Abordagem Cirúrgica. *Implant News* 2006;3(1):30-5.

14. NYSTROM, E.; AHLQVIST, J.; GUNNE, J.; KAHNBERG, K.E. 10-year follow-up of onlay bone grafts and implants in severly resorbed maxillae. *Int J Oral Maxillofac Surg* 2004 Apr;33(3):258-62.

15. OSTMAN, P.O.; HELLMAN, M.; SENNERBY, L. Direct implant loanding in the edentolous maxilla using a bone density-adapted surgical protocol and primary implant stabilitycriteria for inclusion. *Clin Implant Dent Relat Res* 2005;7 Suppl 1:S60-9.

16. PAREL, S.M.; BRÅNEMARK, P.-I.; OHRNELL, L.O.; SVENSSON, B. Remote implant anchorage for the rehabilition of maxillary defects. *J Prosthet Dent* 2001 Oct;86(4):377-81.

17. PEÑARROCHA, M.; URIBE, R.; GARCIA, B.; MARTI, E. Zygomatic implants using the sinus slot technique: clinical report of a patient series. *Int J Oral Maxillofac Implants* 2005 Sep-Oct;20(5):788-92.

18. SCHNITMAN, P.A.; WOHRLE, P.S.; RUBENSTEIN, J.E.; DA SILVA, J.D.; WANG, N.H. Ten-year results for Branemark implants immediately loaded with fixed prostheses at implant placement. *Int J Oral Maxillofac Implants* 1997 Jul-Aug:12(4):495-503.

19. STELLA, J.P.; WAENER, M.R. Sinus slot technique for simplification and improved orientation of zygomaticus dental implants: a tchnical note. *Int J Oral Maxillofac Implants* 2000;15(6):889-93.

20. VAN STEENBERGHE, D.; GLAUSER, R.; BLOMBACK, U.; ANDERSSON, M.; SCHUTYSER, F.; PETTERSSON, A.; WENDELHAG, I. A computed tomographic scan-derived customized surgical template and fixed prosthesis for flapless surgery and immediate loading of implants in fully edentulous maxillae: a prospective multicenter study. *Clin Implant Dent Relat Res* 2005;7 Suppl 1:S111-20.

15

FRANCISCHONE´S CLASSIFICATION FOR IMPLANT PROSTHESES

Carlos Eduardo Francischone
Renato Savi de Carvalho
Carlos Eduardo Francischone Jr.

The observation and confirmation of the phenomenon known as osseointegration by Brånemark in the middle of 1960s created a new rehabilitation method for people with severe body impairment. Congenital defects, tumor resections and trauma are a challenge to prosthetic treatment. However, osseointegration provides a safety and reliable anchorage system to several intra and extra-oral prostheses.

At the same time, total edentulous patients condemned to the poor prognosis of a mucous tissue-supported total prosthesis (complete denture) could envisage the use of a fixed prosthesis, anchored or retained on titanium fixtures installed in the residual bone. This therapeutic approach represented an invaluable progress since individuals retrieve their masticatory function (the main focus of edentulous patients) satisfactorily, otherwise compromised in the mucous tissue-supported complete prostheses, where retention and stability do not afford adequate functional conditions.

Fixed prostheses with a metallic infra-structure, associated to porcelain or artificial acrylic teeth constitutes the main type of prosthetic rehabilitation for patients with osseointegrated implants. Nevertheless, the scientific success of osseointegration motivated clinicians to expand its prosthetic applications. Thus, several prosthetic designs have been tested worldwide, not only to benefit patients with partial or single tooth losses, but also for cases of considerable soft and hard tissue compromise.

Based on these facts, it is necessary to consider a classification for implant-supported prostheses, which must attend clinicians and patient's expectations. The objective is to facilitate communication and comprehension among dental surgeons and laboratory technicians over the planning and manufacturing of an implant prosthesis. Also, patients will be able to understand advantages and drawbacks of their proposed treatment.

This classification is divided in eight groups, comprising from total, removable to partial and single-fixed prosthesis. We use from F1 to F8 (F means Francischone) which subdivisions for each group given the chance of another modalities. Also, it can be applied regardless of materials and methods used for infra-structure confection, as well as in pros-thesis fabrication (artificial teeth, porcelain, ceromers, etc.).

In addition, this classification can be used for several surgical anchorage or reconstruction techniques that aim implant installation.

Groups

Currently, implant-supported prostheses can be classified into the following groups.

FI – Fixed prosthesis with artificial gingival tissue

This is the primary design for implant-supported prostheses, which were used during the pre-osseointegration period over laminate, blade, subperiosteal, and transosteal implants. Composed of a metallic infra-structure veneered by acrylic or porcelain

Table 15-1. Francischone's classification for implant prostheses

Type	Description
F1	Fixed prosthesis with artificial gingival tissue
F2	Fixed prosthesis without artificial gingival tissue (long teeth)
F3	Fixed prosthesis with detachable gingival tissue (epithesis)
F4	Fixed prosthesis with individualized crowns
F5	Removable prosthesis
F6	Overdentures
F7	Fixed prosthesis with subgingival emergence profile
F8	Single-tooth implant crowns

teeth adapted over 4 to 6 fixtures, it represented an incredible improvement for completely edentulous patients who could not cope with their mucous tissue-supported total prosthesis. Also, artificial gingiva is provided to prevent air and salivary escape during speech, as well as to give muscular support to the lips and cheeks, improving patient's facial aspect. It is indicated for patients with high lip lines in their maxillary arches. On the other hand, the role of the mandibular arch is not too significant in esthetics and phonetics, and the artificial gingiva must be primarily design for oral hygiene procedures. Surgical and prosthetic procedures for the *All on Four* concept belong to the F1 group. It is not necessary to install fixtures according to the original position of tooth in the dental arch. The prefabricated abutments are positioned above the gingival tissue (Figs. 15-1A to D).

This type of dentogingival prosthesis is the most frequently used to rehabilitate completely edentulous upper and lower arches.

Fig. 15-1

15-1A. Occlusal view. Implant abutments installed to anchor a fixed prosthesis in the completely edentulous maxilla.

15-1B. Occlusal view. Implant abutments installed to anchor a fixed prosthesis in the completely edentulous mandible.

15-1-C. Fixed prosthesis with artificial gingival tissue installed over the implant abutments. Observe prosthesis overcontouring to compensate for the lack of maxillary alveolar bone.

15-1-D. This option provided good muscular support and excellent esthetics for a patient with high lip line.

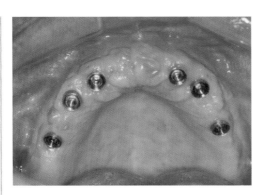

15-1A

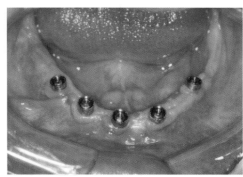

15-1B

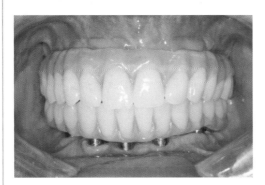

15-1C

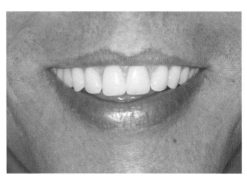

15-1D

Discussion over the need of prosthetic compensation – epithesis, artificial gingiva or long teeth – must be a common practice among clinicians and patients. The first should explain the advantages and disadvantages of each prosthetic modality. In some cases, to create a false expectation that artificial teeth will have the same emergence profile of natural teeth is no good practice since compensation can be impossible. Certainly, patients will not be satisfied at the final appointment.

The frequency of prosthetic compensation (dentogingival fixed prosthesis) was verified at the Francischone's private practice, InterClínica and the postgraduate courses at the USC (University of Sagrado Coracao – Bauru – Sao Paulo – Brazil) in patients with atrophied maxillae rehabilitated with implant-fixed prostheses. These patients were divided in three groups: 1. Total osseous reconstruction with autogenous bone graft, 2. Inclined implants, and 3. Zygomatic fixtures (Table 15-2).

Thus, the professional must explain, show and predict the final product (prosthesis) for the patient. Most patients are first concerned over what type of prosthesis they will receive and how the prosthesis will retrieve their esthetic and phonetic demands; fewer are interested in mechanical or functional benefits.

Values depicted in Table 15-2 show a high incidence of prosthetic compensation (dentogingival prostheses), being these worthwhile data during patient counseling and prosthetic treatment planning. Interestingly, data is not related to the surgical treatment provided.

F2 – Fixed prosthesis without artificial gingival tissue (long teeth)

This type is indicated for patients with low lip line and lesser alveolar ridge loss, suppressing the pink gingival portion, where possible dark spaces are resolved by cervico-incisal lengthening of teeth. Also, patients with little or no loss of lip support can be benefited since the lack of artificial gingival tissue cannot prevent considerable areas of soft and hard deficiencies. It is important to bear in mind that these modalities do not recommend that the implants be positioned exactly in the original root position. Again, prefabricated abutments are positioned above the gingival tissue (Figs. 15-2A to D).

Fig. 15-2

15-2A. Frontal view of both edentulous arches. Implants and prosthetic abutments were chosen as retentive elements for a fixed prosthesis.

15-2B. Diagnostic wax-up which determines the Occlusal Centric Relation (ORC) position, the dimensions of proposed teeth, the need for muscular and lip support, phonetics and adequate spaces for oral hygiene.

15-2C. Final prostheses installed. Observe long teeth that in the maxillary arch without overcontouring and pink porcelain. This option is indicated for patients with good muscular support and a low lip line. It facilitates access for oral hygiene procedures.

15-2D. The patient smile does not display excessive gingival tissue. There is good labial support from this prosthesis type.

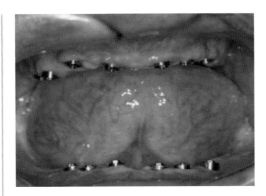

15-2A

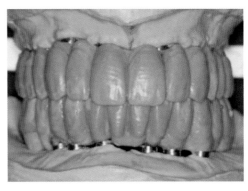

15-2B

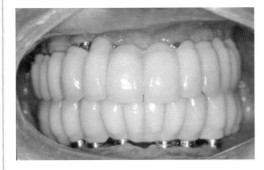

15-2C

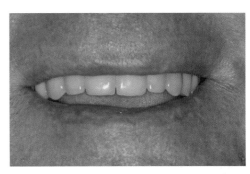

15-2D

F3 – Fixed prosthesis with detachable gingival tissue (epithesis)

When is not adequate to provide an artificial gingival tissue adhered to the implant prosthesis or to lengthen teeth cervico-incisal dimensions, a detachable gingival tissue is a good alternative. Known as "epithesis", it greatly improves esthetics (severe loss of lip and muscular support) and phonetics (air escape). It is highly recommended for patients with severe bucco-lingual volume deficiencies. Also, a detachable gingiva facilitates cleaning of the fixed prosthesis and the home-care hygiene of the implant abutments.

The main indication is for patients with limited motor skills that wish a fixed prosthesis. A detachable tissue here is considered a biological-esthetic-phonetic convenience form (Figs. 15-3A to E).

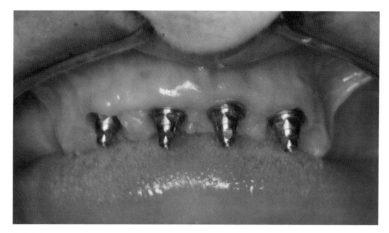

15-3A

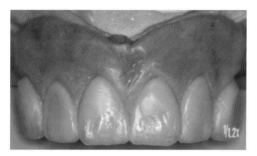

15-3B

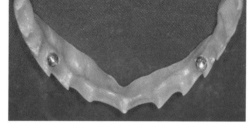

15-3C

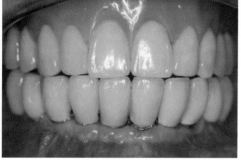

15-3D

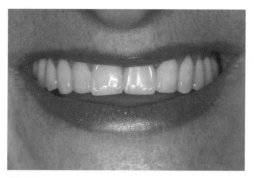

15-3E

Fig. 15-3

15-3A. Frontal view of the maxillary arch with four osseointegrated implants to support a fixed prosthesis.

15-3B. Due to the great maxillary bone deficiency, a detachable gingival tissue (epithesis) was chosen in the diagnostic wax-up phase.

15-3C. Intaglio surface of the detachable gingival tissue, which corresponds to the buccal bone loss in the maxilla (another example of epithesis).

15-3D. The epithesis and the fixed prosthesis already installed.

15-3E. Frontal view of the patient's smile showing good muscular/lip support and esthetics (*Cortesy of Dr. Ronaldo Brum*).

Table 15-2. Clinical evaluation of fixed prostheses used in atrophic maxillae.

Groups	Number of patients	Without prosthetic compensation (without gingiva)	With prosthetic compensation (with gingiva)
Total osseous reconstruction with autogenous bone graft	40	5 (12.5%)	35 (87.5%)
Anchorage:			
• inclined implants	52	7 (13.4%)	46 (86.6%)
• zygomatic implants	44	2 (5.0%)	42 (95%)
Total	136	14 (10.3%)	83 (89.7%)

F4 – Fixed prosthesis with individualized crowns

Any fixed prosthesis is subjected to porcelain fracture. This fact is aggravated in large crown and bridgework because even the most single repair can compromise overall esthetic appearance. In worst cases, all veneering material has to be removed.

On the other hand, the mechanism of fixation initially created to secure the prosthesis to the implant abutment (screw) warranted its retrievability, an impossible feat in the conventional cemented fixed prosthesis. However, for porcelain restorations, laboratory technicians sometimes have to sacrifice the intact portion of the veneering material and start all over again.

To overcome this problem, it is possible to design the metallic infra-structure of an extensive fixed prosthesis with individualized abutments. These abutments would have the same characteristics of prepared teeth for conventional fixed prosthesis. It still does facilitate repair because only crowns and not the metallic infra-structure is removed. Also, patients' acceptance is high because they receive a new ceramic crown and not an acrylic resin repair. The clinician can either use all-ceramic (Procera, In-Ceram, IPS Empress, ceromers), metalloceramic or acrylic resin veneer systems to fabricate single crowns.

This design offers minimal vertical and horizontal distortions during porcelain firing because crowns are directly seated on the metallic-infra-structure that will be connected to the implant abutments (Figs. 15-4A to H).

Fig. 15-4

15-4A. Panoramic radiograph showing osseointegrated implants for prosthesis anchorage and a temporary splint.

15-4B. Metallic framework specially designed for individualized cemented crowns.

15-4C. Detailed view of the prepared segment with a chamfer finish line.

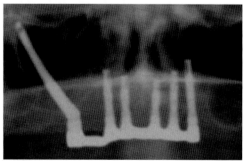
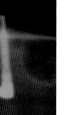

15-4A

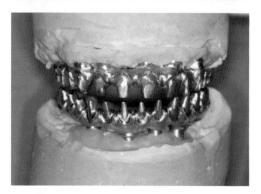

15-4B

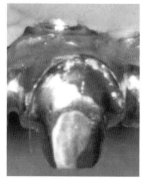

15-4C

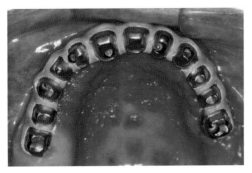

15-4D

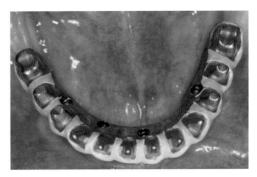

15-4E

15-4D-E. Occlusal view of the titanium framework (Procera Implant Bridge) screwed onto the implant abutments that will receive individualized cemented crowns.

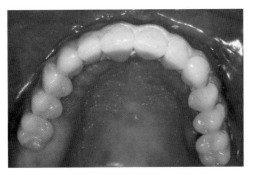

15-4F

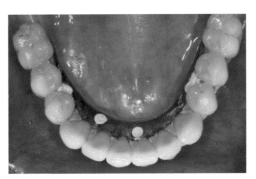

15-4G

15-4F-G. Occlusal view of Procera AllCeram crowns cemented over the individualized prepared segments.

15-4H. Patient's smile showing good muscular and lip support, as well as adequate esthetics. (Cortesy of Drs. Hugo Nary Filho, Luís Guilhermo Peredo-Paz, and Maurício B. Rigolizzo.)

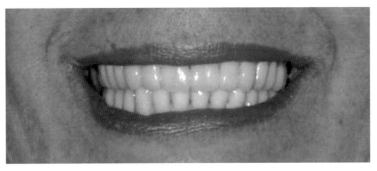

15-4H

F5 – Removable prosthesis

Although rather used, it is necessary to classify this modality because an implant-supported removable prosthesis is quite different from the widespread, conventional removable restoration made over natural abutments.

It consists of a fixed prosthesis over the implants in the pre-maxillary region, with an implant-tissue-supported removable distal extension. It is indicated when implants cannot be installed in the posterior region of the alveolar ridges. Conventional fixed bridgework with large distal cantilevers would overload the prosthesis and the osseointegration. Retention mechanisms for the removable prosthesis varied from conventional clasps to precision or semi-precision attachments. Nowadays, due to a better comprehension of the osseointegration process and surgical techniques, is possible to avoid removable prostheses; implants can be installed in strategic positions to construct a fixed prosthesis (Figs. 15-5A to C).

Fig. 15-5

15-5A. Occlusal view of fixed prosthesis installed in the anterior maxillary region. Observe the attachments that will receive the removable prosthesis.

15-5B. Panoramic radiograph showing the implants and the well-adapted prostheses.

15-5C. Removable prosthesis installed over the implant-supported fixed prosthesis.

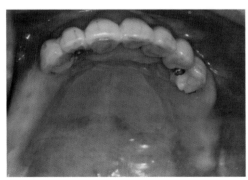

15-5A

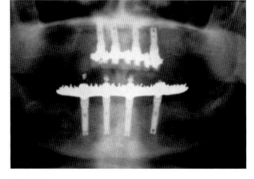

15-5B

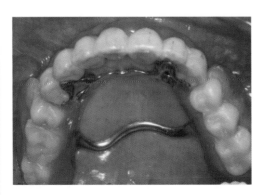

15-5C

F6 – Overdentures

There are situations where an Overdenture is better indicated than a fixed prosthesis. Again, Osseointegration can have a decisive role in retention and stability.

Overdentures are made according to the biomechanical principles of a conventional tissue-supported complete denture, with two or more implants serving as retentive elements. Most often, the edentulous region is the load-bearing area, and hence the name tissue-supported or implant-retained overdenture.

Main indications for overdentures are:

❑ patients with limited motor skills and inadequate oral hygiene;
❑ muscular and lip support for considerable soft tissue deficiencies due to trauma or severe ridge resorption;
❑ great maxillomandibular discrepancies;
❑ bucco-sinusal communications, tumor resection or congenital palatal fissure.

Overdentures can be retained by several attachment mechanisms: ball anchors, bar-clip or magnets. Also, it has been widespread used due to its cost and easy of fabrication.

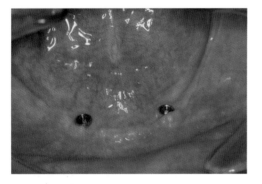

15-6A

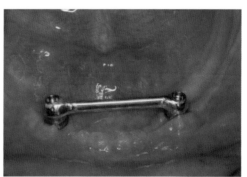

15-6B

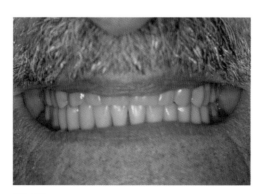

15-6C

Fig. 15-6

15-6-A and B. Completely edentulous mandible with two installed implants that will receive an overdenture.

15-6B. Rigid metallic bar joining the two implants.

15-6C. Overdenture in position, showing good muscular and lip support.

F7 – Fixed prosthesis with subgingival emergence profile

The search for more esthetic rehabilitations is related to the emergence profile obtained in prosthetic crowns. Conventional fixed prostheses supported by dental abutments present technical difficulties at the soft tissue-pontic area, since the lack of a dental element demands an over-contouring in the bucco-cervical region to simulate the emergence profile.

In the implant-supported prosthesis, an artificial root (implant) at the edentulous area helps to create the crown's emergence profile.

After soft tissue management, the gingival tissue can have its original configuration reestablished, e.g., presence of interproximal papillae and the scalloped contour.

Fixed prosthesis are preferred over individual crowns when the number of installed implants does not coincide with the number of artificial crowns to be created, or when long and short implants are connected to improve biomechanical aspects. Cases with an acceptable emergence profile in partial or total fixed prosthesis show mild or no vertical bone loss after tooth extraction. From the prosthetic aspect, they are the element of choice, although being less frequent among patients.

Fig. 15-7

15-7A. Esthetic abutments that will receive a fixed prosthesis with subgingival emergence profile. The aspect of the gingival tissue was achieved through previous tissue conditioning with the provisional prosthesis.

15-7B. A two-unit fixed prosthesis to replace elements 36 and 37.

15-7C. Bitewing radiograph showing correct fit between prosthesis and implant abutment, and between abutment and the osseointegrated implant.

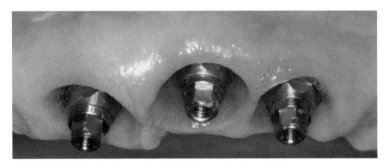
15-7A

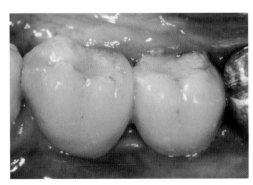
15-7B

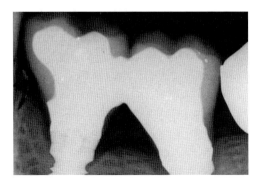
15-7C

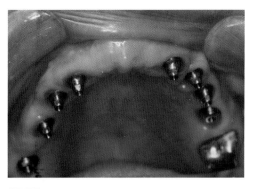

15-7D

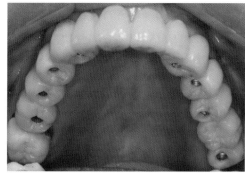

15-7E

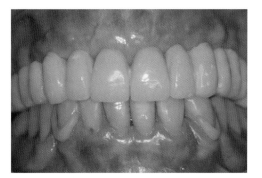

15-7F

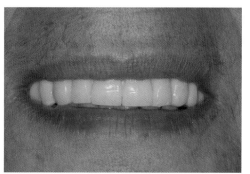

15-7G

15-7D. Esthetic abutments that will receive a fixed prosthesis with ideal emergence profile.

15-7E. Occlusal view of definitive prosthesis, demonstrating that the implants are well-positioned through the access holes.

15-7F. Frontal view of the fixed prosthesis with subgingival emergence profile.

15-7G. Final esthetics with adequate muscular and lip support.

F8 – Single-tooth implant crowns

This is the last option of implant-supported prosthesis, being adequate for single tooth loss. The avoidance of vital adjacent teeth as prepared abutments motivated clinicians and researchers to develop customized prosthetic components. This conservative option has been used and approved by clinicians and patients.

Another important aspect is that individual elements can be created, otherwise impossible in the partial fixed prosthesis situation, where the connection area between abutment and pontic prevented adequate esthetic corrections. Also, the presence of caries, root/porcelain fracture often resulted in failure and removal of the prosthesis.

An esthetic improvement was achieved with single-tooth implant prosthesis because in the normal situation the alveolar ridge becomes flat and papillae are lost after tooth extraction, with the pontic being overcontoured in the cervical region. Also, the alveolar ridge resorption continues throughout life and the soft tissue aspect can even be more compromised in patients with high lip line. Implants installed soon after tooth extraction can maintain adequate bone volume and the height of buccal cortical plate. Still, oral hygiene procedures are facilitated.

Fig. 15-8

15-8A. Buccal view of gingival and papillary architecture obtained through a provisional restoration.

15-8B. Customized esthetic zirconia abutment over the implant.

15-8C. Procera AllCeram crown cemented over the zirconia abutment. Observe excellent gingival contouring, papillae, adequate emergence profile, and harmonious transition between white (crown) and red (soft tissue) esthetics.

15-8D. Periapical radiograph showing osseointegration and the correct adaptation of the esthetic abutment over the implant fixture.

15-8E. Nobel Direct implant installed on the 24 region and immediately loaded.

Fig. 15-8F. AllCeram crown already cemented showing excellent gingival contour. (Cortesy of Drs. Renato Savi de Carvalho and Carlos Eduardo Francischone Jr.)

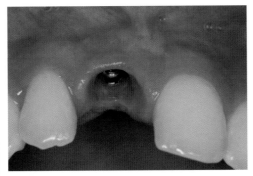

15-8A

15-8B

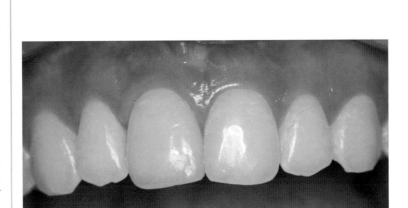

15-8C

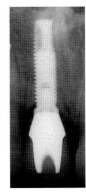

15-8D

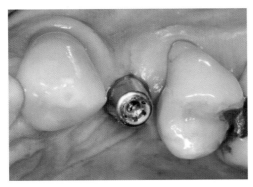

15-8E

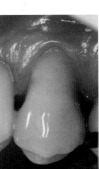

15-8F

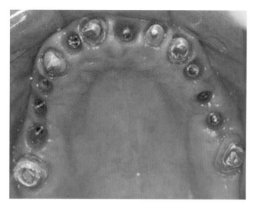

15-8G

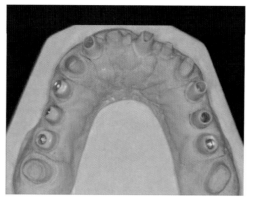

15-8H

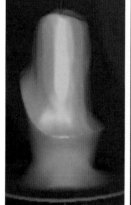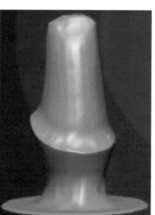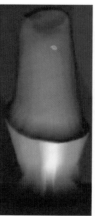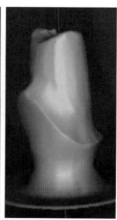

15-8I

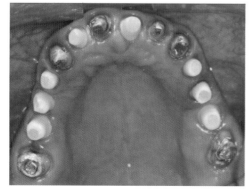

15-8J

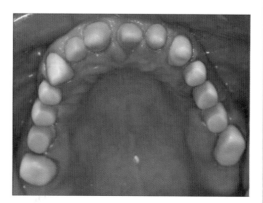

15-8K

15-8G. Maxillary occlusal view with prepared teeth and implant abutments that will receive single crowns.

15-8H. Wax-up of customized esthetic abutments to be scanned.

15-8I. Three-dimensional images of the scanned prosthetic abutments. Observe different designs according to the need for tooth replacement.

15-8J. Occlusal view of the customized zirconia abutments over the implants. Note the gingival contours and the correct design of the abutments that determine and adequate emergence profile for an ideal fixed prosthesis.

15-8K. Alumina oxide copings seated and adapted over teeth and implants.

15-8L. All porcelain crowns cemented over teeth and implants.

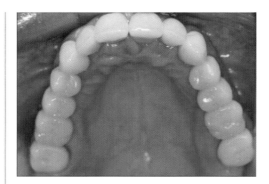

15-8L

15-8M. Adequate prosthetic aspects and the patient's smile.

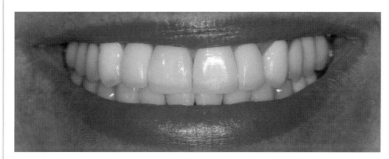

15-8M

Conclusions

Based on the classification proposed above, the following conclusions can be drawn:

1. The F7 and F8 conceptions demand implants placed in the same dental positions, since the aim is to create adequate subgingival emergence profile. These are considered ideal constructions under the esthetic aspect;

2. Concepts F1, F2, F3, F4, F5 and F6 do not demand implants in the same dental positions, since the objective here is to diminish the effects of alveolar atrophy, with prostheses having some degree of overcontouring;

3. An understanding of patient's desires and expectations (type of prosthetic treatment) is the key of a successful osseointegration treatment;

4. This classification was created to facilitate communication among clinicians and laboratory technicians, as well as to improve patient's comprehension over the prosthetic planning that will be afforded in the osseointegration treatment.

References

1. BRÅNEMARK, P.-I.; ZARB, G.A.; ABREKTSSON, T. *Tissue-integrated prostheses: Osseointegration in clinica dentistry.* Chicago: Quintessence, 1985.

2. BRÅNEMARK, P.-I. et al. *The Osseointegration Book.* Berlim: Quintessence, 2006.

3. FRANCISCHONE, C.E. et al. *Osseointegração e o Tratamento Multidisciplinar.* São Paulo: Quintessence, 2006.

4. FRANCISCHONE, C.E. et al. *Osseointegração and the multidisciplinary treatment.* São Paulo: Quintessence, 2007.

5. FRANCISCHONE, C.E. Classificação de Francischone para próteses sobre implantes – Nota Prévia. *Implant News,* v.2; n.5; set-out, 2005.

6. NEVES, J.B. *Estética em Implantologia.* São Paulo: Quintessence, 2006.

7. MISCH, CE. *Implantes dentários contemporâneos.* São Paulo: Ed. Santos, 2000.

8. RUFENACHT, C.R. *Principles of esthetics integration.* Berlim: Quintessence, 2000.